Delmar's
Practice Questions
for
NCLEX-PN®

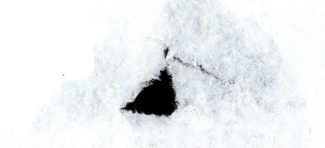

Delmar's Practice Questions for NCLEX-PN®

Judith C. Miller
MS, RN
President, Nursing Tutorial and
Consulting Services

THOMSON

DELMAR LEARNING

Australia Canada Mexico Singapore Spain United Kingdom United States

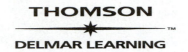

Delmar's Practice Questions for NCLEX-PN®
Judith C. Miller

Vice President,
Health Care Business Unit:
William Brottmiller

Editorial Director:
Cathy L. Esperti

Senior Acquisitions Editor:
Matthew Kane

Editorial Assistant:
Erin Silk

Marketing Director:
Jennifer McAvey

Marketing Coordinator:
Kip Summerlin

Art and Design Coordinator:
Jay Purcell

Project Editor:
Bryan Viggiani

Production Coordinator:
Kenneth McGrath

Library of Congress
Cataloging-in-Publication Data
Miller, Judith C.
  Delmar's practice questions for NCLEX-PN /
Judith C. Miller
    p. ; cm.
  ISBN 1-4018-0403-9
  1. Practical nursing—Examinations, questions,
etc.
  [DNLM: 1. Nursing, Practical—Examination
Questions. 2. Nursing Care—Examination
Questions. WY 18.2 M648da 2004] I. Title:
Practice questions for NCLEX-PN. II. Title.
  RT62.M557 2004
610.73'06'93076—dc22   2003055590

NOTICE TO THE READER

Contents

Contributors

TEST ITEM WRITERS

Lenore Boris, RN, BSN, MS, JD
New York State Public Employees Federation Organizer
Albany, New York

Teresa Burkhalter, RN, BS, MSN
Nursing Faculty
Technical College of the Lowcountry
Beaufort, South Carolina

Judith M. Hall, RNC, MSN, IBCLC, ICCE, FACCE
Lactation Consultant and Childbirth Educator
Fredericksberg, Virginia

Carol Nelson, RN, BSN, MSN
Spokane Community College
Spokane, Washington

REVIEWERS

Terry Ardoin, RN, CCM
Louisiana Technical College
Charles B. Coreil Campus
Ville Platte, Louisiana

Mary E. Arnold, RN, BSN, MA
Director VOCN Program
Blinn College Bryan Campus
Bryan, Texas

Gyl Ann Burkhard, RN, BSN, MS
Instructor
OCM BOCES
Syracuse, New York

Teresa Burkhalter, RN, BS, MSN
Nursing Faculty
Technical College of the Lowcountry
Beaufort, South Carolina

Esther Gonzales, RN, MSN, MSEd.
Del Mar College
Corpus Christi, Texas

Bonnie Grusk, RN, MSN
Continuing Education Coordinator for Health Professions
Illinois Valley Community College
Oglesby, Illinois

Sheila Guidry, RN, LPN, BSN, DSN, PhD.
Wallace Community College
Dothan, Alabama

Carol Nelson, RN, BSN, MSN
Spokane Community College
Spokane, Washington

Linda Walline
Associate Dean of Instruction
Central Community College
Grand Island, Nebraska

Unit I

Overview of Practical/Vocational Nursing

UNIT OUTLINE

Chapter 1

How to Prepare for NCLEX-PN®

QUESTIONS YOU MIGHT HAVE ABOUT THE EXAMINATION

The practice of nursing is regulated by the states to assure the public that only those nurses who have the necessary knowledge and skills are licensed to practice. One requirement for becoming a *licensed practical/vocational nurse* (LPN/LVN) is graduation from an approved school of practical/vocational nursing. Another requirement is passing an examination. All of the states have agreed to use the same examination, NCLEX-PN®. The NCLEX-PN® is designed to assess the candidate's ability to apply the knowledge needed for entry-level practical/vocational nursing. Once a candidate passes NCLEX-PN® and meets any other requirements the individual state might have, he or she can become licensed as an LPN/LVN.

WHAT IS THE NATIONAL COUNCIL OF STATE BOARDS OF NURSING?

The National Council of State Boards of Nursing is a council made up of state boards of nursing from all of the states and territories of the United States. The members of this group have decided to use the same examination as one of the requirements for state licensure. The examination is developed by nurses who are experts in nursing and item writing and who have an in-depth understanding of what practical/vocational nurses need to know.

Every three years, the National Council of State Boards of Nursing studies LPN/LVNs who are newly licensed to see what tasks they are doing and what knowledge and skills are required for them to do their jobs. The blueprint or outline for the licensure examination is developed after analyzing the results of the study. The examination is developed to ensure that new graduates have the knowledge and judgment-making ability that is necessary to function in the workplace as an LPN/LVN.

WHAT IS THE CURRENT TEST PLAN?

The current test plan went into effect April 1, 2002. The test plan, or blueprint, for the examination determines what percent of questions will be in each area. The test plans are available to the public and can be obtained from the National Council of State Boards of Nursing. The framework for the test plan revolves around *client needs* because it provides a universal structure for nursing competencies and actions for a variety of clients in a variety of settings. Integrated concepts and processes are threaded throughout the categories of client needs because they are basic to nursing. Table 1.1 lists the basic categories, subcategories, and integrated concepts and processes.

The first category, Safe, Effective Care Environment has been divided into two sections. The first is called coordinated care and includes items related to legal and ethical concerns such as informed consent, client rights, confidentiality, advance directives, ethical practice, and organ donation. Coordinated care also includes practice concerns such as case management, setting priorities, consultation with health care team members, referral process, resource management (making client care assignments), supervision,

incident/irregular occurrence reports, and continuous quality improvement. The second section under Safe, Effective Care Environment is called safety and infection control and includes such topics as accident and error prevention, medical and surgical asepsis, standard (universal) and other precautions, handling hazardous and infectious materials, proper use of restraints, and disaster planning.

The Health Promotion and Maintenance category is also divided into two sections. The first is growth and development through the life span and contains questions relating to growth and development from the fetus to older adult including pregnancy, labor and delivery, post-partum and newborn care. It also includes normal growth and development of infants, children, and adults, including the elderly. Family planning and human sexuality are included. The second section under Health Promotion and Maintenance is prevention and early detection of disease. Questions related to disease prevention may include immunization and health promotion efforts such as life-style changes and health screening such as self-breast examination and self-testicular exam. Also included are questions on techniques for collecting physical data.

The third category, Psychosocial Integrity, has two sections. The first is coping and adaptation. This category includes questions that relate to the client's ability to cope with and adapt to illness or stressful

Table 1.1 NCLEX-PN® Test Plan

A. Safe, effective care environment
    1. Coordinated care (6–12% of total questions)
    2. Safety and infection control (7–13% of total questions)
B. Health promotion and maintenance
    3. Growth and development through the life span (4–10% of total questions)
    4. Prevention and early detection of disease (4–10% of total questions)
C. Psychosocial integrity
    5. Coping and adaptation (6–12% of total questions)
    6. Psychosocial adaptation (4–10% of total questions)
D. Physiological integrity
    7. Basic care and comfort (10–16%) of total questions
    8. Pharmacological and parenteral therapies (5–11% of total questions)
    9. Reduction of risk potential (11–17% of total questions)
    10. Physiological adaptation (13–19% of total questions)

Integrated concepts and processes include
clinical problem solving (nursing process)   caring
communication and documentation   cultural awareness
teaching/learning   self-care

Adapted from the NCLEX-PN® Test Plan for the National Council Licensure Examination for Practical/Vocational Nurses, April 2001.

events. Questions might be related to grief and loss, situational role changes, unexpected body image changes (such as amputation, mastectomy, or colostomy). Therapeutic communication, mental health concepts, and behavior management are included. End-of-life issues and religious and spiritual influences on health are also included in this section. The second section under Psychosocial Integrity is psychosocial adaptation. This section includes concepts related to the care of clients with acute or chronic mental illness and cognitive psychosocial disturbances. Questions may relate to the care of clients who have been victims of elder or child abuse/neglect or sexual abuse. There also might be questions related to chemical dependency. Crisis intervention and therapeutic environment can also be included.

The fourth and largest category is Physiological Integrity (four sections). The first is basic care and comfort. Questions might relate to helping clients with activities of daily living, using assistive devices (canes, crutches, walkers, or a Hoyer lift); caring for clients who have contact lenses, hearing aids, or artificial eyes; providing personal hygiene; providing for rest and sleep; positioning clients; and transfer techniques, body mechanics, and concepts related to mobility and immobility. Also included are questions on nutrition, oral hydration and tube feedings, and elimination including catheters and enemas. There might be questions on palliative care, nonpharmacological pain interventions, and teaching self-care, such as ostomy care and pain management techniques. The second section under Physiological Integrity is pharmacological and parenteral therapies. This section includes administering medications and monitoring clients who are receiving parenteral therapies. Questions might relate to the actions of medications as well as expected effects, side effects, and untoward effects. The third section is reduction of risk potential. These questions relate to reducing the client's potential for developing complications or health problems related to treatments, procedures, or existing conditions. In order to answer these questions correctly, you need to understand basic pathophysiology. This knowledge includes topics such as diagnostic tests, therapeutic procedures, surgery, health alterations, how to prevent related complications, lab values, and the care of clients with drainage tubes, closed wound drainage, and water

seal systems. The fourth and final section is physiological adaptation. Questions relate to caring for clients with acute, chronic, or life-threatening physical health conditions. In order to correctly answer questions in this area, you need to understand alterations in body systems, basic pathophysiology, fluid and electrolyte imbalances, radiation therapy, and hemodynamics. There might be questions relating to respiratory care, suctioning, oxygen, infectious diseases, an unexpected response to therapies, medical emergencies, and CPR. Other topics that might be included are heat and cold, dialysis, wound and pressure ulcer care, newborn phototherapy, the application of dressings, and vital signs.

Concepts and processes integrated throughout the exam questions include the clinical problem-solving process (nursing process), caring, communication and documentation, cultural awareness, self-care, and teaching/learning.

HOW DO I APPLY TO TAKE THE EXAMINATION?

You will need to apply to the state board of nursing in the state in which you wish to be licensed. This process involves completing the application forms, having your school of nursing send transcripts, and sending the required fees to the state board of nursing and the testing service. A passport photo is required. When the State Board of Nursing gives approval, the testing service will be notified. If you have paid your fees to the testing service, the testing service sends you an Authorization To Test (ATT) notice along with your identification number. Your authorization to test is valid for several months. The exact time varies from state to state so check your notice very carefully. If you do not test within the authorization period, you must apply and pay fees all over again.

The exam is administered at Pearson Professional Centers. It is your responsibility to call the testing service and schedule the exam. Note that you do not need to take the exam at a testing center located in the state in which you wish to be licensed. The computer sends the results to the state to which you have sent your credentials. The first time candidate is guaranteed to be given a testing date within 30 days.

Those who are repeating the exam may sometimes have to wait longer to be scheduled. During peak testing times most testing centers will be open evenings and weekends. You should not wait until the day before you wish to test. If, after you have scheduled the test, you find that you need to change the date you may do so without penalty up to 24 hours before the scheduled appointment.

WHAT TYPES OF QUESTIONS ARE ON THE EXAM?

At least 98% are multiple-choice questions with only one correct answer. There is no credit for the second best answer. Each item stands alone. The scenario that describes the client situation and the answer choices are all on the same computer screen. There are three new types of questions on the exam. The first is a question in which you will be asked to select one or all of the answers that apply. In order for the answer to be correct, all of the correct responses and no others must be selected. The second new question type is one in which the candidate types in the answer. An example is a calculation question in which the correct answer is typed. The third new item type is to locate a structure on a diagram. An example is locating the spot to place the stethoscope to listen to an apical pulse.

DO I HAVE TO KNOW A LOT ABOUT COMPUTERS TO TAKE THE TEST?

It is not necessary to be a computer expert to take the exam. You are oriented to the computer and given a few practice questions before taking the test. You can successfully take the test if you have never seen a computer. When you select an answer choice you will be asked to confirm that this is the answer you want to record. You may change your answer at this time. When you confirm your choice, your answer is recorded. After that, you may not go back to that question. You may use the drop-down calculator on the computer for math problems. You do not have to use the calculator. You may not bring your own calculator to the testing center.

HOW IS THE EXAM SCORED?

The exam is administered on a computer using a program called *computerized adaptive testing*. You will get questions that are tailored to how you are performing. Each candidate, therefore, takes a unique test. The questions, however, are drawn from the same test pool and conform to the test plan as described earlier.

The specific questions you are given depend upon the answers you gave to the previous question. As you answer questions correctly, you are given more difficult questions to determine your ability level. When you can successfully answer questions at the "passing" level, the test terminates. The test also terminates if you show clearly that you cannot answer questions at the "passing" level. If you can successfully answer questions that are well above the passing level, you will answer fewer questions; conversely, if you cannot successfully answer questions that are well below the passing level, you will also answer fewer questions.

You will answer between 85 and 205 questions depending on how well you perform, which includes 25 experimental ("try out") questions. The purpose of the experimental questions is to be sure that all questions that count for your license are good questions that are accurate and statistically correct. These experimental questions are mixed in with real questions. You have no way of knowing which questions are experimental and which questions are real, so you must do your best on all of the questions.

The minimum number of questions that a candidate can take is 85. There is no minimum amount of time. The exam can take a maximum of 5 hours or 205 questions. Most candidates will not take the maximum time or the maximum number of questions. If you are answering questions that are close to the passing level, either just above or just below, you will answer more questions until you prove that you can consistently answer questions well above or well below the passing level or until you run out of questions or time.

CAN I TAKE A BREAK?

After two hours, you will be asked if you want to take a 10-minute break. At the end of three-and-a-half hours, you will be given an option to take another break. You may choose to take breaks, or not, depending on how you feel. If necessary, you may take a break during the test. The clock keeps running during your breaks, however.

WHEN WILL I KNOW IF I PASSED?

The State Board of Nursing should receive notification of your results within three business days of the day you take the test. You are notified by the State Board of Nursing, usually within a couple of weeks. You will not know whether you passed when you leave the testing center. Most candidates feel very unsure after taking the test. This is a normal reaction. Some states have web sites or special telephone lines that will verify licensure. If your state has these services, you must enter your social security number for verification as a licensed nurse.

Tips for Test Taking

Read and review the tips that follow to help you do your best on the examination.

LOOK FOR KEY CONCEPTS

Read the question carefully to determine the key concepts. Key concepts include determining who the client is, what the problem is, what specifically is asked about the problem, and what the time frame is.

An elderly woman who has senile dementia is admitted to the long-term care facility by her son. During the admission process, the son says to the nurse, "Did I do the right thing to bring my mother here?" Which initial response by the nurse will be most helpful?
1. Say to the woman, "You will like it here. We will take very good care of you."
2. Ask the woman if she is comfortable or if there is anything that can be done to make her feel more at home.
3. Tell the son, "You made the right decision. We will take good care of her."
4. Say to the son, "It must have been very difficult to make this decision."

In this question, *the client is the son* of the elderly woman. *The problem is the son's concern* about whether he should have brought his mother to the long-term care facility. What is *asked about the problem is which initial response by the nurse is most helpful.* The *time frame is the day of admission.* All of these factors must be considered when choosing the correct answer.

Look at the answer choices in light of the key concepts in the question. The client is the son; therefore, answers 1 and 2 cannot be correct. The time is during the admission process. The questions asks for an initial response. Initially, the goal is to open communication. Choice 3 does not open communication. Choice 4 is an empathic answer that will open communication.

LOOK FOR KEY WORDS

Look for words in the question that focus on the issue. There might be words such as *early* or *late* symptoms; *most* or *least* likely to occur. These words are critical to understanding the question and are very easy to miss unless you practice looking for them.

When the question asks for the *initial* nursing action, remember that initial means first—and think of the first step in the nursing process, which is assessment. Assess before acting. Sometimes you will have been given enough assessment data that you can take an action. When the question asks for an initial action, always ask yourself whether there is any relevant assessment data needed. Then, ask whether there is an emergency action you should take.

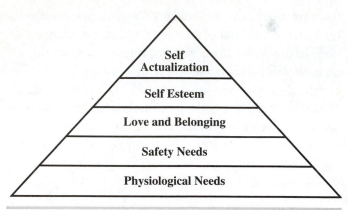

FIGURE 1.1 Maslow's Hierarchy of Needs

When the question asks what action is *essential* for the nurse to take, think safety. Essential means that you must do it, and it cannot be left undone. When setting priorities, remember Maslow's hierarchy of needs (Figure 1.1). Remember, "Keep them breathing, keep them safe." It is also important to consider which actions will help prevent complications.

UTILIZE TEST-TAKING STRATEGIES

Using the following test-taking strategies will also maximize your success.

The Odd Man Wins

The option that is most different in length, style, or content is usually correct. The correct answer is often the longest or the shortest. Remember also that if two or three answers say the same thing in different words, they cannot both be correct—so neither one is correct (poor appetite and anorexia, for example).

Opposites

When two answers are opposites, such as hypotension and hypertension or tachycardia and bradycardia, the answer is usually one of the two.

An adult is admitted in shock. Which assessment finding would the nurse most expect to find in this client?
1. Elevated blood pressure
2. Blood pressure below normal
3. Slow pulse
4. Flushed color

Note that choices 1 and 2 are opposites. The answer will most likely be one of these. The answer is 2.

Repeated Words

Words from the question are repeated in the answer. Frequently, the same word or a synonym will be in both the question and the answer.

An adult client is to have a liver scan. Which explanation is most appropriate for the nurse to give the client?
1. You will be given a radiopaque substance to swallow before x-rays are taken.
2. You will be given a laxative the night before the x-rays are taken.
3. You will be given a radioisotope that will be picked up by the liver and can be measured by a scanner.
4. An iodine dye will be injected into your vein and will outline the liver.

Note that the question asks about a liver *scan,* and the third choice talks about a *scanner.* Also note that the correct answer is the longest. It takes more words to make the answer correct.

Absolutes

Absolutes tend to make answers wrong. Always, never, all, and none are usually not correct statements. Qualified answers such as usually, frequently, and often are usually correct statements.

A 65-year-old man stopped taking high blood pressure medication because he no longer had headaches. What is most important for the nurse to teach him about the symptoms of hypertension?
The symptoms
1. occur only when there is danger of a stroke.
2. are sometimes not evident.
3. occur only when there is kidney involvement.
4. occur only with malignant hypertension.

In the question, answers 1, 3, and 4 are absolutes and 2 is much more qualified. The correct answer is 2. You might also note that 2 is the shortest answer.

Becoming aware of the structure of questions and utilizing these test-taking strategies can help you answer questions more accurately. You will still need to study, however, and you should still understand the material. These test-taking strategies are not a substitute for knowing the material.

Read the Question Carefully

Read the entire question and all of the answers carefully before selecting the correct response. If the answer does not appear obvious to you, note the key words and use these test-taking strategies. Eliminate answers that cannot be correct. From the responses left, look at the data in the question and see which answer most correctly relates to the data. Remember, the answer must relate to the question. If you really do not know the answer, make an educated guess and move on to the next question. You cannot go back to any question.

You will be given something to write on during the test—most likely a dry erase board. When you get into the exam room, write on the board any things you are trying to remember, such as lab values, conversion facts (lbs to Kg; oz to ml, and so on). Use the writing board for any calculations and to write down key words for a question if necessary.

Tips on How to Prepare for NCLEX-PN®

You have completed a nursing program, so you should already be familiar with the material. You will need to review the material and practice many multiple choice questions before you are ready to take the exam, however.

REVIEW CONTENT

You will need to review content in an organized fashion. This book will help you do that. As you review the material in the book, note any areas that are particularly difficult for you or that you do not remember well. You will need to put more effort into these topics. As you are reviewing, remember to relate pathophysiology to nursing care. Be sure to understand the "whys" of procedures, treatments, and nursing actions. Consider priorities when reviewing nursing care. Ask yourself which of the actions listed is of highest priority.

Prepare a calendar and schedule for review. On a calendar, schedule which content areas you will review on which days. Allow time for both content review and multiple-choice questions.

Try to study in an environment where you can concentrate. If you cannot study in your home, go to the public library. You need uninterrupted study time.

PRACTICE MULTIPLE-CHOICE QUESTIONS

The examination consists of multiple-choice questions. You need two things to pass the examination. One is knowledge of nursing care. The second is the ability to answer multiple-choice questions concerning that knowledge.

You should plan to practice several thousand multiple-choice questions as part of your preparation before taking the examination. You should be consistently answering correctly 75 percent of the questions in the review books. Answering many multiple-choice questions not only increases your skill in answering multiple-choice questions, but it also helps you review the content and look at the same information from different perspectives. Be sure to read all the answers and rationales, even for the questions you answered correctly. You need to be sure that you chose the correct answer for the right reasons. You can learn a lot from reading the rationales. If you notice that you are missing several questions on the same subject, then you should review the subject again, clarifying any areas about which you are confused.

If you have a computer available, you might want to practice at least a few questions on the computer. Answering questions on the computer might make you more comfortable with the computer and the screen. It is not essential to practice on a computer, however. The key point is that you practice thousands of questions before you go to the exam. You want to be well prepared.

PRACTICE STRESS-REDUCTION STRATEGIES

When taking the exam, you might find that you become anxious. You should practice a stress-reduction technique to use during the exam. Some candidates find that closing their eyes and taking several slow, deep breaths help clear the mind when stress is rising. Some candidates have found that closing the eyes and taking a "mini vacation" to the beach or the mountains or to their favorite rose garden might help reduce anxiety during the exam. Another technique that candidates have found helpful is getting up and taking a short walk when stress is building and the mind does not seem to function well.

The key to implementing these stress-reduction techniques is first learning to recognize the signs of anxiety that will keep you from thinking well and secondly to practice whatever technique you choose during your study sessions. As with any skill, you need to practice it before you become good at it.

When you are practicing multiple-choice questions, note when you start to miss a lot of questions. What sensations are you experiencing at this time? How many questions have you done already? How long have you been sitting? Learn to recognize the clues that your body and mind are giving you that suggest you need to take a brief break. Utilize a stress-reduction strategy. Practice several techniques and see which one works best for you and then use that one when your mind starts to wander during study.

Do not use alcohol and sedatives as a way to reduce stress before or during the exam. These substances might reduce stress, but they also interfere with thinking and problem solving.

EXAM DAY

Plan to spend all five hours at the exam. If you do not take the maximum time, consider it a gift and do something special for yourself. Do not have someone waiting for you outside the testing center because it might make you feel as if you have to hurry during the test. You want to be able to take as much time as you need to read the questions carefully before answering them.

Eat breakfast. Remember that your brain needs fuel. You cannot think well if your brain cells do not have any fuel.

Dress in layers. The room might be cooler or warmer than you like, and the temperature might change. Dress comfortably.

Bring two forms of identification with you to the testing center—one of which is a picture ID. Also bring your authorization to test letter from the testing service.

When you get to the testing center, you will be asked for a picture ID. They will take two finger prints and your picture. This picture goes with your exam results (it does not go on your license).

Chapter 2

Essential Concepts

Sample Questions

1. When caring for a client in hemorrhagic shock, how should the nurse position the person?

   1. Flat in bed with legs elevated
   2. Flat in bed
   3. Trendelenburg position
   4. Semi-Fowler's position

2. An adult woman has been in an automobile accident. She sustained numerous lacerations, a fractured tibia set by closed reduction, and a mild concussion. She has no apparent renal injuries and is conscious. An indwelling catheter is inserted for which of the following purposes?

   1. To measure urine flow as an indicator of shock
   2. To prevent contamination of her cast
   3. For her comfort
   4. To prevent renal complications

3. An adult is admitted with chronic renal failure. Strict intake and output is ordered. The client is sometimes incontinent, so it is impossible to obtain an accurate record of output. How can the nurse best assess the client's fluid status?

   1. Estimate the amount voided each time.
   2. Observe her skin turgor.
   3. Weigh the client daily.
   4. Record the number of voidings.

4. A client has Crohn's disease with chronic diarrhea. Which nursing diagnosis is most likely to be appropriate for this client?

   1. Alteration in acid-base balance (metabolic acidosis) related to loss of intestinal fluids
   2. Alteration in potassium balance (hyperkalemia) related to renal potassium retention with bicarbonate
   3. Alteration in acid-base balance (metabolic alkalosis) related to excessive chloride losses in diarrhea
   4. Alteration in calcium balance (hypercalcemia) related to loss of phosphorus in diarrhea

5. The nurse is assessing a woman upon admission. Which data should be recorded as subjective data?

   1. Her weight is 142 pounds.
   2. She has a red rash covering the backs of her hands.
   3. She states, "My hands itch so bad, I can hardly stand it."
   4. Her temperature is 99.8°F.

6. The LPN/LVN working in a long-term care facility is supervising a CNA. Which observation indicates that the CNA needs further instruction in performing hygienic care?

   1. The CNA washes the client's face before washing the rest of the body.
   2. The CNA puts one foot at a time into the basin of warm water when bathing the client's feet.
   3. The CNA applies lotion and powder liberally after bathing the client.
   4. The bath water contains only a small amount of soap.

7. The nurse is taking vital signs on a very obese individual and uses an extra-wide cuff. What is the primary reason for using an extra-wide cuff?

   1. A regular-size cuff is not going to be long enough to go around the client's arm.
   2. Blood pressure taken with a cuff that is too narrow gives an artificially high reading.
   3. A regular cuff is too tight and causes discomfort to the client.
   4. A narrow cuff causes the client's pulse to be elevated.

8. The LPN/LVN notes that an apical-radial pulse is ordered for a client. Which is the correct way to obtain this reading?

   1. Have another nurse take the radial pulse while the LPN takes the apical pulse.
   2. Take the apical pulse and immediately take the radial pulse.
   3. The LPN should listen to the apical pulse and ask the client to take the radial pulse.
   4. Take the radial pulse and then take the apical pulse.

9. Which behavior by a CNA in a long-term care facility indicates a need for further instruction?

   1. Placing bed linens at the bedside prior to giving morning care.

2. Using the same wash basin for both residents in the semi-private room.
3. Washing hands after caring for one resident and before starting care for the next.
4. Wearing unsterile gloves to clean a resident who is soiled with feces.

10. There is blood on the floor. How should the nurse clean up the spill?

    1. Wipe up the spill and then clean the area with alcohol.
    2. Use a 1:10 solution of chlorine bleach to clean the spill.
    3. Wipe up the spill and clean the area with water.
    4. Use an iodine solution to clean up the spill.

11. The nurse is changing a dressing. Which behavior, if observed, would indicate a break in technique?

    1. The nurse opens a package of 4 × 4s away from the sterile field and then drops them onto the sterile field.
    2. The sterile field is at waist height.
    3. The nurse opens the first flap of a sterile package away from his or her body.
    4. While pouring sterile saline into a sterile basin on the sterile field, the saline splatters onto the cloth backing.

12. The nurse is caring for a woman who had a CVA and has right-sided hemiplegia. Which action is least appropriate?

    1. Performing ROM exercises when bathing her
    2. Changing her position every two hours
    3. Positioning the client supine and pulling the bed sheets tightly across her feet
    4. Placing her in the prone position for one hour three times a day

13. The nurse is caring for an adult who had abdominal surgery this morning. Which action

will do the most to prevent vascular complications?

1. Turn the client every two hours.
2. Encourage deep breathing and coughing every two hours.
3. Have the client move her legs and make circles with her toes every two hours.
4. Dangle the client as soon as she is awake and alert.

14. The nurse observes that an elderly man who is bedridden has a reddened area on his coccyx. The skin is not broken. The nurse most correctly interprets this pressure ulcer to be which stage?

1. Pre-ulcer
2. Stage one
3. Stage two
4. Stage three

15. An older adult who has a stage one pressure ulcer asks the nurse why a clear dressing has been put over the site when the skin is not broken. What should the nurse include when replying?

1. This dressing is a preventive measure to protect the skin from injury.
2. Covering it so the area is moist makes it heal faster.
3. Covering the area makes it more comfortable for you.
4. The clear dressing is designed to let light through and promote healing.

16. An adult is now alert and oriented following abdominal surgery. What position is most appropriate for the client?

1. Semi-Fowler's
2. Prone
3. Supine
4. Sims

17. The LPN has delegated the task of taking vital signs to an unlicensed assistive personnel (UAP). Which instruction is most appropriate?

1. Take all the vital signs at 10 A.M.
2. Report any abnormalities to me.
3. Tell me if any blood pressure readings are over 140/90 or under 100/70.
4. I am available if you have any problems.

18. The LPN/LVN delegates the task of performing hygienic care of a bedridden client to a UAP. What responsibility does the LPN/LVN have regarding the performance of the care?

1. The LPN/LVN should check to be sure the task is performed correctly.
2. The UAP is solely responsible for his or her own actions.
3. The LPN/LVN should observe all of the care.
4. The UAP has the responsibility to ask for assistance if needed.

19. Following a craniotomy, the nurse positions a client in a semi-reclining position for which reason?

1. To promote comfort
2. To promote drainage from the operative area
3. To promote thoracic expansion
4. To prevent circulatory overload

20. The nurse is to help a client who has had a CVA and has right-sided hemiplegia get up into a wheelchair. How should the nurse place the wheelchair?

1. On the left side of the bed facing the foot of the bed
2. On the right side of the bed facing the head of the bed
3. Perpendicular to the bed on the right side
4. Facing the bed on the left side of the bed

21. The nurse is observing two UAPs log roll a client who had a laminectomy yesterday. Which observation indicates the procedure is being incorrectly performed?

   1. One person moves the head and shoulders and the second person moves the hips and legs at the same time.

   2. The UAPs use a turning sheet to help turn the client.

   3. One person keeps the client from falling out of bed while the other person moves first the head and shoulders and then the hips and legs.

   4. The UAPs place the bed in the highest position prior to turning the client.

22. An elderly adult has a *nasogastric* (NG) tube and an *intravenous* (IV) line. The client is confused and attempts to remove both the NG tube and the IV. How should the nurse assure the client's safety?

   1. Apply four-point restraints.

   2. Ask the physician for an order for wrist restraints.

   3. Request a sitter to stay with the client.

   4. Suggest that the family stay with the client at all times.

23. The client has just returned to the nursing care unit following a hemorrhoidectomy. What order should the nurse expect?

   1. A sitz bath stat and qid

   2. Warm compresses to the surgical area prn

   3. A hot water bottle to the surgical area prn

   4. An ice pack to surgical area

24. Warm compresses are ordered for an open wound. Which action is appropriate for the nurse?

   1. Use sterile technique when applying the compresses.

   2. Leave the compresses on continually, pouring warm solution on the area when it cools down.

   3. Alternate warm compresses with cool compresses.

   4. Apply a wet dressing to the wound and cover with a dry dressing.

25. An adult returned from the *Post Anesthesia Care Unit* (PACU) following abdominal surgery. At 2 P.M., he asks for pain medication. He has an order for meperidine (Demerol) 75 mg I.M. q 3–4 hr prn for operative site pain. He was last medicated at 10:30 A.M. What is the best initial action for the nurse?

   1. Administer 75 mg of meperidine.

   2. Ask the client to tell you where he hurts.

   3. Listen to the client's bowel sounds and breath sounds before administering the meperidine.

   4. Inform the client he has to wait a half hour before receiving pain medication.

26. The family of an adult who is terminally ill with advanced metastatic cancer asks the nurse to "let him die in peace." The client is alert and oriented and in severe pain. What response is appropriate for the nurse?

   1. Ask the family member to sign a release form for a DNR order.

   2. Encourage the family to talk with the client and the physician.

   3. Suggest that not doing all that is possible for the client is unethical.

   4. Ask the doctor for a DNR order.

27. An adult who is terminally ill says to the nurse, "Am I going to die soon?" What is the best response for the nurse to make?

   1. "No one can tell for sure when the end will come."

   2. "Are you afraid of dying?"

3. "You are concerned about when you will die?"

4. "Everyone has to die sometime."

28. An adult has just died. How should the nurse prepare the body for transfer to the mortuary?

1. Leave the body as is; no preparation is necessary.

2. Bathe the body and put identification tags on it.

3. Remove dentures before bathing the body.

4. Position the body with its head down and arms folded on its chest.

29. A cooling blanket is ordered for an adult who has a temperature of 106°F. Which nursing action is appropriate?

1. Place a sheet over the cooling blanket before putting the client on the blanket.

2. Maintain the client in a supine position on the blanket.

3. Apply powder to the skin that is in contact with the blanket.

4. Turn the client every 10 minutes and assess for frostbite.

30. An adult is admitted to the hospital after several days of vomiting. Her breathing is now slow and shallow. What acid-base imbalance does the nurse suspect?

1. Respiratory acidosis with metabolic compensation

2. Respiratory alkalosis with little metabolic compensation

3. Metabolic alkalosis with respiratory compensation

4. Metabolic acidosis with little respiratory compensation.

Answers and Rationales

1. (1) The shock position is flat in bed with the legs elevated to increase venous return. The head can be placed on a pillow. The Trendelenburg position, with the head lower than the chest, is no longer the recommended position because the abdominal organs can put pressure on the diaphragm and interfere with breathing and heart function. The semi-Fowler's position would make the client worse by increasing venous return.

2. (1) 25% of the cardiac output goes to the kidneys. If cardiac output goes down, as it will in shock, the kidneys will produce less urine. Most trauma victims will be catheterized to help determine whether there is shock caused by possible internal bleeding. A urinary catheter does not prevent kidney damage; it merely measures urine output.

3. (3) Daily weights are the best way to assess fluid balance. Estimations of the amount voided are usually not accurate. Skin turgor can give some information about fluid status but is not the best way to assess it. Recording the number of voidings gives some indication of fluid status but does not indicate how much urine is in each voiding. When unable to measure output, the best assessment measure is daily weights.

4. (1) Loss of alkaline intestinal fluid causes metabolic acidosis. Hyperkalemia is unlikely because intestinal fluids are high in potassium. Sodium, not potassium, is resorbed with bicarbonate. Chloride is retained as bicarbonate is lost, contributing to metabolic acidosis. Calcium levels do increase as phosphorus is lost, but diarrhea does not cause a loss of large amounts of phosphorus.

5. (3) Subjective data is data from the client's perspective, something that the client tells you. Weight and temperature are measured and are objective data. A rash is observed and is objective data.

6. (3) Powder tends to cake and dry the client's skin. Powder applied following the application of lotion makes a sticky mess. The bath should start with the eyes and face first. Putting the feet into warm water when bathing the feet is a very good thing to do. It is comforting and soothing to the client and helps soften any tough skin on the feet. The bath water should contain only small amounts of soap; too much soap dries the skin.

7. (2) A too-narrow cuff gives an artificially high reading. A cuff that is too wide will give a reading that is too low. The pulse will not be affected. It is not the length of the cuff that is the concern, it is the width of the cuff.

8. (1) When an apical radial pulse is taken, two nurses are needed. One listens to the apical pulse while the other nurse takes the radial pulse. The nurse should not ask the client to take his or her own radial pulse.

9. (2) Each person should have their own wash basin which is used exclusively for them. Bed linens can be placed at the bedside prior to morning care so that the needed materials are close at hand. Hands should be washed before and after all client contact. Feces are full of bacteria. Protective barriers should be working when the health care worker is at risk for exposure to body fluids. Gloves are appropriate when cleaning up feces.

10. (2) Blood should be cleaned with a solution of bleach at a 1:10 dilution. Alcohol and iodine are not appropriate because they do not kill HIV, which might be in the blood. Sometimes soap and water are used, but just plain water does not kill microorganisms.

11. (4) Moisture carries organisms through a barrier. If moisture spills on a cloth or paper sterile field, the field is no longer sterile. Sterile packages should be opened away from the sterile field. Items below the waist on a sterile field are not considered sterile. The first flap of a sterile package should be opened away from the nurse so that the last flap will come toward the nurse. Reaching across a sterile field is not appropriate.

12. (3) The bed sheets should not be drawn tightly over the feet, because this action might cause foot drop—especially with the client in the supine position. ROM exercises should be performed during the bath and several other times during the day. The client's position should be changed every two hours. Placing a person who has had a CVA in the prone position for an hour three times a day will help prevent hip flexion contractures. Note that the question asked which action is LEAST appropriate.

13. (3) Moving the legs and drawing circles with the toes promotes venous return and helps prevent venous stasis and thrombophlebitis. Turning the client every two hours will help prevent respiratory complications and skin breakdown. Deep breathing and coughing help to prevent respiratory complications. Dangling the client is not related to preventing vascular complications. In fact, it promotes venous stasis. Not enough information is given as to whether dangling the client as soon as she is alert is appropriate.

14. (2) Pressure areas that have color changes and changes in skin texture with no break in the skin are assessed as stage one pressure ulcers. Stage two ulcers have a break in the skin with involvement of the dermis. Stage three pressure ulcers involve the subcutaneous tissue. Pressure ulcers are not classed as pre-ulcers.

15. (2) Moist skin will heal better than skin that is dried out. There is some truth to the idea that covering the area helps to prevent further injury, but answer 2 is more correct. Comfort is not the primary reason for covering the area. The dressing is not primarily designed to let light in.

16. (1) The semi-Fowler's position is the position of choice following abdominal surgery. This position allows for greater thoracic expansion and puts less pressure on the suture line. Supine puts pressure on the suture line and is

very uncomfortable for persons who have had abdominal surgery. Prone is contraindicated for someone who has abdominal surgery. The Sims position is a semi-lateral, semi-prone position and would put too much pressure on the suture line.

17. (3) The nurse should give specific instruction to the UAP. This answer choice is the most specific of the instructions. The other choices are all very vague. The UAP might not know the norms.

18. (1) The LPN/LVN can delegate tasks that are delegatable to the UAP. The responsibility for making sure that the task is correctly performed, however, rests with the LPN/LVN. The UAP has responsibility, but the delegator also retains responsibility for the care given by those to whom it has been delegated. It is not necessary to directly observe all care given by the UAP. While the UAP should ask for help if needed, it is the responsibility of the delegator to be sure that assistance is not needed.

19. (2) The semi-reclining position will promote drainage from the operative area and prevent cerebral edema without putting undue pressure on the cerebral structures. The major goal post-craniotomy is to prevent cerebral edema and increased intracranial pressure. The position might or might not promote comfort. Comfort is not the major reason for placing the client in the semi-reclining position, however. Semi-reclining allows for moderate thoracic expansion (not as much as semi-sitting), but that is not the reason for using a semi-reclining position in a client who had a craniotomy. Semi-reclining position will help a little in preventing circulatory overload (not as much as semi-sitting), but that is not the reason for using semi-reclining position in a client who has had a craniotomy.

20. (1) The wheelchair should be placed on the unaffected side of the bed, facing the foot of the bed. The client can then stand on the unaffected leg and pivot and sit in the chair.

21. (3) Log rolling is used when the spine must be kept straight. The head and shoulders and hips and legs should be moved as a unit at the same time. Log rolling can be correctly performed by using a turning sheet. The bed should be placed in the highest position before turning the client to protect the backs of the personnel.

22. (2) The client is at risk for injuring himself or herself, so restraints are indicated. The nurse should ask the physician for an order for wrist restraints. The least restraint possible should be used. Four-point restraints are not indicated by the data in the question. A sitter does not appear to be necessary in this situation. There is no data to support that need. The nurse and the staff should be able to ensure the client's safety without requiring the family to be present at ALL times.

23. (4) The client will have an ice pack applied to the surgical area on the day of surgery. Sitz baths will probably be ordered for the following day. The rule is cold for the first 24 hours to prevent edema followed by warmth to promote healing. The day after surgery, the client will start taking sitz baths.

24. (1) The nurse should use sterile technique when applying compresses to an open wound. Warm compresses are not left in place continually. Moist heat is left on for 15–25 minutes at a time. Alternating warm compresses and cool compresses is not what is ordered for the client. Option 4 describes a wet to dry dressing.

25. (2) The question states that the client asks for pain medication. There is no indication of where the pain is. The nurse cannot assume that the pain is in the operative area. The time frame is adequate, so if the client's pain is in the operative area, the nurse should administer the medication. Listening to bowel and breath sounds is not a criteria for administering pain medication.

26. (2) Because the client is alert, he should be involved in making the decision. This matter should be discussed with the client and with the physician who will need to write any

orders. Suggesting that such a request is unethical is not appropriate. Clients have the right to refuse treatment and have advance directives. The alert client should be involved in the process.

27. (3) This response is the most therapeutic. It focuses on what the client asked and opens the lines of communication. The first answer might be true but does not encourage the client to discuss his concerns. The second choice is not appropriate because it focuses on fear, which is not in the client's question. The third response is much better than choice 2. Choice 4 closes communication and is not appropriate.

28. (2) The body should be bathed, a clean gown put on, and it should have identification tags placed on it. Dentures, if normally used by the client, should be placed in the mouth. The body should be flat with extremities straight. If the head is down, the blood will go to the head and discolor the skin, making viewing difficult.

29. (1) There should always be a sheet between the client and the cooling blanket to protect from frostbite. The position of the client should be changed every two hours. Powder is not applied to the skin; it will cause the skin to be dry. If necessary oil could be applied to the skin. The client should be checked for frostbite and should be turned every two hours, not every 10 minutes.

30. (3) A client who is vomiting is losing acid and will go into metabolic alkalosis. The slow, shallow breathing is evidence of trying to hold on to CO_2, which is acid, thus compensating for the alkalosis.

Unit II

Medical-Surgical Nursing

UNIT OUTLINE

Chapter 3

Cardiovascular System

Sample Questions

1. The nurse counts an adult's apical heart beat at 110 beats per minute. The nurse describes this as:

   1. Asystole
   2. Bigeminy
   3. Tachycardia
   4. Bradycardia

2. A client has an elevated AST 24 hours following chest pain and shortness of breath. This is suggestive of which of the following?

   1. Gall bladder disease
   2. Liver disease
   3. Myocardial infarction
   4. Skeletal muscle injury

3. An adult has a coagulation time of 20 minutes. The nurse should observe the client for:

   1. Blood clots
   2. Ecchymotic areas
   3. Jaundice
   4. Infection

4. A prothrombin time test should be performed regularly on persons who are taking which medication?

   1. Heparin
   2. Warfarin
   3. Phenobarbital
   4. Digoxin

5. Which prothrombin time value would be considered normal for a client who is receiving warfarin (coumadin)?

   1. 12 seconds
   2. 20 seconds
   3. 60 seconds
   4. 98 seconds

6. The nurse is caring for a client who is receiving heparin. What drug should be readily available?

   1. Vitamin K
   2. Caffeine
   3. Calcium gluconate
   4. Protamine sulfate

7. An adult who is receiving heparin asks the nurse why it cannot be given by mouth. The nurse responds that heparin is given parenterally because:

   1. It is destroyed by gastric secretions.
   2. It irritates the gastric mucosa.
   3. It irritates the intestinal lining.
   4. Therapeutic levels can be achieved more quickly.

8. An adult who is admitted for a cardiac catheterization asks the nurse if she will be asleep during the cardiac catheterization. What is the best initial response for the nurse to make?

   1. "You will be given a general anesthesia."
   2. "You will be sedated but not asleep."
   3. "The doctor will give you an anesthetic if you are having too much pain."
   4. "Why do you want to be asleep?"

9. During the admission interview, a client who is admitted for a cardiac catheterization says, "Every time I eat shrimp I get a rash." What action is essential for the nurse to take at this time?

   1. Notify the physician.
   2. Ask the client if she gets a rash from any other foods.
   3. Instruct the dietary department not to give the client shrimp.
   4. Teach the client the dangers of eating shrimp and other shellfish.

10. The nurse is preparing a client for a cardiac catheterization. Which action would the nurse expect to take?

    1. Administer a radioisotope as ordered.
    2. Give the client a cleansing enema.
    3. Locate and mark peripheral pulses.
    4. Encourage high fluid intake before the test.

11. A young adult with a history of rheumatic fever as a child is to have a cardiac catheterization. She asks the nurse why she must have a cardiac catheterization. The nurse's response is based on the understanding that cardiac catheterization can accomplish all of the following EXCEPT:

    1. Assessing heart structures
    2. Determining oxygen levels in the heart chambers
    3. Evaluating cardiac output
    4. Obtaining a biopsy specimen

12. When a client returns from undergoing a cardiac catheterization, it is most essential for the nurse to:

    1. Check peripheral pulses.
    2. Maintain NPO.
    3. Apply heat to the insertion site.
    4. Start range of motion exercises immediately.

13. A male client with angina pectoris has been having an increased number of episodes of pain recently. He is admitted for observation. During the admission interview, he tells the nurse that he has been having chest pain during the last week. Which statement by the client would be of greatest concern to the nurse?

    1. "I had chest pain while I was walking in the snow on Thursday."
    2. "We went out for a big dinner to celebrate my wife's birthday, but I couldn't enjoy it because I got the pain before we got home from the restaurant."
    3. "I had chest pain yesterday while I was sitting in the living room watching television."
    4. "I felt pain all the way down my left arm after I was playing with my grandson on Monday."

14. The nurse responds to the call light of a client who has a history of angina pectoris. He tells the nurse that he has just taken a nitroglycerin tablet sublingually for anginal pain. What action should the nurse take next?

    1. If the pain does not subside within five minutes, place a second tablet under his tongue.

    2. Position him in the Trendelenburg position.

    3. Administer a prn narcotic for pain if he still has pain in 10 minutes.

    4. Call his physician and alert the code team for possible intervention.

15. The nurse is teaching an adult who has angina about taking nitroglycerine. The nurse tells him he will know the nitroglycerine is effective when:

    1. He experiences tingling under the tongue.

    2. His pulse rate increases.

    3. His pain subsides.

    4. His activity tolerance increases.

16. A client with angina will have to make lifestyle modifications. Which of the following statements by the client would indicate that he understands the necessary modifications in lifestyle to prevent angina attacks?

    1. "I know that I will need to eat less, so I will only eat one meal a day."

    2. "I will need to stay in bed all the time so I won't have the pain."

    3. "I'll stop what I'm doing whenever I have pain and take a pill."

    4. "I will need to walk more slowly and rest frequently to avoid the angina."

17. A client who has been treated for angina is discharged in stable condition. On a clinic visit, he tells the nurse he has anginal pain when he has sexual intercourse with his wife. The best response for the nurse to make is:

    1. "Do you have ambivalent feelings toward your wife?"

    2. "Many persons with angina have less pain when their partner assumes the top position."

    3. "Be sure that you attempt intercourse only when you are well rested and relaxed."

    4. "You might try having a cocktail before sexual activity to help you relax."

18. A low-sodium, low-cholesterol weight-reducing diet is prescribed for an adult with heart disease. The nurse knows that he understands his diet when he chooses which of the following meals?

    1. Baked chicken and mashed potatoes

    2. Stir-fried Chinese vegetables and rice

    3. Tuna fish salad with celery sticks

    4. Lean steak with carrots

19. An adult client is admitted with a diagnosis of left-sided congestive heart failure. Which assessment finding would most likely be present?

    1. Distended neck veins

    2. Dyspnea

    3. Hepatomegaly

    4. Pitting edema

20. Digoxin (Lanoxin) and Lasix (Furosemide) are ordered for a client who has congestive heart failure. Which of the following would the nurse also expect to be ordered for this client?

    1. Potassium

    2. Calcium

    3. Aspirin

    4. Coumadin

21. When the nurse is about to administer digoxin to a client, the client says, "I think I need to see the eye doctor. Things seem to look kind of green today." The nurse takes his vital signs, which are B.P. 150/94; P 60; R. 28. What is the most appropriate initial action for the nurse to take?

1. Administer the medication and record the findings on his chart.
2. Withhold the digoxin and report to the charge nurse.
3. Request an appointment with the ophthalmologist.
4. Reassure the client that he is having a normal reaction to his medication.

22. An adult client is admitted to the hospital with peripheral vascular disease of the lower extremities. He has several ischemic ulcers on each ankle and lower leg area. Other parts of his skin are shiny and taut with loss of hair. A primary nursing goal for this client should be to:

1. Increase activity tolerance
2. Relieve anxiety
3. Protect from injury
4. Help build a positive body image

23. An adult client who has peripheral vascular disease of the lower extremities was observed smoking in the waiting area. What is the most appropriate response for the nurse to make in regards to the client's smoking?

1. "Smoking is not allowed for patients with blood diseases."
2. "Smoking causes the blood vessels in your legs to constrict and reduces the blood supply."
3. "Smoking increases your blood pressure and strains your heart."
4. "Smoking causes your body to be under greater stress."

24. An adult client with peripheral vascular disease tells the nurse he is afraid his left leg is not improving and may need to be amputated. How should the nurse respond?

1. "You and your wife should discuss your feelings before surgery."
2. "You sound concerned about your leg and possible surgery."
3. "It is better to have an amputation when the ulcers are not improving."
4. "You don't need to be afraid of surgery."

25. An adult is diagnosed with hypertension. He is prescribed chlorothiazide (Diuril) 500 mg po. What nursing instruction is essential for him?

1. Drink at least two quarts of liquid daily.
2. Avoid hard cheeses.
3. Drink orange juice or eat a banana daily.
4. Do not take aspirin.

26. A low-sodium diet has been ordered for an adult client. The nurse knows that the client understands his low-sodium diet when the client selects which menu?

1. Tossed salad, carrot sticks, and steak
2. Baked chicken, mashed potatoes, and green beans
3. Hot dog, roll, and coleslaw
4. Chicken noodle soup, applesauce, and cottage cheese

27. A female client is admitted to the hospital with obesity and deep vein thrombophlebitis (DVT) of the right leg. She weighs 275 pounds. Which of the following factors is least related to her diagnosis?

1. She has been taking oral estrogens for the last three years.
2. She smokes two packs of cigarettes daily.
3. Her right femur was fractured recently.
4. She is 30 years old.

28. Which assessment finding would most likely indicate the client has thrombophlebitis in the leg?

1. Diminished pedal pulses
2. Color changes in the extremities when elevated
3. Red, shiny skin
4. Pain when climbing stairs

29. What should be included in the teaching plan for an adult who has hypertension?

1. Reduce dietary calcium.
2. Avoid aerobic exercise.
3. Reduce alcohol intake.
4. Limit fluid intake.

30. The nurse is caring for an elderly client who has congestive heart failure and is taking digoxin. The client should be monitored for which of the following signs of toxicity?

1. Disorientation
2. Weight gain
3. Constipation
4. Dyspnea

31. The LPN is assisting the RN in developing the nursing care plan for an older adult who has congestive heart failure. Which nursing diagnosis is most likely to be included?

1. Fluid volume deficit
2. Impaired verbal communication
3. Chronic pain
4. Activity intolerance

32. The nurse is caring for a client who is being evaluated for arteriosclerosis obliterans. Which complaint is the client most likely to have?

1. Burning pain in the legs that wakens him/her at night

2. Numbness of the feet and ankles with exercise
3. Leg pain while walking that becomes severe enough to force him/her to stop
4. Increasing warmth and redness of the legs when they are elevated

33. An adult is admitted with venous thromboembolism. What treatment should the nurse expect during the acute stage?

1. Application of an elastic stocking
2. Ambulation three times a day
3. Passive range of motion exercises to the legs
4. Use of ice packs to control pain

34. The nurse is observing a client who is learning to perform Buerger-Allen exercises. The nurse knows that the client is performing these exercises correctly when the client is observed:

1. Alternately dorsiflexing and plantar flexing the feet while the legs are elevated
2. Massaging the legs beginning at the feet and moving toward the heart
3. Alternately walking short distances and resting with the legs elevated
4. Elevating the legs, then dangling them, then lying flat for three minutes

35. What should be included in foot care for the client who has a peripheral vascular disorder?

1. Soaking the feet for 20 minutes before washing them
2. Walking barefoot only on carpeted floors
3. Applying lotion between the toes to avoid cracking of the skin
4. Avoiding exposure of the legs and feet to the sun

36. An adult male is being evaluated for possible dysrhythmia and is to be placed on a Holter monitor. What instructions should the nurse give him to ensure that this test provides a comprehensive picture of his cardiac status?

1. Remove the electrodes intermittently for hygiene measures.
2. Exercise frequently while the monitor is in place.
3. Keep a diary of all your activities while being monitored.
4. Refrain from activities that precipitate symptoms.

37. An older adult is scheduled for coronary arteriography during a cardiac catheterization. Which nursing intervention will be essential as she recovers from the diagnostic procedure on the hospital unit?

1. Encouraging frequent ambulation to prevent deep vein thrombosis.
2. Limiting fluid intake to prevent fluid overload.
3. Assessing bowel sounds at frequent intervals.
4. Assessing the arterial puncture site when taking vital signs.

38. An older adult is admitted to the hospital with symptoms of severe dyspnea, orthopnea, diaphoresis, bubbling respirations, and cyanosis. He states that he is afraid "something bad is about to happen." How should the nurse position this client?

1. Sitting upright
2. Trendelenburg
3. Supine
4. Prone

39. An adult male has a high level of high-density lipoproteins (HDL) in proportion to low-density lipoproteins (LDL). How does this relate to his risk of developing coronary artery disease (CAD)?

1. His risk for CAD is low.
2. There is no direct correlation.
3. His risk may increase with exercise.
4. His risk will increase with age.

40. A 72-year-old man had a total hip arthroplasty eight days ago. He suddenly develops tenderness in his left calf, a slight temperature elevation, and a positive Homan's sign. Which of the following will be included in the initial care of this man?

1. Warm packs to the left leg
2. Vigorous massage of the left leg
3. Placing the left leg in a dependent position
4. Performing range of motion exercises to the left leg

Answers and Rationales

1. (3) Tachycardia in an adult is defined as a heart rate above 100 beats per minute. Asystole is cardiac arrest. There is no heart beat. Bigeminy means that the heart beats are coming in pairs. Bradycardia in an adult is defined at a heart rate of 60 beats or less per minute.

2. (3) AST is an enzyme released in response to tissue damage. The symptoms are suggestive of myocardial damage. AST rises 24 hours after a myocardial infarction. It will also rise when there is liver damage and skeletal muscle injury. This client has symptoms typical of myocardial infarction; however, gall bladder disease may present with pain in the right scapula (shoulder blade) region but would not have an elevated AST.

3. (2) The normal clotting time is 9–12 minutes. A prolonged clotting time would suggest a bleeding tendency; the client should be observed for signs of bleeding, such as ecchymotic areas. Blood clots would occur with a clotting time that is less than normal. Jaundice occurs with liver damage or rapid breakdown of red blood cells, such as is seen in

sickle cell anemia. Too few white blood cells put the client at risk for infection. Too many white blood cells indicate an infection is present.

4. (2) A prothrombin time test is done to determine the effectiveness of warfarin. A partial thromboplastin time test is done for persons taking heparin. Phenobarbital and digoxin do not require regular clotting tests. Serum levels of these drugs may be done if the client is on long-term therapy.

5. (2) When a client is receiving coumadin, the prothrombin time should be 1½ to 2 times the normal value, which is 11–12.5 seconds. Twenty seconds falls within that range. Twelve seconds is normal for someone who is not receiving coumadin. Sixty seconds is normal for a PTT test. Ninety-eight seconds on a PTT would be acceptable for a client who is receiving heparin. It should be 1½ to 2 times the normal range of 60 to 70 seconds.

6. (4) The antidote for heparin is protamine sulfate. Vitamin K is the antidote for coumadin. Calcium gluconate is the antidote for magnesium sulfate. Caffeine is a central nervous system stimulant and will increase alertness and heart rate.

7. (1) Heparin is a protein and is destroyed by gastric secretions. It is given either IV or subcutaneously for that reason.

8. (2) Persons who are undergoing cardiac catheterization will receive a sedative but are not put to sleep. Their cooperation is needed during the procedure. Asking "why" makes the client defensive and is not appropriate for this client at this time. Give the client the information asked for.

9. (1) Allergy to shellfish is indicative of an allergy to iodine. The dye used in a cardiac catheterization is an iodine dye. Anaphylactic reactions can occur. Because the exam is scheduled for the morning, the nurse should notify the physician immediately. The other actions might have relevance but are not essential (safety related) at this time.

10. (3) It is essential to monitor peripheral pulses after the procedure. They should be assessed before the procedure to determine location and baseline levels. An iodine dye is used during a cardiac catheterization, not a radioisotope. There is no need to give the client an enema. Fluids may be encouraged after the test. The client will be NPO for eight hours before the test.

11. (4) A biopsy specimen cannot be obtained during a cardiac catheterization. Heart structures can be assessed; oxygen levels in the heart chambers can be determined; and cardiac output can be measured during a cardiac catheterization.

12. (1) Checking peripheral pulses is of highest priority. The complications most likely to occur are hemorrhage and obstruction of the vessel. The client is NPO before the procedure, not after. Cold may be applied to the insertion site to vasoconstrict. Heat vasodilates and is contraindicated because it might cause bleeding. Range of motion exercises might cause bleeding. The extremity used for the insertion site is kept quiet immediately following a cardiac catheterization.

13. (3) This answer indicates pain at rest, which suggests a progression of the angina. The other answers all indicate pain with known causes of angina—exercise, cold environment, or eating.

14. (1) Nitroglycerine can be given at five-minute intervals for up to three doses if the pain is not relieved. The Trendelenburg position (head lower than feet) increases cardiac work load and would make the client worse. PRN narcotics are not usually ordered for clients who have anginal pain. Nitroglycerine, a vasodilator, is usually the medication of choice. At some point, the physician will need to be called, but there is no need to alert the code team for possible intervention.

15. (3) Pain relief is the expected outcome when taking nitroglycerine. Vasodilation of coronary vessels will increase the blood supply to the heart muscle, decreasing pain caused by

ischemia. Tingling under the tongue and a headache indicate that the medication is potent. His pulse rate should decrease when the pain is relieved. Increase in activity tolerance is nice, but nitroglycerine is given to relieve anginal pain.

16. (4) Walking more slowly and resting decreases energy expenditure and *prevents* an attack. Answer #3 *treats* an attack. By the time he has pain, he is experiencing angina. To prevent angina, he needs to walk slowly and rest frequently. He should eat small, frequent meals—not one large meal. He should exercise within his tolerance level. Staying in bed predisposes the client to the complications of immobility, such as clots and pneumonia.

17. (2) Reducing his physical activity reduces the cardiac workload. This response suggests a way he can engage in sexual activity with minimum strain on the heart. Ambivalent feelings toward his wife are unlikely to cause anginal pain. There is some truth to being well rested and relaxed, but telling him this is the only time he should have intercourse is not realistic. The nurse should not advise the client to have an alcoholic beverage before sexual activity.

18. (1) Chicken is lower in sodium than beef or seafood. Baking adds no sodium to the chicken. Barbecuing adds sodium and fat, and frying adds fat and usually sodium. Mashed potatoes contain little sodium. Chinese food is usually high in sodium. Tuna fish is high in sodium; so is celery. Steak is high in sodium; so are carrots.

19. (2) Dyspnea occurs with left-sided heart failure. Distended neck veins, hepatomegaly and pitting edema are signs of right-sided heart failure.

20. (1) Lasix is a potassium-depleting diuretic. Digoxin toxicity occurs more quickly in the presence of a low serum potassium. Potassium supplements are usually ordered when the client is on a potassium-depleting diuretic. There is no indication for supplemental

calcium. Aspirin and coumadin are anticoagulants and not indicated because the client is taking Lasix and digoxin.

21. (2) Disturbance in green and yellow vision is a sign of digoxin toxicity. A pulse of 60 is borderline for digoxin toxicity. When there is any possibility of digoxin toxicity, withhold the medication and report to the charge nurse. Once a person takes digoxin, it stays in the system for nearly a week. The LPN will of course record the findings, but withholding the medication is essential. The client needs to have serum digoxin levels done, not be seen by an ophthalmologist. Visual disturbances are a sign of digoxin toxicity, but these are not normal.

22. (3) Because the client has such poor blood supply to his legs, the nurse must be very careful to protect him from injury. Increasing activity tolerance might be desirable but is certainly not the primary nursing goal. Note that the question does not indicate that he has poor exercise tolerance. There is no data in the question to indicate that the client is anxious. He may need help in building a positive body image because his legs are disfigured, but this is certainly not a high priority.

23. (2) This is an accurate answer that relates his behavior to his illness. All of the other statements are true about smoking but do not relate to his current health problem.

24. (2) This response opens communication and allows him to talk about his feelings. The other answers do not allow him to discuss his feelings with the nurse now.

25. (3) Chlorothiazide (Diuril) is a potassium-depleting diuretic. Orange juice and bananas are good sources of potassium. It is not necessary to increase fluids to two quarts when the client is taking a diuretic. Hard cheeses should be avoided when the client is taking monamine oxidase inhibitors. MAOIs are antidepressants. People who take coumadin should not take aspirin.

26. (2) Chicken is low in sodium, as are mashed potatoes and green beans. Carrot sticks, steak,

hot dogs, soup, and cottage cheese are all high in sodium.

27. (4) Age is least related to DVT. Oral estrogens, smoking, and a broken leg are all risk factors for DVT.

28. (3) Red, shiny skin suggests inflammation. Diminished pedal pulses, pain when climbing stairs, and color changes in the extremities when elevated are indicative of arterial insufficiency, not a clot in the vein.

29. (3) High alcohol intake contributes to increases in blood pressure. Hypertensive clients are usually advised to limit alcohol intake to the equivalent of two glasses of wine or less per day. Dietary sodium should be limited in people with hypertension; however, dietary calcium is not a contributing factor in hypertension. Aerobic exercise is helpful in controlling high blood pressure. It may also contribute to weight reduction, which can help decrease blood pressure. Restriction of fluid intake is a medical order and is not appropriate advice for a nurse to give. Fluid restriction is avoided unless other measures are not successful.

30. (1) Disorientation and confusion are often the first signs of digitalis toxicity in the elderly. Weight gain and dyspnea are not signs of digoxin toxicity. They might indicate exacerbation of congestive heart failure. Diarrhea, not constipation, is a sign of digoxin toxicity. Constipation could occur if the client has restricted activity.

31. (4) Dyspnea and impaired oxygenation of tissues reduce the client's ability to tolerate exercise. Fluid volume excess, manifested by edema, is much more likely to occur with CHF than fluid volume deficit. Impaired verbal communication would describe dysphasia, which occurs with CVA, not CHF. Acute pain may occur with CHF when exacerbations occur. Chronic pain does not usually occur with CHF.

32. (3) Severe leg pain while walking describes intermittent claudication, which is the most common symptom of arteriosclerosis obliterans. Pain at rest develops in the late stages of the disease. Pain is much more likely than numbness with exercise. Paresthesias (including numbness) do occur, but they are likely at rest. The legs and feet of the client with arteriosclerosis obliterans become cool and pale when elevated because there is not enough blood flow to the extremities.

33. (1) Compression bandages or stockings help prevent edema and promote adequate venous blood flow and are a major element in the treatment of venous thromboembolism. Bed rest is appropriate in the acute stage of venous thromboembolism. Any form of exercise to the legs would increase the risk of pulmonary emboli. Heat is appropriate in the treatment of venous thromboembolism. Ice causes vasoconstriction, which decreases blood flow to the extremities.

34. (4) In Buerger-Allen exercises, the feet are elevated until they blanch, then dangled until they redden, then stretched out while the client is lying flat. This promotes arterial circulation to the feet. Dorsiflexing and plantar flexing the feet help to maintain range of motion but are not Buerger-Allen exercises. The client with peripheral vascular disease should never massage the legs because of the high risk of dislodging a thrombus if one is present. Walking promotes venous circulation but is not a Buerger-Allen exercise.

35. (4) Sunburn would damage the already fragile skin, increasing the risk of ulceration and infection. Feet should not be soaked. Soaking leads to maceration, predisposing to skin breakdown or infection. The client with a peripheral vascular disorder should never walk barefoot. Small sharp objects such as pins may not be visible in carpet and could be stepped on. Lotion may be applied to dry areas of the legs and feet but must be avoided between the toes, where the excess moisture causes maceration. Ingredients in lotion provide a nutrient source for bacteria and fungi, increasing the infection risk if cracks in the skin occur.

36. (3) The client should function according to his normal daily schedule unless directed to do otherwise by the physician. Keeping a diary or log of these daily activities is necessary so that it can be correlated with the continuous ECG monitor strip to determine whether the dysrhythmia occurs during a certain activity or at a particular time of day. The Holter monitor is usually worn for only 24 hours, so it is not necessary to change the leads. Activities that precipitate symptoms may be correlated with a dysrhythmia that can be treated, preventing further symptoms from occurring. Therefore, it would be helpful if the patient were symptomatic while attached to the Holter monitor.

37. (4) Following a cardiac catheterization in which an arterial site is used for access, the puncture or cutdown site should be assessed at least as often as vital signs are monitored. The client is at risk for development of bleeding, hemorrhage, hematoma formation, and arterial insufficiency of the affected extremity. When the arterial access site is used, the client is on strict bed rest for at least several hours. Fluids are encouraged after catheterization to increase urinary output and flush out the dye used during the procedure. It is not necessary to assess bowel sounds frequently. The client is not given a general anesthetic during a cardiac catheterization.

38. (1) The client's symptoms suggest pulmonary edema. Any client with severe dyspnea, orthopnea, and bubbling respirations needs to be in an upright position. Sitting upright decreases venous return to the heart by allowing blood to pool in the extremities. Decreasing venous return lowers the output of the right ventricle and decreases lung congestion. Sitting upright also allows the abdominal organs to fall away from the diaphragm, easing breathing. The Trendelenburg position would not promote venous pooling in the extremities and would increase venous return and pulmonary congestion. The supine position also would contribute to increased pulmonary congestion. The prone position, lying on the abdomen, does not decrease venous return—which is what this client desperately needs.

39. (1) While elevated LDL levels in proportion to HDL levels are positively correlated with CAD, elevated HDL levels in proportion to LDL levels may decrease the risk of developing CAD. HDL levels may increase with exercise, thereby decreasing a client's risk of CAD. Age is not a predictor of HDL and LDL levels.

40. (1) Warm, moist heat applied to the extremity reduces the discomfort associated with thrombophlebitis. Vigorous massage of the leg is contraindicated in any client because it may cause a thrombus to become dislodged and possibly cause a pulmonary embolus. The leg should be elevated to prevent venous stasis. Leg exercises are used to prevent thrombophlebitis; once a client has thrombophlebitis, the leg is not exercised to prevent the thrombus from becoming an embolus.

Chapter 4

Hematologic System

Sample Questions

1. The nurse is discussing dietary sources of iron with a client who has iron deficiency anemia. Which menu, if selected by the client, indicates the best understanding of the diet?

   1. Milkshake, hot dog, and beets
   2. Beef steak, spinach, and grape juice
   3. Chicken salad, green peas, and coffee
   4. Macaroni and cheese, coleslaw, and lemonade

2. Ferrous Sulfate is prescribed for a client. She returns to clinic in two weeks. Which assessment by the nurse indicates that she has NOT been taking iron as ordered?

   1. The client's cheeks are flushed.
   2. The client reports having more energy.
   3. The client complains of nausea.
   4. The client's stools are light brown.

3. A Schilling test has been ordered for a client suspected of having pernicious anemia. What is the nurse's primary responsibility in relation to this test?

   1. Collect the blood samples.
   2. Collect a 24-hour urine sample.
   3. Assist the client to X-ray.
   4. Administer an enema.

4. A client who receives a diagnosis of pernicious anemia asks why she must receive vitamin shots. What is the best answer for the nurse to give?

   1. "Shots work faster than pills."
   2. "Your body cannot absorb Vitamin B_{12} from foods."
   3. "Vitamins are necessary to make the blood cells."
   4. "You can get more vitamins in a shot than a pill."

5. A woman who has been diagnosed as having pernicious anemia asks how long she will have to take shots. What is the best answer for the nurse to give?

   1. "Until your blood count returns to normal."
   2. "Until you are feeling better."
   3. "For the rest of your life."
   4. "That varies with each person. Ask your doctor."

6. A toddler has been treated for sickle cell crisis. The crisis subsides and the child improves. Which statement is essential for the nurse to include in the discharge teaching?

   1. Your child will bruise easily. Do not let your child bump into things.
   2. Notify the physician immediately if your child develops a fever.
   3. Your child will need special help with feeding.
   4. Observe your child frequently for difficulty breathing.

7. Which statement made by the parent of a child newly diagnosed with sickle cell anemia indicates a need for more teaching?

   1. "We are going to the mountains for our vacation this year."
   2. "It's a good thing she likes to drink juices."
   3. "If she needs something for pain, I will give her baby acetaminophen."
   4. "I will make sure that she doesn't get chilled when it is cold outside."

8. A five-year-old boy is admitted because he bled profusely when he lost his first baby tooth. After a workup, he is diagnosed as having classic hemophilia. His mother asks the nurse if his two younger sisters will also develop hemophilia. The best answer for the nurse to give is:

   1. "They will not develop the disease."
   2. "Statistically, one of them is likely to develop the disease."
   3. "They are unlikely to get the disease, but they may be carriers."
   4. "If it doesn't show up by the time they start school, they are unlikely to develop the condition."

9. The nurse has been teaching the parents of a child with hemophilia about the care he will

need. Which statement by the parents indicates a need for more instruction?

   1. "If my child needs something for pain or a fever, I will give him acetaminophen instead of aspirin."
   2. "I will take my child to the dentist for regular checkups."
   3. "I will keep my child in the house most of the time."
   4. "My son's medic-alert bracelet arrived."

10. A college student who is diagnosed as having infectious mononucleosis asks how the disease is spread. The nurse's response is based on the knowledge that the usual mode of transmission is through:

    1. Skin
    2. Genital contact
    3. Contaminated water
    4. Intimate oral contact

11. A young man who has infectious mononucleosis asks what the treatment is for his condition. The best response for the nurse to make is:

    1. "You will receive large doses of antibiotics for the next 10 days."
    2. "Rest and good nutrition are the best things you can do."
    3. "You will be given an antiviral agent that will help to control the symptoms."
    4. "You will probably be given steroid medications for several months."

12. An 8-year-old boy is admitted to the unit with a diagnosis of acute lymphocytic leukemia. During a routine physical exam, numerous ecchymotic areas were noted on his body. The parents reported that the child had been more tired than usual lately. The parent says that the child has had a cold for the last several weeks and asks if this is related to the leukemia. The

nurse's response is based on the knowledge that:

1. Leukemia causes a decrease in the number of normal white blood cells in the body.
2. A chronic infection such as the child has had makes a child more likely to develop leukemia.
3. The virus responsible for colds is thought to cause leukemia.
4. Having an infection prior to the onset of leukemia is merely a coincidence.

13. A child with leukemia bruises easily. This is most likely due to:

1. Decreased fibrinogen levels
2. Excessive clotting elsewhere in the body
3. Decreased platelets
4. Decreased erythrocytes

14. A child who is being treated for leukemia develops stomatitis. Which of the following nursing care measures is essential?

1. Using dental floss to clean the teeth
2. Frequent cleaning of the mouth with an astringent mouth wash
3. Use of an overbed cradle
4. Swabbing the mouth with moistened cotton swabs.

15. When planning care for a client who is HIV positive, the nurse should:

1. Teach persons coming in contact with the client to wear a gown and mask at all times.
2. Teach persons to wear gloves when handling any of the client's body fluids.
3. Restrict visitors to immediate family.
4. Encourage the client to stay away from other persons as much as possible.

16. Which action should the nurse expect to perform after a client has a bone marrow biopsy taken from the iliac crest?

1. Apply pressure to the site for 1 minute.
2. Administer a narcotic analgesic.
3. Apply an adhesive bandage to the site.
4. Place the client in a recumbent position.

17. Which of the following would be the most appropriate snack for a client who has iron deficiency anemia?

1. A half grapefruit
2. A carrot raisin salad
3. A cup of yogurt
4. Apple slices and cheese

18. Which of the following assessment findings should alert the nurse that the elderly client should be evaluated for pernicious anemia?

1. Clubbing of the nails
2. Bloody stools
3. Beefy-red tongue
4. Enlarged lymph nodes

19. An elderly client who is being treated for pernicious anemia needs to be monitored periodically for which of the following conditions?

1. Lactose intolerance
2. Stomach cancer
3. Dementia
4. Hearing loss

20. Which of the following would be the best lunch for a client with folic acid deficiency anemia?

1. Bologna sandwich and vegetable soup
2. Grilled cheese sandwich and tomato soup
3. Coleslaw and cream of mushroom soup
4. Spinach salad and bean soup

21. The nurse administers iron using the Z track technique. What is the primary reason for administering iron via Z track?

    1. To prevent adverse reactions
    2. To prevent staining of the skin
    3. To improve the absorption rate
    4. To increase the speed of onset of action

22. The nurse is caring for a client who is thought to have pernicious anemia. What signs and symptoms would the nurse expect in this person?

    1. Easy bruising
    2. Beefy-red tongue
    3. Fine red rash on the extremities
    4. Pruritus

23. A one-year-old is admitted to the hospital with sickle cell anemia in crisis. Upon admission, which therapy will assume priority?

    1. Fluid administration
    2. Exchange transfusion
    3. Anticoagulant
    4. IM administration of iron and folic acid

24. A toddler is diagnosed with sickle cell anemia. Her mother is four months pregnant with her second child. The mother asks if there is any chance the new baby will have sickle cell anemia. She says that neither she nor her husband have sickle cell anemia. What is the best response for the nurse to make?

    1. "No. Sickle cell anemia is not inherited."
    2. "Yes. The new baby will also have sickle cell anemia."
    3. "There is a 25% chance that each child you have will have the disease."
    4. "Because neither of you have the disease, another child will not have it. You should ask your physician."

25. A child who has hemophilia is admitted to the hospital with a swollen knee joint. He is complaining of severe pain. What is the priority of nursing care for this child upon admission?

    1. Maintain joint function
    2. Use a bed cradle
    3. Administer aspirin prn for pain
    4. Encourage fluids

26. The nurse is caring for a child who has hemophilia. He is admitted with a bleeding episode. Which of the following should the nurse expect will be given to stop the bleeding?

    1. Heparin
    2. Cryoprecipitate
    3. Packed cells
    4. Whole blood

27. A 19-year old-college student reports to the health service with a sore throat, malaise, and fever of four days duration. Examination shows cervical lymphadenopathy and splenomegaly. Temperature is 103°F. Blood is positive for heterophil antibody agglutination test. Which condition does the nurse expect this student has?

    1. Streptococcal sore throat
    2. Infectious mononucleosis
    3. Rubella
    4. Influenza

28. The nurse knows that infectious mononucleosis is caused by which of the following?

    1. Cytomegalovirus
    2. Beta hemolytic streptococcus
    3. Epstein-Barr virus
    4. Herpes simplex virus I

29. A child who has leukemia is to have a bone marrow biopsy performed. How will the child be positioned for this procedure?

   1. On his side with the top knee flexed
   2. Prone
   3. Modified Trendelenburg
   4. On his back with his head elevated 30 degrees

30. A child is being evaluated for possible leukemia. Which assessment finding is most likely to be present?

   1. Numerous bruises on the child's body
   2. Ruddy complexion
   3. Diarrhea and vomiting
   4. Chest pain

Answers and Rationales

1. (2) Beef, spinach, and grape juice contain iron. Milk contains no iron.

2. (4) Iron turns stool black. The other answers all indicate compliance with the medication regime.

3. (2) The client is given radioactive Vitamin B_{12} orally, and a 24-hour urine sample is collected to see if Vitamin B_{12} is absorbed from the GI tract into the blood stream and excreted in the urine.

4. (2) Injections of Vitamin B_{12} will be necessary, because without intrinsic factor her body cannot absorb Vitamin B_{12} from foods.

5. (3) Because she is deficient in intrinsic factor and cannot absorb Vitamin B_{12} from foods, she will have to take Vitamin B_{12} shots for life.

6. (2) Fevers cause dehydration and sickling, which may result in a crisis.

7. (1) The mountains are high in altitude and have less oxygen saturation, which may precipitate an attack. Drinking juices is good because

it will help to prevent dehydration. Acetaminophen is better for the child than aspirin, which may cause acidosis. The child should be protected from extremes in temperature.

8. (3) Hemophilia is carried on the X chromosome and causes disease when it appears in combination with the Y chromosome in the male. Number 1 is a true statement, but it is not complete and, therefore, not the best answer.

9. (3) Parents of children with hemophilia tend to overprotect them. A goal is to have the child lead as normal a life as possible. Number 1 is correct. He should not receive aspirin because it is an anti-coagulant. Number 2 indicates good knowledge. Prophylactic dental care is important, so he will not need dental work or extractions. Number 4 indicates good knowledge. He should always wear a medic-alert bracelet in case he is injured.

10. (4) The virus is spread through intimate oral contact. It is called the "kissing disease." It can also be spread by sharing eating and drinking utensils and by coughing and sneezing.

11. (2) Rest and good nutrition are the hallmarks of treatment for mononucleosis. Recovery may take several months. Because it is caused by a virus, antibiotics are not indicated. He would receive antibiotics only if he develops a secondary infection. There are no effective antiviral agents for this condition. Steroids are not indicated.

12. (1) Leukemia causes a decrease in normal white cells. White blood cells are the infection fighting cells. Infections occur because of the decrease in WBCs due to leukemia. Infections do not cause leukemia.

13. (3) In leukemia, there is bone marrow failure. In addition to producing abnormal, immature WBCs, the bone marrow fails and does not produce stem cells from which RBCs and platelets develop.

14. (4) Stomatitis is a frequent complication of chemotherapy for leukemia. The client has a

tendency to bleed because of his decreased platelets. Dental floss might cause bleeding. An astringent mouth wash is too strong for his tender mouth. An overbed cradle does not relate to stomatitis. Moistened cotton swabs are a gentle means of cleaning the mouth.

15. (2) Universal precautions are indicated. Number 1 is not correct. It is not necessary to wear a gown and mask unless there is a risk of exposure to body fluids. Number 3 is not correct. There is no reason to limit visitors. Number 4 is not correct. The client is HIV positive. There is no indication that the client is immunocompromised and at an increased risk of infection from others. The client will not transmit the disease unless there is contact with body fluids.

16. (4) The client should lie in bed in a recumbent position on top of a pressure dressing that has been applied to the site. Hemorrhage poses a slight risk after this procedure. Pressure should be applied to the site for several minutes. A pressure dressing should then be applied for one hour to reduce the chances of bleeding or hemorrhage. An analgesic may be ordered and administered prior to the procedure. Use of deep breathing and relaxation techniques may also be helpful. There is seldom any pain after the biopsy, although the site may ache for a few days.

17. (2) Carrots and raisins are both high in iron. Red meats and spinach are other good iron sources. Citrus fruits such as grapefruit are high in folic acid, vitamin C, and potassium but not iron. Dairy products such as yogurt and cottage cheese provide calcium but no iron. Apples are not good sources of iron.

18. (3) Early in the course of pernicious anemia, the tongue becomes beefy red and painful. Later, the tongue atrophies and becomes smooth. Nail clubbing is associated with respiratory and cardiac disorders. Numbness and tingling of the hands and feet are more common with pernicious anemia. Mild diarrhea is associated with pernicious anemia, whereas bloody stools

usually are not. Colorectal bleeding is likely to lead to iron deficiency anemia. Enlarged lymph nodes are associated with leukemia, not anemia.

19. (2) The incidence of stomach cancer is increased in clients with deficiency of gastric acid. Intrinsic factor is in gastric acid. Treatment of pernicious anemia corrects the deficiency of Vitamin B_{12} but does not alter the gastric acid production, so the client remains at risk for stomach cancer. Both lactose intolerance and hearing loss occur more commonly with aging, as does pernicious anemia. The presence of pernicious anemia does not alter the risk for either lactose intolerance or hearing loss, however. Dementia does occur in the late stages of untreated pernicious anemia, but for a client who is receiving treatment, there is no increased risk of dementia.

20. (4) Leafy green vegetables and dried beans are good sources of folic acid. Nuts and citrus fruits are other good sources. The other options do not contain foods high in folic acid.

21. (2) Iron is black and stains the skin. The Z track method of pulling the skin to one side before injecting the medications prevents staining of the skin. It also reduces pain from the medication. It does not prevent adverse reactions, improve the absorption rate, or increase the speed of onset of action.

22. (2) A beefy-red tongue is characteristic of pernicious anemia. Easy bruising would be seen in a clotting disorder such as hemophilia or in leukemia or in bone marrow depression. Pruritus is characteristic of Hodgkin's disease. Pernicious anemia does not present a fine, red rash on the extremities.

23. (1) Dehydration causes sickling. Sickling causes clumping and pain. First priority of care upon admission should be the administration of fluids. Exchange transfusion, if done, is not the first priority. Anticoagulants are not the first priority. Iron and folic acid may be given but are not the first priority. They will not help stop

the sickling. Folic acid and iron are necessary to make RBC.

24. (3) Sickle cell anemia is a recessive gene that is transmitted, giving a 25% chance that each child will have the disease. To have a child with the disease, both parents must be carriers for the disease even though neither one has the disease.

25. (2) Hemarthrosis (bleeding into a joint) is very painful. A bed cradle will keep the bed covers off of his sore joint. Moving a bleeding joint will increase bleeding and should not be done. Aspirin is an anticoagulant and contraindicated for a hemophiliac. Fluid administration is not the priority nursing action.

26. (2) Cryoprecipitate is frozen clotting factor and replaces the factors that the child is missing. Heparin is an anticoagulant and contraindicated for this child. Packed cells might be given after a severe hemorrhage but do not contain any clotting factors. Whole blood does not contain clotting factors.

27. (2) The findings are characteristic of infectious mononucleosis. The heterophil antibody agglutination test is diagnostic for mononucleosis. A throat culture would identify a streptococcal sore throat. Rubella (German measles) typically has a rash. The fever and sore throat are not typical of rubella. Influenza might have similar symptoms but would not have a positive heterophil agglutination test.

28. (3) The Epstein-Barr virus is the causative organism for infectious mononucleosis.

29 (1) The iliac crest is the site usually used for a bone marrow biopsy.

30. (1) The child with leukemia has a large number of immature white blood cells and not enough red blood cells and platelets. He is likely to have numerous bruises because of the low platelet count. He is likely to have a pale, not ruddy, complexion because he is deficient in red blood cells. Diarrhea and vomiting are possible if he had an intestinal virus, but bruises are much more common. Chest pain is unlikely.

Chapter 5

The Respiratory System

Sample Questions

1. An adult client is to have a sputum for culture. When is the best time for the nurse to collect the specimen?

   1. In the morning right after he awakens
   2. Immediately after breakfast
   3. Two hours after eating
   4. Shortly before he retires for the evening

2. A thoracentesis was performed on an adult client. After the procedure, the client has hemoptysis and a pulse of 80, respirations of 28 and temperature of 99°F. Which of these is of greatest concern to the nurse?

   1. Hemoptysis
   2. Respirations of 28
   3. Pulse of 80
   4. Temperature of 99

3. An adult client is to have postural drainage qid. In developing the care plan, the nurse should schedule this for:

   1. 7 A.M.; 11 A.M.; 4 P.M.; 10 P.M.
   2. 10 A.M.; 2 P.M.; 6 P.M.; 10 P.M.
   3. 6 A.M.; 12 noon; 6 P.M.; 12 mid.
   4. 6 A.M.; 10 A.M.; 2 P.M.; 6 P.M.

4. An adult man has a tracheostomy tube in place. Which of the following actions is most appropriate for the nurse to take when suctioning the tracheostomy?

   1. Use a sterile tube each time and suction for 30 seconds
   2. Use sterile technique and turn the suction off as the catheter is introduced
   3. Use clean technique and suction for 10 seconds
   4. Discard the catheter at the end of every shift

5. During suctioning of a tracheostomy tube, the catheter appears to attach to the tracheal wall and creates a pulling sensation. What is the best action for the nurse to take?

   1. Release the suction by opening the vent
   2. Continue suctioning to remove the obstruction
   3. Increase the pressure
   4. Suction deeper

6. A client comes to the clinic with a bloody nose. Which instruction is most appropriate?

   1. "Sit up with your head tilted forward. Grasp the soft part of your nose firmly between your thumb and forefinger."

   2. "Lay down and tilt your head backward. Grasp the end of your nose between your fingers."

   3. "Sit up and lean backwards. Put pressure on the side of your nose with your hand."

   4. "Lie down with your head lower than your feet. Grasp as much of your nose as possible between your fingers."

7. A client is admitted with a diagnosis of cancer of the larynx. Which statement made by the client is most likely related to the cause of his illness?

   1. "I have always enjoyed hot Mexican-style food."

   2. "I have smoked three packs of cigarettes a day for the last 40 years."

   3. "I used to work in a factory that burned coal."

   4. "I sang in the church choir every Sunday until my voice got hoarse last year."

8. During the preoperative period, which nursing action will be of greatest priority for a person who is to have a laryngectomy?

   1. Establish a means of communication.

   2. Prepare the bowel by administering enemas until clear.

   3. Teach the client to use an artificial larynx.

   4. Demonstrate the technique for suctioning a laryngectomy tube.

9. A 62-year-old man is admitted with emphysema and acute upper-respiratory infection. Oxygen is ordered at 2 liters per minute. The reason for low-flow oxygen is to:

   1. Prevent excessive drying of secretions

   2. Facilitate oxygen diffusion of the blood

3. Prevent depression of the respiratory drive

4. Compensate for increased airway resistance

10. An adult is admitted with COPD. The nurse notes that he has neck vein distention and slight peripheral edema. The practical nurse notifies the registered nurse and continues frequent assessments because the nurse knows that these signs signal the onset of:

    1. Pneumothorax

    2. Cor pulmonale

    3. Cardiogenic shock

    4. Left-sided heart failure

11. A 79-year-old is admitted to the hospital with a diagnosis of pneumococcal pneumonia. The client has dyspnea. The client's temperature is 102°F; respirations are 36; and pulse is 92. Bed rest is ordered. This position is ordered for this client primarily to:

    1. Promote thoracic expansion

    2. Prevent the development of atelectasis

    3. Decrease metabolic needs

    4. Prevent infection of others

12. An adult is to have a tracheostomy performed. What is the nursing priority?

    1. Shave the neck

    2. Establish a means of communication

    3. Insert a Foley catheter

    4. Start an IV

13. Which nursing action is essential during tracheal suctioning?

    1. Using a lubricant such as petroleum jelly

    2. Administering 100% oxygen before and after suctioning

    3. Making sure the suction catheter is open or on during insertion

    4. Assisting the client to assume a supine position during suctioning

14. An adult has a chest drainage system. Several hours after the chest tube was inserted, the nurse observes that there is no bubbling in the water seal chamber. What is the most likely reason for the absence of bubbling?

   1. His lungs have re-expanded.
   2. There is an obstruction in the tubing coming from the client.
   3. There is a mechanical problem in the pump.
   4. Air is leaking into the drainage apparatus.

15. An adult has a chest drainage system. The client's wife reports to the nurse that her husband is restless. The nurse enters the room just in time to see him pull out his chest tube. The most appropriate initial action for the nurse to take is:

   1. Go get petrolatum gauze and apply over the wound.
   2. Place her hand firmly over the wound.
   3. Apply a sterile 4 × 4 dressing.
   4. Reinsert the chest tube.

16. An adult had a negative PPD test when he was first employed two years ago. A year later, the client had a positive PPD test and a negative chest X-ray. This indicated that at that time the client:

   1. Was less susceptible to a tuberculosis infection than the year before
   2. Had acquired some degree of passive immunity to tuberculosis
   3. Had fought the mycobacterium tuberculosis but had not developed active tuberculosis
   4. Was harboring a mild tuberculosis infection in an organ other than the lung

17. An adult is being treated with Isoniazid (INH) and streptomycin for active tuberculosis. Which of the following symptoms would suggest a toxic effect of Isoniazid?

   1. Paroxysmal tachycardia
   2. Erythema multiforma

   3. Peripheral neuritis
   4. Tinnitus and deafness

18. An adult is being treated with Isoniazid (INH) and streptomycin for active tuberculosis. He is also receiving pyridoxine (Vitamin B_6). Why is this medication prescribed for him?

   1. Pyridoxine is bacteriostatic against the mycobacterium tuberculosis.
   2. To enhance his general nutritional status
   3. To prevent side effects of Isoniazid
   4. Pyridoxine acts to increase the effects of streptomycin.

19. The wife of a client with active tuberculosis has a positive skin test for tuberculosis. She is to be started on prophylactic drug therapy. What drug is the drug of choice for prophylaxis of tuberculosis?

   1. Streptomycin
   2. Para-amino-salicylic acid (PAS)
   3. Isoniazid (INH)
   4. Ethambutol (Myambutol)

20. A farmer who has had a cough for several months has noticed a lack of energy lately. He is being tested for histoplasmosis. Which factor reported by the client would be most related to the diagnosis of histoplasmosis?

   1. He drinks raw milk.
   2. He cleans chicken houses.
   3. He handles fertilizer frequently.
   4. He stepped on a rusty nail recently.

21. The nurse is caring for a client who is admitted with histoplasmosis. What drug is most likely to be prescribed for this client?

   1. Penicillin
   2. Chloromycetin
   3. Streptomycin
   4. Amphotericin B

22. An adult is to have a thoracentesis performed. What should the nurse do while preparing the client for this procedure?

1. Keep him NPO for 8 hours.

2. Prepare him to go to the operating room.

3. Explain the procedure to him.

4. Administer anticholinergic and analgesic as ordered.

23. The nurse is planning care for a client who has COPD. Which statement is the client most likely to say about activity tolerance?

1. "The most difficult time of the day for me is the first hour after waking up in the morning."

2. "I feel best in the morning after a good night's sleep."

3. "I seem to have more energy after eating a big meal."

4. "I don't know why, but I get my 'second wind' at night and don't want to go to bed."

24. The nurse is caring for a woman who is admitted with pneumonia. On admission, the client is anxious and short of breath but able to respond to questions. One hour later, the client becomes more dyspneic and less responsive, answering only yes and no questions. What is the best action for the nurse to take at this time?

1. Stimulate the client until the client responds.

2. Increase the oxygen from the ordered 6 liters to 10 liters.

3. Assess the client again in 15 minutes.

4. Notify the charge nurse of the change in the client's mental status.

25. A client's PPD test is positive, and a chest X-ray is negative. What is the best interpretation of these data?

1. The client's resistance to tuberculosis is low.

2. The client has been exposed to the organism but has not developed the disease.

3. The client has tuberculosis, but it is not serious.

4. The client has active tuberculosis.

26. An adult with tuberculosis has started taking Rifampin (Rimactane). Which side effect is the client most likely to experience when taking this drug?

1. Reddish-orange color of urine, sputum, and saliva

2. Erythema and urticaria

3. Tinnitus and deafness

4. Peripheral neuritis

27. Which laboratory tests should the client receive before prophylactic drug therapy for tuberculosis is started?

1. Serum creatinine and BUN

2. SGOT (AST) and SGPT (APT)

3. CBC and hematocrit

4. WBC and urinalysis

28. A client who had a laryngectomy is nearly ready for discharge. Which instruction is most appropriate for the nurse to give?

1. "Always be sure you have a buddy with you when you go swimming or boating."

2. "You may take a tub bath, but you should not take a shower."

3. "Be sure to have only liquids for another three weeks."

4. "Never cover your stoma with anything."

29. The client asks the nurse why inspiration through the nose is preferable to inspiring through the mouth. What is the best response?

1. It produces greater blood oxygen levels.

2. It is easier to breathe through the nose.

3. The nares humidify, warm, and filter the air.

4. Mouth breathing dilutes the air and reduces the amount of air entering the lungs.

30. While the nurse is suctioning a tracheostomy tube, the client starts to cough. What is the best action for the nurse to take?

   1. Suction deeper to pick up secretions.

   2. Gently withdraw suction tubing to allow suction or coughing out of mucus.

   3. Remove the suction as quickly as possible.

   4. Put the suction tube in and out several times to pick up secretions.

Answers and Rationales

1. (1) The sputum has collected during the night. It is most concentrated early in the morning.

2. (1) Hemoptysis is the only abnormal finding. All of the others are within normal range for someone who has undergone an invasive procedure.

3. (1) Postural drainage should be scheduled between meals and close to bedtime.

4. (2) Suctioning should be done under sterile technique for no more than 10 seconds. The suction should be off as the tube is inserted and applied intermittently as it is withdrawn.

5. (1) Suction should not be applied as the suction tube is inserted, because this will cause the suction tube to appear to attach to the tracheal wall and create a pulling sensation.

6. (1) This position will help to stop bleeding without causing aspiration of any blood dripping down the back of the throat.

7. (2) Cigarette smoking is the greatest risk factor for development of laryngeal cancer.

8. (1) Establishing a means of communication is the highest priority. Teaching the client to use an artificial larynx is a postoperative task. Because the laryngectomy tube will be temporary, the client will not need to learn to suction. That is a nursing function.

9. (3) The stimulus to breathe in a person with COPD is a low O_2 level rather than a CO_2 level, as in normal persons. If high-flow oxygen were given, the O_2 level would increase and the respiratory drive would cease.

10. (2) Distended neck veins and peripheral edema are signs of right-sided heart failure or cor pulmonale-heart failure due to pulmonary causes.

11. (3) Bed rest will reduce metabolic needs in this client who has pneumonia and is having difficulty meeting oxygenation needs. A semi-sitting (semi-Fowler's) position, not bed rest, will promote thoracic expansion. Isolation prevents infection of others. Deep breathing will help to prevent the development of atelectasis.

12. (2) The nursing priority is to establish a means of communication, because she will not be able to speak after the tracheostomy is performed.

13. (2) 100% oxygen is given before and after suctioning to help prevent hypoxia. Petroleum-based lubricants are not water-soluble and should never be used near an airway. Saline is used as a lubricant. The suction catheter is off during insertion to avoid traumatizing the tissues. She should be in semi-Fowler's position during suctioning. Supine predisposes to aspiration.

14. (2) Cessation of bubbling in the water seal bottle means either an obstruction in the tubing or re-expansion of the lung. This is the night of insertion of the tube. It takes at least 24 hours and often two to three days for the lung to re-expand.

15. (2) The nurse's primary goal has to be to stop air from entering the thoracic cavity and causing the lung to collapse again. Placing a hand firmly over the wound will accomplish this. Number 1 is wrong, because the nurse should not leave the client. Petrolatum gauze would be ideal but the nurse should not leave the

client. Number 3 is wrong because a sterile 4 × 4 dressing allows air to enter the thoracic cavity. The nurse should not reinsert the chest tube.

16. (3) A positive PPD test indicates that the client has come in contact with the organism and fought it. A negative chest X-ray says that the client won the fight and does not at that time have active tuberculosis.

17. (3) Peripheral neuritis is a toxic effect of INH. Tinnitus and deafness are side effects of streptomycin.

18. (3) Pyridoxine (Vitamin B_6) prevents the development of peripheral neuritis toxicity of INH.

19. (3) INH is the drug of choice for chemoprophylaxis. All of the other drugs listed can be used in the treatment of tuberculosis.

20. (2) Histoplasmosis is a fungus that grows in chicken and pigeon manure. Drinking raw milk might cause "milk fever." Handling fertilizer could cause "white lung," a COPD illness. Stepping on a nail might cause tetanus.

21. (4) Amphotericin B is the drug of choice to treat histoplasmosis.

22. (3) The nurse should explain the procedure to the client and obtain a permit if one has not already been signed. Thoracentesis is usually done at the bedside. NPO is not necessary. Anticholinergics and analgesics are not ordered.

23. (1) Morning is a difficult time for persons with COPD because secretions have accumulated during the night. They have to do a great deal of hacking and coughing to clear their air passages in the morning. The client with COPD is apt to be short of breath after a big meal because he is an abdominal breather. Most clients with COPD do not get a "second wind" at night. They need a lot of rest.

24. (4) The change in the client's status is significant and indicates hypoxia. The charge nurse or physician must be notified quickly. Stimulating a severely hypoxic client is not

appropriate. Increasing the oxygen from 6 liters to 10 liters is not likely to change the client's status. The LPN should notify the charge nurse now, not in 15 minutes.

25. (2) A positive PPD test indicates antibodies against tuberculosis. A positive PPD test and a negative X-ray indicate that the client has been exposed to tuberculosis but has not developed the disease. These findings do not give information regarding the client's resistance. The negative X-ray indicates that the client does not have active tuberculosis.

26. (1) Rifampin (Rimactane) causes body secretions to turn reddish-orange. Erythema and urticaria are not likely to be seen. Tinnitus and deafness is a side effect of streptomycin. Peripheral neuritis is a side effect of isoniazid (INH).

27. (2) SGOT (AST) and SGPT (APT) are liver function tests. INH can cause liver toxicity. Serum creatinine and BUN are renal function tests and would test for toxicity to streptomycin or kanamycin. CBC and hematocrit might be indicated if bleeding or bone marrow depression were major expected toxicities. WBC and urinalysis might be indicted for urinary tract infections.

28. (2) Showering is not usually allowed, because water will go into the stoma. The client will never be able to swim. The client does not need a liquid diet for three weeks. The stoma should be covered with a special absorbent scarf to filter and warm the air.

29. (3) The purpose of the nares is to humidify, warm, and filter the air before it enters the lungs. Breathing through the nose does not produce greater blood oxygen levels. It is not easier to breathe through the nose. Mouth breathing does not dilute the air.

30. (2) Allow the client to cough. He will frequently cough out the mucus. If he does not, then the nurse can resuction to pick up secretions. The client's cough is more powerful than the suction catheter.

Chapter 6

The Neurosensory System

Sample Questions

1. An adult man fell off a ladder and hit his head and lost consciousness. After regaining consciousness several minutes later, he was drowsy and had trouble staying awake. He is admitted to the hospital for evaluation.

   The nursing care plan will most likely include which of the following?

   1. Elevate head of bed 15–30 degrees.
   2. Encourage fluids to 1000 ml q. 8 hrs.
   3. Assist to cough and deep-breathe every two hours.
   4. Chest physical therapy every four hours while awake.

2. A teenager is admitted following a seizure.

   The next day, the nurse goes into his room and finds him lying on the floor starting to have a seizure. What action should the nurse take at this time?

   1. Carefully observe the seizure and gently restrain him.
   2. Attempt to put an airway in his mouth so he doesn't swallow his tongue and observe the type and duration of the seizure.

   3. Place something soft under his head, carefully observe the seizure, and protect him from injury.
   4. Shout for help so that someone can help you move him away from the furniture.

3. An adult is being treated with phenytoin (Dilantin) for a seizure disorder. Five days after starting the medication, he tells the nurse that his urine is reddish-brown in color. What action should the nurse take?

   1. Inform him that this is a common side effect of phenytoin (Dilantin) therapy.
   2. Test the urine for occult blood.
   3. Report it to the physician because it could indicate a clotting deficiency.
   4. Send a urine specimen to the lab.

4. The nurse is caring for a client who has recently had a CVA. When positioning the client and supporting her extremities, the nurse must remember that when voluntary control of muscles is lost:

   1. The feet will maintain a position of eversion.
   2. The upper extremities will rotate externally.
   3. The hip joint will rotate internally.
   4. Flexor muscles will become stronger than extensors.

5. A stroke victim regains consciousness three days after admission. She has right-sided hemiparesis and hemiplegia and also has expressive aphasia. She becomes upset when she is unable to say simple words. The best approach for the nurse is to:

   1. Stay with her and give her time and encouragement in attempting to speak.

   2. Say, "I'm sure you want a glass of water. I'll get it for you."

   3. Say, "Don't get upset. You rest now and I'll come back later and try to talk to you then."

   4. Encourage her attempts and say, "Don't worry, it will get easier every day."

6. A young man was swimming at the beach when an exceptionally large wave caused him to be drawn under the water. His family members found him in the water and pulled him ashore. He states that he heard something snap in his neck. When a nurse arrives, he is conscious and lying on his back. He states that he has no pain. He is unable to move his legs. How should he be transported?

   1. Position him in a prone position and place on a backboard.

   2. Apply a neck collar and position supine on a backboard.

   3. Log roll him to a rigid backboard.

   4. Position in an upright position with a firm neck collar.

7. A client who is recovering from a spinal cord injury complains of blurred vision and a severe headache. His blood pressure is 210/140.

   The most appropriate initial action for the nurse to take is:

   1. Check for bladder distention.

   2. Place him in the Trendelenburg position.

   3. Administer prn pain medication.

   4. Position him on his left side.

8. A 27-year-old woman is admitted to the hospital complaining of numbness in both legs, difficulty walking, and double vision of one week duration. Multiple sclerosis is suspected. Orders include: bed rest with bathroom privileges, brain scan, EEG, Lumbar puncture, ACTH 40 Units I.M. bid 33 days, then 30 Units I.M. bid 33 days, then 20 Units I.M. bid 33 days; and passive ROM progressing to active ROM as tolerated. In planning care for this client, which activity is most important to include?

   1. Encouraging her to perform all care activities for herself

   2. Frequent ambulation to retain joint mobility

   3. Scheduling frequent rest periods between physical activity

   4. Feeding the client to reduce energy needs

9. The doctor orders a Tensilon test for a woman suspected of having myasthenia gravis.

   Which statement is true about this test?

   1. A positive result will be evident within one minute of injection of Tensilon if she has myasthenia gravis.

   2. This is of diagnostic value in only 25% of patients with myasthenia gravis.

   3. Administration of Tensilon causes an immediate decrease in muscle strength for about an hour in persons with myasthenia gravis.

   4. Tensilon works by blocking the action of acetylcholine at the myoneural junction.

10. When planning care for a woman with myasthenia gravis, the nurse asks her what time of day she feels strongest. The nurse would expect which of the following replies?

    1. "I can wash up and comb my hair before breakfast because I feel best in the morning."

    2. "I only feel good for about an hour after I take my medication."

3. "I feel strongest in the evening, so I would prefer to take a shower before bedtime."

4. "I feel best after lunch after I've been moving around a little."

11. Which of the following would not be included in the nursing care plan for a client with Parkinson's disease?

1. Restricting his intake of oral fluids

2. Range-of-motion exercises

3. Allowing him to carry out activities of daily living by himself even though he is very slow

4. Providing him with diversionary tasks that require motor coordination of hands

12. The nurse is caring for a client admitted with Guillain-Barré syndrome. On day three of hospitalization, his muscle weakness worsens and he is no longer able to stand with support. He is also having difficulty swallowing and talking. The priority in his nursing care plan should be to prevent:

1. Aspiration pneumonia

2. Decubitus ulcers

3. Bladder distention

4. Hypertensive crisis

13. An adult client is admitted for removal of a cataract from her right eye. Which of the following would the client likely have experienced as a result of the cataracts?

1. Acute eye pain

2. Redness and constant itching of the right eye

3. Gradual blurring of vision

4. Severe headaches and dizziness

14. The client has had a cataract extraction performed. Which statement that the client makes indicates a need for more teaching?

1. "I will take a stool softener daily."

2. "I'm going to start doing calisthenic exercises as soon as I get home."

3. "I'm going to my daughter's for a few weeks until I am recovered."

4. "I am looking forward to watching television during my recovery period."

15. The client is a 50-year-old admitted with the diagnosis of open-angle glaucoma. Which of the following symptoms would the nurse expect the client to have?

1. Severe eye pain

2. Constant blurred vision

3. Severe headaches, nausea, and vomiting

4. Reports of seeing halos around objects

16. The nurse is administering eye drops to a client. Which action is correct?

1. Ask the client to report any blurring of vision and difficulty focusing that occurs after the administration of eye drops.

2. Apply gentle pressure to the naso-lacrimal canal for 1 to 2 minutes after instillation to prevent systemic absorption.

3. Have the client lie down with eyes closed for 45 minutes after giving drops.

4. Gently pull the lower lid down and place medicine in the center of the eye.

17. A 10-year-old boy comes to the school clinic holding his broken pair of glasses. He says that he got hit in the face playing ball and his eye hurts and feels like there's something in it.

What should the nurse do before taking him to the emergency room?

1. Thoroughly examine his eyes.

2. Put a pressure dressing on his right eye.

3. Cover both eyes lightly with gauze.

4. Flush his right eye with water for 20 minutes.

18. How should a nurse walk a client who is blind?

    1. Stand slightly behind and tell her when to turn.

    2. Stand slightly behind and to the side and guide her by holding her hand.

    3. Walk slightly ahead with the client's arm inside the nurse's arm.

    4. Walk beside the client and gently guide her by grasping her elbow.

19. The client is a 60-year-old man who had a stapedectomy. He is to ambulate for the first time. Which nursing action should be taken?

    1. Encourage him to walk as far as he comfortably can.

    2. Suggest that he practice bending and stretching exercises.

    3. Walk with him.

    4. Tell him to take deep breaths while he is ambulating.

20. A client complains of tinnitus and dizziness and has a diagnosis of Meniere's Disease.

    She asks the nurse what the cause of Meniere's disease is. What is the nurse's best response?

    1. "Meniere's Disease is caused by a virus."

    2. "The cause of Meniere's Disease is unknown."

    3. "Meniere's Disease frequently follows a streptococcal infection."

    4. "It is hereditary. Both of your parents carried the gene for Meniere's Disease."

21. An adult man fell off a ladder and hit his head. His wife rushed to help him and found him unconscious. After regaining consciousness several minutes later, he was drowsy and had trouble staying awake. He is admitted to the hospital for evaluation. When the nurse enters the room, he is sleeping. While caring for the client, the nurse finds that his systolic blood pressure has increased, his pulse has

decreased, and his temperature is slightly elevated. What does this suggest?

    1. Increased cerebral blood flow

    2. Respiratory depression

    3. Increased intracranial pressure

    4. Hyperoxygenation of the cerebrum

22. The physician has ordered Mannitol IV for a client with a head injury. What should the nurse closely monitor because the client is receiving Mannitol?

    1. Deep tendon reflexes

    2. Urine output

    3. Level of orientation

    4. Pulse rate

23. A 17-year-old had one generalized convulsion several hours prior to admission to the medical unit for a neurological workup. Physician's orders include Dilantin 100 mg po tid and Phenobarbital 100 mg po qd. He tells the nurse, "I can't believe I really had a seizure. My mom says she was in the room when it happened, but I don't even remember it." What is the best interpretation of his comments?

    1. They indicate an initial denial mechanism, but he will begin to remember the seizure later.

    2. Anoxia suffered during the seizure has damaged part of his cerebral cortex.

    3. Inability to remember the seizure is a normal response of a person who has had a seizure.

    4. They are an indication that he would rather not talk about his seizure at this time.

24. What should the nurse include when teaching the client with Parkinson's disease?

    1. He should try to continue working as long as he can remain sitting most of the day.

    2. Drooling may be reduced somewhat if he remembers to swallow frequently.

    3. He should return monthly for lab tests, which will predict the progression of the disease.

4. Emotional stress has no effect on voluntary muscle control in clients with Parkinson's disease.

25. A 68-year-old woman is brought to the emergency room by ambulance. She was found by her husband slumped in her chair, unresponsive. Tentative diagnosis is cerebrovascular accident (CVA). The physician orders a 15% solution of Mannitol IV. The nurse knows that this drug is given for what purpose?

    1. To increase urine output
    2. To dissolve clots
    3. To reduce blood pressure
    4. To decrease muscle spasms

26. An older woman has had a CVA. The nurse notes that she seems to be unaware of objects on her right side (right homonymous hemianopia). Which nursing action is most important in planning to assist her to compensate for this loss?

    1. Place frequently used items on the affected side.
    2. Position her so that her affected side is toward the activity in the room.
    3. Encourage her to turn her head from side to side to scan the environment on the affected side.
    4. Stand on the affected side while assisting her in ambulating.

27. A client asks the nurse what causes Parkinson's disease. The nurse's correct reply would be based on which of the following statements?

    Parkinson's disease is thought to be due to:
    1. A deficiency of dopamine in the brain
    2. A demyelinating process affecting the ~MS central nervous system
    3. Atrophy of the basal ganglia
    4. Insufficient uptake of acetylcholine in the body

28. The nurse is caring for a client who is very hard of hearing. How should the nurse communicate with this person?

    1. Speak loudly and talk in his best ear.
    2. Stand in front of him and speak clearly and distinctly.
    3. Yell at him using a high-pitched voice.
    4. Write all communication on a note pad or magic slate.

29. The day following a stapedectomy, the client tells the nurse that he cannot hear much in the operative ear and thinks the stapedectomy was a failure. What is the best response for the nurse to make?

    1. "There is packing in your ear. You will not hear well for a few days."
    2. "The doctors have not yet turned on the stapes replacement."
    3. "You may not have hearing, but you will now be free of pain."
    4. "You seem upset that you aren't hearing well."

30. A cataract extraction is performed on the client's right eye. What is the priority nursing care immediately postoperative?

    1. Assist her to turn, cough, and deep-breathe q 2 hrs.
    2. Keep her NPO for four hours.
    3. Assist her in moving her arms and legs in ROM.
    4. Position client on her right side.

Answers and Rationales

1. (1) The head of the bed should be slightly elevated to allow gravity drainage of fluid and reduce cerebral edema. Coughing and forcing fluids are contraindicated because they may raise intracranial pressure. Chest physical

therapy would be apt to raise intracranial pressure.

2. (3) Protect his head from injury and observe the seizure. Never try to restrain a seizing person. Current thinking says do not put an airway in the mouth. Placing something soft under his head will help to protect his head from injury. The question does not indicate that the client is in danger from the furniture.

3. (1) He is receiving Dilantin, which frequently causes the urine to turn reddish-brown in color. There is no indication for testing the urine or notifying the physician. The finding should be recorded on the client's chart.

4. (4) Flexor muscles are stronger than extensors, causing flexion contractures. The hip joint tends to rotate externally.

5. (1) Offering help is always therapeutic. This approach will help her to express herself. The nurse should not routinely anticipate her needs because this does not encourage attempts at speech. Telling her not to get upset is not therapeutic. Encouraging her attempts to speak is therapeutic but telling her not to worry is not therapeutic.

6. (2) He may have a neck or spinal cord injury. The neck and back should be supported and maintained in a rigid position. He should be transported in the position in which he was found. He should not be turned.

7. (1) The symptoms suggest autonomic hyperreflexia, which is usually caused by bladder distention. The patient will need to be catheterized and the physician notified. Autonomic hyperreflexia is a medical emergency. The head is usually elevated to reduce blood pressure.

8. (3) She will need rest periods between activities. She may be too weak to perform all self activities. Her orders include bed rest, not ambulating ad lib. Feeding her is not necessary and is likely to cause her to be upset.

9. (1) Tensilon works almost immediately to cause an increase in muscle strength by increasing

the amount of acetylcholine at the myoneural junction. The test is of value in almost all clients suspected of having myasthenia gravis.

10. (1) Muscle strength is best early in the day. Weakness usually progresses during the day and is at its worst in the evening.

11. (1) Fluids should be encouraged because he has a tendency to drool and lose fluid. Encouraging the client to perform activities of daily living is desirable. He should be encouraged to move frequently to prevent joint contractures. Activities requiring hand coordination will help him to retain function.

12. (1) Because he is having difficulty swallowing and talking, he is at high risk for aspiration pneumonia. He is also at risk for decubitus ulcers, but this is of lesser priority than the airway. Bladder distention is a possibility but not as high a priority as the risk of aspiration pneumonia. There is no evidence that he is at risk for hypertensive crisis.

13. (3) Cataracts are characterized by a gradual blurring of vision. Acute eye pain is characteristic of acute glaucoma or foreign objects in the eye. Redness and itching are more characteristic of an eye infection. Severe headaches and dizziness are not characteristic of cataracts.

14. (2) Bending, stooping, and lifting should be avoided for several weeks following eye surgery. A stool softener is recommended so that the client will not strain at stool. Television and reading are not restricted following cataract extraction. Eye movement is restricted following surgery for detached retina.

15. (4) Chronic glaucoma is characterized by halos around objects. Severe eye pain and severe headaches, nausea, and vomiting are more characteristic of acute glaucoma. Constant blurred vision is characteristic of cataracts.

16. (2) This action will prevent systemic absorption of eye medication and prevent the nose from running. Blurred vision and difficulty focusing is normal immediately after administering eye

drops. There is no need to lie down after eye drops are given. Eye drops should be placed in the conjunctival sac, not the center of the eye.

17. (3) Covering both eyes lightly with gauze prevents tracking by the affected eye, which would occur if the unaffected eye was not covered. Examining the eyes should be done only at the emergency room by a physician. A pressure dressing would further damage the eye if broken glass is in the eye. Flushing is appropriate for chemical spills in the eye.

18. (3) Walking slightly ahead of the client allows the nurse to see what is in the way. The client feels more in control if her arm is through the nurse's rather than the other way around.

19. (3) The client is apt to be dizzy after ear surgery. For safety, the nurse should be with him.

20. (2) The cause of Meniere's Disease is unknown. Glomerulonephritis and rheumatic fever follow a streptococcal infection. As far as is known, Meniere's Disease is not hereditary nor is it caused by a virus.

21. (3) These are classic manifestations of increased intracranial pressure.

22. (2) Mannitol is an osmotic diuretic. Urine output should increase. He must be on intake and output.

23. (3) People seldom remember a seizure; this is a normal response.

24. (2) Swallowing may reduce drooling. Sitting most of the day causes stiffness. There is no lab test to determine disease progression. Emotional stress can aggravate the symptoms.

25. (1) Mannitol is an osmotic diuretic which increases urine output and will decrease intracranial pressure. Streptokinase and tPA dissolve clots and might be ordered for this client. Antihypertensive medications may also be ordered for this client.

26. (3) Encouraging her to turn her head from side to side will do the most to help her learn a skill that will compensate for loss of the visual field. With homonymous hemianopia, the client does not see on the affected or paralyzed side. Choices 1 and 2 will make life more difficult for her. If the nurse stands on the affected side, the client will be unaware of the nurse.

27. (1) A deficiency of dopamine is thought to be the cause of Parkinson's. Multiple Sclerosis is caused by demyelination of the central nervous system. Alzheimer's Disease involves atrophy of the basal ganglia. Myasthenia Gravis is caused by insufficient uptake of acetylcholine in the body.

28. (2) Standing in front of him and speaking clearly and distinctly will allow him to read lips. Speaking loudly is usually not the best approach. Most persons with difficulty hearing hear low-pitched sounds better than high-pitched ones; yelling and speaking loudly tend to raise the pitch of the voice. Written communication might become necessary for some persons. However, that would only be a last resort after all other methods of communication had failed.

29. (1) Packing in the ear will reduce sound wave transmission. Hearing will be muffled until the packing is removed. The stapes replacement does not need to be turned on. The purpose of a stapedectomy is to restore some hearing. Otosclerosis for which the stapedectomy was performed is not a painful condition. It is more appropriate to give the client the information that he needs regarding hearing rather than to focus on the client's feelings.

30. (3) Of these answers, moving arms and legs is the best as it will help to prevent thrombophlebitis. The client should not cough because this will increase intraocular pressure. There is no need to keep her NPO. She should not be positioned on the operative side because this will increase intraocular pressure.

Chapter 7

The Gastrointestinal System

Sample Questions

1. A client is admitted to the hospital with a gnawing pain in the mid-epigastric area and black stools for the past week. A diagnosis of chronic duodenal ulcer is made. During the initial nursing assessment, the client makes all of the following statements. Which is most likely related to his admitting diagnosis?

   1. "I am a vegetarian."
   2. "My mother and grandmother have diabetes."
   3. "I take aspirin several times a day for tension headaches."
   4. "I take multivitamin and iron tablets every day."

2. An upper GI series is ordered for a client. Which action is essential for the nurse before the test?

   1. Check to see if the client has an allergy to shellfish.
   2. Instruct the client to have nothing to eat after midnight before the test.
   3. Encourage the client to drink plenty of liquids before the test.
   4. Be sure he does not eat fat-containing foods for 18 hours before the test.

3. The client with a duodenal ulcer is ready for discharge. Which statement made by the client indicates a need for more teaching about his diet?

   1. "It's a good thing I gave up drinking alcohol last year."
   2. "I will have to drink lots of milk and cream every day."
   3. "I will stay away from cola drinks after I am discharged."
   4. "Eating three nutritious meals and snacks every day is okay."

4. The client, admitted with appendicitis, overhears the physician say that the pain has reached McBurney's point. She becomes very frightened and asks the nurse to explain what this means. Which is the best response?

   1. "The next time the doctor comes in, we should ask him what he meant by that."
   2. "I've felt that I don't understand the doctor at times either."
   3. "That is the term used to indicate that the pain has traveled to the right lower side."
   4. "McBurney's point refers to severe pain for which surgery is the only treatment."

5. Which blood test results would confirm a diagnosis of appendicitis?

   1. WBC of 13,000
   2. RBC of 4.5 million
   3. Platelet count of 300,000
   4. Positive Heterophil antibody test

6. The nurse is admitting a client with the diagnosis of appendicitis to the surgical unit. Which question is it essential to ask?

   1. "When did you last eat?"
   2. "Have you had surgery before?"
   3. "Have you ever had this type of pain before?"
   4. "What do you usually take to relieve your pain?"

7. The client with appendicitis asks the nurse for a laxative to help relieve her constipation. The nurse explains to her that laxatives are not given to persons with possible appendicitis. What is the primary reason for this?

   1. Laxatives will decrease the spread of infection.
   2. Laxatives are not given prior to any type of surgery.
   3. The patient does not have true constipation. She only has pressure.
   4. Laxatives could cause a rupture of the appendix.

8. A child with appendicitis is scheduled for surgery this evening. The nurse enters the room and sees the child's mother starting to place hot, wet washcloths on her daughter's abdomen so that "she will feel better."

   The nurse explains that this action is contraindicated because heat:

   1. Can cause the appendix to rupture and cause peritonitis
   2. Can mask symptoms of acute appendicitis

3. Will increase peristalsis throughout the abdomen
4. Will arrest progression of the disease

9. A client returns from having had abdominal surgery. Her vital signs are stable. She says she is thirsty. What should the nurse give her initially?

   1. Orange juice
   2. Milk
   3. Ice chips
   4. Mouth wash

10. The client who has had an appendectomy and has a penrose drain in place has recovered from anesthesia. The nurse places her in semi-Fowler's position. What is the primary reason for selecting this position?

    1. To promote optimal ventilation
    2. To promote drainage from the abdominal cavity
    3. To prevent pressure sores from developing
    4. To reduce tension on the suture line

11. The client is admitted to the hospital complaining of malaise, abdominal discomfort, and severe diarrhea. The diagnosis is possible Crohn's Disease. The client says that he has lost 27 pounds in the last four months even though he has not been dieting. To plan nursing care, which assessment data is most essential for the nurse to obtain?

    1. Approximate number and characteristics of stools each day
    2. Amount of liquid consumed daily
    3. History of previous gastric surgery
    4. Bowel sounds in the right lower quadrant

12. The nurse is preparing a client with Crohn's Disease for discharge. Which statement he makes indicates that he needs further teaching?

1. "Stress can make it worse."

2. "Since I have Crohn's Disease I don't have to worry about colon cancer."

3. "I realize I shall always have to monitor my diet."

4. "I understand there is a high incidence of familial occurrence with this disease."

13. A low-residue diet is ordered for a client. Which food would be contraindicated for this person?

    1. Roast beef

    2. Fresh peas

    3. Mashed potatoes

    4. Baked chicken

14. The client is to have a sigmoidoscopy in the morning. Which activity will be included in the care of this client?

    1. Give him an enema one hour before the examination.

    2. Keep him NPO for eight hours before the examination.

    3. Order a low-fat, low-residue diet for breakfast.

    4. Administer enemas until the returns are clear this evening.

15. The client had a barium enema. Following the barium enema, the nurse should anticipate an order for which of the following?

    1. An antacid

    2. A laxative

    3. A muscle relaxant

    4. A sedative

16. The client is found to have colon cancer. An abdomino-perineal resection and colostomy is scheduled. Neomycin is ordered. The nurse explains to the client that the primary purpose for administering this drug is to:

    1. Decrease peristalsis in the intestines

    2. Decrease the bacterial content in the colon

    3. Reduce inflammation of the bowel

    4. Help prevent post-operative pneumonia

17. The day after surgery in which a colostomy was performed, the client says "I know the doctor did not really do a colostomy." The nurse understands that the client is in an early stage of adjustment to the diagnosis and surgery. What nursing action is indicated at this time?

    1. Agree with the client until the client is ready to accept the colostomy.

    2. Say, "It must be difficult to have this kind of surgery."

    3. Force the client to look at his colostomy.

    4. Ask the surgeon to explain the surgery to the client.

18. The nurse is irrigating the client's colostomy when the client complains of cramping. What is the most appropriate initial action by the nurse?

    1. Increase the flow of solution.

    2. Ask the client to turn to the other side.

    3. Pinch the tubing to interrupt the flow of the solution.

    4. Remove the tube from the colostomy.

19. A 32-year-old female is admitted for a hemorrhoidectomy. During the nursing assessment, all of the following factors are elicited. Which one is most likely to have contributed to the development of hemorrhoids? The client:

    1. States that she usually cleans herself from back to front after a bowel movement

    2. Says her mother and grandmother had hemorrhoids

    3. Has had four pregnancies

    4. Eats bran every day

20. Following a hemorrhoidectomy, the nurse is instructing the client in self care. Which statement is especially important to include in these instructions?

    1. "Wash the anal area with water after defecation and pat it dry."

    2. "Gently wipe the anal area after defecation from back to front."

    3. "Do not drink more than three glasses of fluid per day until after you have had the first bowel movement."

    4. "When you first feel the need to defecate, call me and I will give you the enema the doctor has ordered."

21. The client who has had a hemorrhoidectomy wants to know why she cannot take a sitz bath immediately upon return from the operating room. The nurse's response is based upon which of the following concepts?

    1. Heat can stimulate bowel movement too quickly after surgery.

    2. Patients are generally not awake enough for several hours to safely take sitz baths.

    3. Heat applied immediately postoperatively increases the possibility of hemorrhage.

    4. Sitting in water before the sutures are removed may cause infection.

22. Following a hemorrhoidectomy, the nurse assesses the client's voiding. What is the reason for this concern?

    1. The client has been NPO before and during surgery.

    2. Urinary retention is frequently seen after a hemorrhoidectomy.

    3. The client has a long history of hemorrhoids, making her prone to voiding problems.

    4. The client had several pregnancies, which can make voiding difficult.

23. The client has had a hemorrhoidectomy. Which statement she makes indicates a need for more teaching?

    1. "I'll decrease the amount of fiber in my diet."

    2. "I should drink more liquids at home."

    3. "There seems to be a relationship between bowel regularity and diet."

    4. "Establishing a routine for bowel movements is important."

24. A client with pancreatitis tells the nurse that he fears nighttime. Which of the following statements most likely relates to the client's concerns?

    1. The pain is aggravated in the recumbent position.

    2. The client has fewer distractions at night.

    3. The mattress is uncomfortable.

    4. The pain increases after a day of activity.

25. Warm Aveeno baths are ordered for a client with cancer of the pancreas. What is the chief purpose of this procedure for this client?

    1. Relief of paralytic ileus

    2. Alleviate pruritus associated with jaundice

    3. Relief of bloating and fullness after eating

    4. Reducing the fever associated with the disease

26. A distal pancreatectomy and splenectomy is performed on a client with cancer of the pancreas. He is returned to his room post-operatively. The client is sleepy but can answer simple questions appropriately. His dressing is dry and intact. Vital signs are within normal limits. Which of the following nursing measures must be done before the nurse leaves the room?

    1. Inform his wife that he has returned to his room.

2. Check to see if the indwelling urinary catheter bag is correctly attached to the bed frame.

3. Assess to be sure he is not experiencing any discomfort.

4. Put all four side rails in the high position.

27. The client's temperature rises to 100.4°F (38°C) on the first post-operative day following abdominal surgery. The nurse interprets this to be:

1. Indicative of a wound infection

2. A normal physiologic response to the trauma of surgery

3. Suggestive of a urinary tract infection

4. An indication of over-hydration

28. The client asks how he contracted hepatitis A. He reports all of the following. Which one is most likely related to hepatitis A?

1. He ate home-canned corn.

2. He ate oysters his roommate brought home from a fishing trip.

3. He stepped on a nail two weeks ago.

4. He donated blood two weeks before he got sick.

29. The client has had a liver biopsy. The nurse should position him on his right side with a pillow under his rib cage. What is the primary reason for this position?

1. To immobilize the diaphragm

2. To facilitate full chest expansion

3. To minimize the danger of aspiration

4. To reduce the likelihood of bleeding

30. A client with cirrhosis is about to have a paracentesis for relief of ascites. Which activity is essential prior to the procedure?

1. Administer thorough mouth care.

2. Ask the client to empty his bladder.

3. Be sure his bowels have moved recently.

4. Have the client bathe with betadine.

31. The client has severe liver disease. Which of the following observations is most indicative of serious problems? The client:

1. Has generalized urticaria

2. Is "confused" and can no longer write his name legibly

3. Is jaundiced

4. Has ecchymotic areas on his arms

32. An adult has a nasogastric tube in place. Which nursing action will relieve discomfort in the nostril with the NG tube?

1. Remove any tape and loosely pin the NG tube to his gown.

2. Lubricate the NG tube with viscous lidocaine.

3. Loop the NG tube to avoid pressure on the nares.

4. Replace the NG tube with a smaller-diameter tube.

33. An adult is being treated for a peptic ulcer. The physician has prescribed cimetidine (Tagamet) for which reason?

1. It blocks the secretion of gastric hydrochloric acid.

2. It coats the gastric mucosa with a protective membrane.

3. It increases the sensitivity of H_2 receptors.

4. It neutralizes acid in the stomach.

34. The nurse is assessing a client who may have a hiatal hernia. What symptom is the client most likely to report?

1. Projectile vomiting

2. Crampy lower abdominal pain

3. Burning substernal pain

4. Bloody diarrhea

35. When an elderly client is receiving cimetidine (Tagamet), it is important that the nurse monitor for which side effect?

   1. Chest pain

   2. Confusion

   3. Dyspnea

   4. Urinary retention

Answers and Rationales

1. (3) Aspirin is very irritating to the gastric mucosa and is known to cause ulcers. Being a vegetarian does not cause ulcers. Ulcers are not known to be inherited. Multivitamins and iron do not cause ulcers.

2. (2) Preparation for an upper GI series is NPO for eight hours. In an upper GI series, the client swallows barium, a radiopaque substance. An iodine dye is not used, so it is not necessary to ask about iodine allergies (shellfish). Fats are restricted before gallbladder X-rays, not for an upper GI series.

3. (2) Milk and cream are now known to cause rebound acidity and are not prescribed for ulcer clients. The other choices all indicate good knowledge. He should not drink alcohol or cola. Three meals and snacks will help keep the stomach from staying empty for long periods.

4. (3) McBurney's point is the area in the right lower quadrant where the appendix is. The client asked for information that the nurse should be able to provide. Answer 4 is not correct. McBurney's point refers to the location of the appendix, not the severity of the pain.

5. (1) An elevated white blood count indicates appendicitis. The RBC and platelet levels given are normal but are not specifically related to appendicitis. A positive Heterophil antibody test indicates infectious mononucleosis.

6. (1) When a person is admitted with possible appendicitis, the nurse should anticipate surgery. It will be important to know when she last ate when considering the type of anesthesia so that the chance of aspiration can be minimized. The other information is "nice to know" but not essential.

7. (4) Laxatives cause increased peristalsis, which may cause the appendix to rupture. Answer 2 is not a true statement. Laxatives may well be given prior to gynecological, rectal, and colon surgery. Answer 3 is true but is not the primary reason why laxatives are not given when a person has appendicitis.

8. (1) Heat can cause drawing of the inflammation and rupture of the appendix, which will cause peritonitis. Heat is not likely to mask the symptoms of appendicitis, increase peristalsis, or arrest progression of the disease.

9. (3) Ice chips can be given to help relieve thirst. Only clear liquids will be given until peristalsis has returned; milk and orange juice are not clear liquids. Mouth wash is not consumed and when used appropriately does not relieve thirst. It may freshen the mouth but does not relieve thirst.

10. (2) The client has a Penrose drain in place. The primary reason for the semi-Fowler's position is to promote drainage. This position may also help reduce tension on the suture line and promote ventilation. Turning will help prevent pressure sores.

11. (1) It is most important for the nurse to know how many stools he has been having each day. Frequent stools are characteristic of Crohn's Disease and may cause dehydration and skin breakdown. The nurse may want to know how much liquid he has been consuming, but that is not the most important. Previous gastric surgery is not usually related to Crohn's Disease. Bowel sounds may be assessed but are not the most important assessment data.

12. (2) Persons with Crohn's Disease are at high risk for the development of colon cancer. The other answers are all correct and therefore do not indicate a need for more instruction.

13. (2) Fresh peas are high in residue. Roast beef, mashed potatoes, and baked chicken are not high in residue. High-residue foods are those that contain skins, seeds, and leaves. Milk products are also to be avoided on a low-residue diet.

14. (1) An enema one hour before the exam will clear the sigmoid colon. A client having an upper GI series will be NPO. A low-fat diet is indicated prior to a gallbladder series. A low-residue diet is part of the preparation for a barium enema. Enemas until clear are sometimes ordered prior to a barium enema or colonoscopy.

15. (2) Barium can be very constipating and may cause blockage of the bowel. Laxatives help to empty the bowel of barium. The other drugs are not appropriate following a barium enema.

16. (2) Neomycin is an antibiotic that is poorly absorbed from the GI tract and will therefore kill the bacteria in the bowel. This must be done before colon surgery to prevent peritonitis. Neomycin is an antibiotic and does not decrease peristalsis or reduce inflammation. Because it is not absorbed from the bowel, it does not kill bacteria outside the GI tract and therefore will not prevent pneumonia.

17. (2) The first stage of adjustment to a major loss is usually denial. The client is denying the colostomy. This empathic response encourages the client to discuss feelings. The nurse should never agree with the client's denial. The denial should not be confronted at this point in time. He needs time to adjust. Notice that the stem of the question focuses on the denial stage.

18. (3) When cramping occurs during a colostomy irrigation or an enema, the nurse should temporarily stop the flow of solution. Having the client take deep breaths may help also. Increasing the flow of solution will increase the cramping. Changing position will not decrease the cramping. It is not necessary to remove the tube; simply stop the flow of the solution briefly.

19. (3) Pregnancy causes increased portal hypertension, which can cause hemorrhoids.

Cleaning from back to front after bowel movements may cause cystitis but not hemorrhoids. There may be some familial tendency toward hemorrhoids; however, pregnancies are more directly related. Bran will promote bowel regularity and would help to prevent constipation, which is a risk factor for hemorrhoids.

20. (1) After hemorrhoid surgery, the anal area should be washed with water, no soap, and patted, not rubbed, dry. Wiping should be from front to back to reduce risk of urinary tract infection. Fluids are encouraged because they will promote a soft stool, which will pass more easily. If an enema is used to promote the first bowel movement, it would be given to promote the urge to defecate, not after the client feels the need to defecate.

21. (3) Heat causes vasodilation. In the immediate post-operative period, this could cause hemorrhaging. Ice packs will be applied for the first 24 hours. Sitz baths are ordered after that.

22. (2) The proximity of the anus and the bladder make urinary retention a frequent complication after hemorrhoidectomy. The client was NPO before and during surgery but received IV fluids during and after surgery. The long history of hemorrhoids and the client's previous pregnancies are not the key factors causing bladder retention immediately following surgery.

23. (1) She should increase fiber in her diet. The other actions all indicate a good understanding of her care.

24. (1) The recumbent position aggravates pancreatic pain. The client will be more comfortable on his side with his knees flexed. While the client may have more to distract his mind from pain during the day, this is not the primary reason why pancreatic pain is worse at night.

25. (2) Aveeno baths are used to reduce itching. Jaundice, seen in pancreatic cancer, causes severe itching. Paralytic ileus is not a major feature of pancreatic cancer, and Aveeno baths

are not the way to relieve paralytic ileus. Aveeno baths do not relieve bloating and fullness or reduce fever.

26. (4) Side rails are safety devices. When the question asks for an essential action, think of an answer related to safety. It is important to check for correct positioning of the urinary catheter drainage bag and to assess for comfort. However, the side rails are essential. The nurse will notify the client's family after leaving the room.

27. (2) A low-grade temperature on the first post-operative day is a normal response to surgery. It takes at least 72 hours for a wound infection to develop. Urinary tract infections take 48 to 72 hours to develop. Dehydration, not over-hydration, may cause a slight temperature increase in the first few hours after surgery. A temperature elevation the day after surgery could also indicate the development of a respiratory infection, but that was not a choice.

28. (2) Hepatitis A is viral hepatitis and is spread via the fecal-oral route. Shellfish that grow in contaminated waters may have the virus. Home-canned corn might cause food poisoning if it was not properly done. Stepping on a nail might cause tetanus. Donating blood will not cause hepatitis. Receiving blood might cause hepatitis B.

29. (4) The liver is a very vascular organ. It is located on the right side. Lying on the right side will put pressure on it and provide hemostasis and reduce the chance of bleeding. There is no reason to immobilize the diaphragm. Lying on the right side does not immobilize the diaphragm or facilitate chest expansion. Aspiration is not a problem following a liver biopsy.

30. (2) Emptying the bladder is essential prior to a paracentesis so that the bladder will not be punctured during the procedure. Mouth care is not related to a paracentesis. It is not necessary to empty the bowels before a paracentesis. Bathing with betadine is not necessary before a paracentesis.

31. (2) This indicates that the client is going into hepatic coma. He will have urticaria from the jaundice, but this is not the most serious. He will have ecchymotic areas on his body due to the decrease in prothrombin, which is made in the liver. It is not the most serious.

32. (3) Looping the NG tube will prevent pressure on the nares that can cause pain and eventual necrosis. Pinning the tube to the client's gown would cause irritation of the nares each time he moved and might cause dislocation of the tube. Prior to insertion of an NG tube, it is proper to lubricate the tip with viscous xylocaine, but this is not applied to the nostril. A smaller tube might not be large enough to drain the stomach contents; it would still irritate the nose; and it may not be changed without a doctor's order.

33. (1) Cimetidine (Tagamet) is a histamine antagonist that blocks the secretion of hydrochloric acid. Sucralfate (Carafate) coats the gastric mucosa. Cimetidine is an H_2 receptor antagonist; it does not increase the sensitivity; it blocks it. Antacids neutralize acid in the stomach and raise the pH.

34. (3) Heartburn, which is a burning substernal pain, is the most common sign of hiatal hernia in clients who have symptoms. Projectile vomiting is more likely to be associated with pyloric obstruction due to scarring from chronic peptic ulcer disease. Crampy pain in the lower abdomen is commonly associated with lactose intolerance. Bloody diarrhea is more likely to be associated with diverticulitis or ulcerative colitis.

35. (2) Drowsiness, confusion, or mood swings may be side effects of cimetidine. Confusion is particularly common in the elderly. Chest pain is more likely to reflect heartburn, which is a symptom that cimetidine is given to relieve. Dyspnea is a sign of an anaphylactic, allergic reaction to any drug. Allergic reactions to cimetidine are very rare. Urinary retention is associated with anticholinergic drugs. Cimetidine is not anticholinergic.

Chapter 8

The Genitourinary System

Sample Questions

1. The nurse is performing a urethral catheterization on a female. After separating the labia, where would the nurse observe the urethral meatus?

    1. Between the vaginal orifice and the anus
    2. Between the clitoris and the vaginal orifice
    3. Just above the clitoris
    4. Within the vaginal cana

2. An adult had an indwelling catheter removed. After she voids for the first time, the nurse catheterizes her as ordered and obtains 200 cc of urine. What is the best interpretation of this finding? The client:

    1. Is voiding normally
    2. Has urinary retention
    3. Has developed renal failure
    4. Needs an indwelling catheter

3. The nurse is preparing to insert an indwelling catheter. What type of technique should the nurse use to perform this procedure?

    1. Clean technique
    2. Medical asepsis
    3. Isolation protocol
    4. Sterile technique

4. After inserting the indwelling catheter, how should the nurse position the drainage container?

    1. With the drainage tubing taut to maintain maximum suction on the urinary bladder
    2. Lower than the bladder to maintain a constant downward flow of urine from the bladder
    3. At the head of the bed for easy and accurate measurement of urine
    4. Beside the patient in his bed to avoid embarrassment

5. The nurse is attempting to pass an indwelling catheter in an adult male and is having difficulty. What is the most appropriate action for the nurse?

    1. Remove the catheter and reinsert it with the client positioned differently.
    2. Try a straight catheter instead.
    3. Try a smaller catheter.
    4. Discontinue the procedure and notify the physician.

6. A client has just had a needle biopsy of the kidney. What should the nurse do immediately following the procedure?

   1. Keep him NPO; take his blood pressure q 5 min for 1 hour and then q 15 min.
   2. Keep him flat for 24 hours; take his blood pressure q 5 min for 1 hour, then q 15 min.
   3. Check his blood pressure q 30 min for 2 hours; monitor I & O; position in the Sims position.
   4. Check I & O; send all urine to lab for analysis; ambulate after 8 hours; position in high-Fowler's position.

7. A five-year-old has been wetting his bed since coming into the hospital. The best approach for the nurse to use to help him regain his voluntary bladder control is to:

   1. Put diapers on him until he promises to stay dry.
   2. Leave him in his wet bed so he will learn he should not wet his bed.
   3. Promise him a lollipop if he will call when he needs to void.
   4. Assist him to the bathroom at regular intervals.

8. An adult client has returned to his room following a cystoscopy. When he voids, his urine is pink-tinged. The most appropriate action for the nurse to take is:

   1. Continue to observe him.
   2. Report it immediately to the physician.
   3. Irrigate the catheter with normal saline.
   4. Take his blood pressure every 15 min.

9. An 18-year-old female is seen in the clinic for a bladder infection. Which of the following signs and symptoms would the nurse expect her to manifest?

   1. Burning upon urination
   2. Flank pain

3. Nausea and vomiting
4. Elevated potassium

10. The nurse instructs a woman in the proper procedure for obtaining a clean-catch urine specimen. What should the nurse tell her to do?

    1. Clean the perineal area with soap and water and then void into the collection container.
    2. Clean around the urethral opening using antibacterial cleaning pads, wiping from front to back. Urinate and let some of the urine go into the toilet; then collect urine in the sterile container.
    3. Wash the area around the urethra and vagina. Insert the end of the sterile catheter into your urethra and collect the urine that is drained.
    4. Use the special cotton balls and clean your perineal area, wiping in circles from outer labia inward. Collect the urine in the sterile container.

11. A urinalysis reveals white cells and bacteria in the urine of a female client suspected of having a bladder infection. The client is instructed to take the prescribed anti-infective. What else should the nurse include when teaching the client?

    1. Limit fluid intake until the pain subsides.
    2. Wipe from back to front after voiding.
    3. Empty her bladder immediately after having sexual relations.
    4. Take the medication until she is pain-free for 48 hours.

12. An adult male is admitted with severe right-flank pain, nausea, and vomiting of four hours duration. The admitting diagnosis is kidney stones. Orders include encourage fluids to 1,000 cc per shift. What is the primary reason for encouraging fluids in this client?

    1. To prevent renal failure
    2. To help the stone pass

3. To prevent infection

4. To relieve his dehydration

13. The nurse is straining the urine of a client admitted with possible renal calculi. A small stone is discovered. What should the nurse do?

    1. Send the stone to the laboratory for analysis.
    2. Immediately test for guaiac.
    3. Test the stone for glucose.
    4. Administer pain medication.

14. A client who has kidney stones complains of pain. The nurse finds him pacing the hall. What is the most appropriate action for the nurse to take?

    1. Tell him to get back in bed where he will be more comfortable.
    2. Encourage him to walk if it helps to relieve the pain.
    3. Remind him to walk only when he has someone with him.
    4. Put him back in bed immediately and position him in semi-Fowler's.

15. The nurse is caring for a client who has acute renal failure. His potassium rises to 7.3 mEq/l. A Kayexalate enema is ordered. What is the primary purpose of the Kayexalate enema?

    1. To remove fluid from the extracellular spaces
    2. To exchange potassium ions for sodium ions
    3. To reduce abdominal pressure
    4. To introduce potassium into the bowel

16. The nurse is caring for a client who is in acute renal failure. Which of the following selections would be best to give for a snack?

    1. A slice of watermelon
    2. Orange juice
    3. A turkey sandwich
    4. A dish of applesauce

17. A 67-year-old man is admitted with dysuria that has gotten worse over the past six months. Rectal examination revealed an enlarged prostate. Following urination, he was catheterized and found to have 250 cc of thick, foul-smelling, residual urine. He is admitted with a diagnosis of benign prostatic hypertrophy. Which symptom is least likely to be present in this client?

    1. Urinary frequency
    2. Pus in the urine
    3. Dribbling
    4. Decreased force of urinary stream

18. The client who has urinary retention has had an indwelling catheter inserted. Which action is **not appropriate** for the nurse to take?

    1. Limit fluid intake.
    2. Monitor blood pressure frequently.
    3. Weigh the client daily.
    4. Assess renal function.

19. The nurse has inserted an indwelling catheter into an adult male. The nurse tapes the urinary drainage tube laterally to the thigh for which of the following reasons?

    1. To insure patient comfort
    2. To prevent reflux of urine
    3. To maintain tension on the balloon of the Foley
    4. To prevent compression at the penoscrotal junction

20. A client who had a transurethral prostatectomy is returned to the unit with continuous bladder irrigation. The nurse understands that the primary purpose of continuous bladder irrigation for this client is to:

    1. Prevent a urinary tract infection
    2. Maintain bladder tone
    3. Flush blood clots from the bladder
    4. Prevent urethral stricture

21. A 35-year-old man asks the nurse about a vasectomy. In discussing a vasectomy with this man, which information is most important to provide?

1. A vasectomy involves tubal ligation done by surgery.
2. This is a permanent method of contraception.
3. The surgery takes approximately one hour.
4. A vasectomy may cause intermittent impotence.

22. A client asks the nurse if he can get his wife pregnant after the vasectomy. What is the best response for the nurse to make?

1. "No. The procedure works immediately and is permanent."
2. "The first few ejaculations after a vasectomy contain active sperm."
3. "Yes. You should continue to practice birth control for six months."
4. "No. The doctor will flush the sperm out after the procedure is completed."

23. A client asks the nurse if he will be able to ejaculate after the vasectomy is done. What is the best response for the nurse to make?

1. "Yes. This procedure does not affect the ejaculate."
2. "No. The purpose of a vasectomy is to prevent ejaculation."
3. "Are you concerned about your sexual identity?"
4. "My husband had a vasectomy and it doesn't bother us."

24. An adult has been on bed rest for several weeks. A nursing care goal is to prevent the formation of renal calculi. Which of the following liquids is it especially important to include in the client's diet?

1. Tomato juice
2. Coffee
3. Cranberry juice
4. Milk

25. The physician has prescribed a diuretic for an adult client. Which nursing intervention is most important in relation to diuretic therapy?

1. Test the urine for sugar and acetone
2. Measure daily weights
3. Maintain accurate intake and output
4. Assess for pedal edema

26. The nurse is caring for an adult who has an indwelling urinary catheter with a continuous bladder irrigation infusing. How should the nurse calculate the urine output when the drainage bag is emptied?

1. Subtract the total drainage from the amount of irrigation solution used.
2. Measure the amount of drainage and subtract the amount of solution infused.
3. Record both the total drainage and the amount of irrigant used on the intake and output record.
4. Calculate the total fluid intake and subtract this amount from the total drainage.

27. The nurse calculates intake and output for an adult client. His intake for the shift is 1,000 ml. The total amount of drainage emptied from the drainage bag is 2,550 ml. During the shift, 1,825 ml of GU irrigant has infused. What is the client's eight-hour urine output?

1. 725 ml
2. 650 ml
3. 825 ml
4. 750 ml

28. The nurse is caring for a client admitted for treatment of acute glomerulonephritis. Which question would the nurse ask when obtaining information about the present illness?

1. "Have you had a sore throat recently?"
2. "Has anyone in your family had chickenpox recently?"

3. "Have you had a bladder infection in the last six weeks?"

4. "Does anyone in your family have a history of kidney disease?"

29. A 78-year-old man is scheduled for a transurethral resection of the prostate (TURP) tomorrow morning for treatment of benign prostatic hypertrophy. What instruction should the nurse give him about the initial post-operative period?

    1. "Void every two hours whether or not you feel the urge to do so."

    2. "Get up and walk to decrease discomfort from bladder spasms."

    3. "Cough and deep-breathe every two hours to prevent clot formation."

    4. "Expect cherry-red urine that will gradually turn pink."

30. A 35-year-old man is admitted with severe renal colic. The nurse should monitor this man for possible complications. Which of the following is a complication of renal colic?

    1. Anemia

    2. Polyuria

    3. Hypertension

    4. Oliguria

31. A woman is being seen in the walk-in clinic for recurrent cystitis. The nurse is teaching her about measures to prevent future episodes of cystitis. What should the nurse include in the teaching?

    1. Drink 1,000 ml of fluid each day, including a serving of cranberry juice at bedtime.

    2. Take a daily bath, and avoid the use of bath oils and soaps.

    3. Take all the medication prescribed, even if you feel better.

    4. Go to the bathroom and void soon after sexual intercourse.

32. A 64-year-old client with late stage chronic renal failure is admitted. What would the nurse expect in the nursing care plan for this client?

    1. Insert a urinary catheter to promote bladder drainage.

    2. Elevate the client's feet when out of bed to promote venous return.

    3. Assess the client's lung sounds each shift to monitor fluid status.

    4. Supplement the client's diet with protein powder shakes to provide essential amino acids to promote healing.

33. The nurse is teaching self-testicular examination to a group of young men on a college campus. Which information should be included in the discussion?

    1. Perform the examination immediately following sexual intercourse.

    2. See your physician for an examination yearly.

    3. A self-testicular exam should be done monthly.

    4. Daily examination of the testicles is recommended.

34. The nurse is caring for an adult who recently received a kidney transplant. Which statement, if made by the client, indicates a lack of understanding of his long-term management?

    1. "I plan to go back to work as soon as I feel strong enough."

    2. "We have started using gloves whenever we are scrubbing things."

    3. "My spouse has helped me work out a schedule for taking all these medications."

    4. "If my face gets puffy or my feet swell, I will stop taking the new medications."

35. An adult is scheduled for an intravenous pyelogram. Which comment by the client is of greatest concern to the nurse?

    1. "I am afraid of needles."

    2. "I get short of breath when I eat crab meat."

    3. "When I had an arteriogram, I felt nauseated when they injected the dye."

    4. "I am allergic to tetanus shots."

Answers and Rationales

1. (2) The urethral meatus is located between the clitoris and the vaginal orifice.

2. (2) After the client has voided, catheterization for retention should yield 50 mL or less. 200 cc indicates a retention of urine.

3. (4) Catheterization is performed by using the sterile technique. Medical asepsis is the clean technique.

4. (2) The drainage bag is positioned below the bladder with tubing angled so that there is a constant downward flow of urine from the bladder. This position helps to prevent ascending infection.

5. (4) Difficulty passing a catheter suggests an obstruction of some nature. The nurse should discontinue the procedure and notify the physician.

6. (2) He should be flat to prevent bleeding from the kidney, a very vascular organ. Blood pressure needs frequent monitoring to determine if he is bleeding. Bleeding is the most common complication following needle biopsy of the kidney.

7. (4) Taking him to the bathroom at regular intervals will help him regain control. Regression is common in children who are hospitalized. Putting diapers on him or leaving him in his wet bed are punitive, which is not therapeutic. Promising him a lollipop is bribing, which is not therapeutic.

8. (1) Pink-tinged urine is normal following a cystoscopy. Bright-red bleeding would need to be reported.

9. (1) Burning upon urination is usually seen in clients with a bladder infection. Flank pain and nausea and vomiting are seen more frequently in persons with kidney infection or stones. Elevated potassium is seen in renal failure.

10. (2) This describes the correct technique for a clean-catch midstream urine collection. Antiseptic wipes, not soap and water, are used.

The container must be sterile for urine for culture. A midstream collection is necessary. The initial urine voided may contain organisms from near the urethral opening. The object of the urine culture is to culture urine in the bladder.

11. (3) Failure to empty the bladder after sexual relations is thought to be a cause of bladder infections. Fluids should be encouraged, not restricted. She should wipe from front to back to prevent rectal organisms from entering the bladder, also thought to be a cause of bladder infections. All of the medication should be taken to adequately treat the infection and to prevent the development of resistant organisms.

12. (2) Encouraging fluids will often help the stone to pass. The client in this question has kidney stones; there is no mention of impending renal failure. High fluid intake is advised for clients who have bladder infections. However, that is not the diagnosis for this client. Increasing fluid intake may be indicated for a client who is dehydrated; however, that is not the diagnosis for this client.

13. (1) The stone should be sent to the laboratory for analysis to determine the type of stone. This will help to determine the diet he should follow. Stones do not usually contain blood or glucose. The laboratory needs to do the analysis. Passing the stone may be painful, but the pain is usually relieved after the stone is passed.

14. (2) Walking often helps to relieve the pain and will help the stone to pass. The nurse would instruct the client to have assistance with walking only if he is sedated from pain medication.

15. (2) The client's potassium is dangerously high. The normal level is 3.5–5.0 mEq/l. Kayexalate is a sodium-potassium exchange resin. It removes potassium from the bloodstream. While it will not correct the underlying problem, it will lower the serum potassium to safer levels and perhaps prevent serious or even fatal cardiac dysrhythmias. Kayexalate does not remove

fluid or reduce abdominal pressure. Kayexalate does not introduce potassium into the bowel. A client who has hyperkalemia does not need additional potassium.

16. (4) A client in acute renal failure is on a low-sodium, low-protein, low-potassium, high-carbohydrate diet. Applesauce is all of these. Watermelon and orange juice are high in potassium. Turkey contains protein, and the bread contains sodium.

17. (2) Benign prostatic hypertrophy (BPH) causes retention, urinary frequency, dribbling, and decreased force of the urinary stream. It does not cause pus in the urine. If pyuria (pus in the urine) is present, this indicates a secondary infection.

18. (1) Fluid intake should be encouraged to help prevent the development of a urinary tract infection. It is not appropriate to limit fluid intake. Following the removal of urine from a distended bladder, there is a risk of shock. The nurse should monitor the blood pressure. The nurse should weigh the client daily to assess for fluid retention. The nurse would assess renal function by monitoring intake and output.

19. (4) Compression of the penoscrotal junction will cause obstruction of urine flow. Taping the catheter to the thigh straightens out the urethra and prevents compression of the penoscrotal junction. Leaving the penis in a dependent position increases pressure at the penoscrotal junction. Taping the catheter to the thigh does not prevent the reflux of urine. Keeping the tubing gently sloping in a downward direction will help to prevent reflux. There is no need to maintain tension on the balloon of the indwelling catheter. If the balloon is inflated and positioned properly, it will stay in position. The client may or may not be more comfortable with the catheter in this position. However, comfort is not the reason for taping the catheter to the thigh.

20. (3) Continuous bathing of the bladder with the irrigating solution will flush clots from the bladder. The primary purpose of continuous

bladder irrigation (CBI) is not to prevent urinary tract infection. CBI does not maintain bladder tone. When a client has CBI, the client has an indwelling catheter. CBI does not prevent urethral stricture formation.

21. (2) A vasectomy is considered a permanent method of contraception even though it is occasionally possible to reverse. A vasectomy is essentially a ligation of the tube (vas Deferens) and is done by surgery, so answer 1 is a true statement. However, the information in answer 2, that this is a permanent method of sterilization, is much more essential. A vasectomy causes sterility but not impotence (inability to maintain an erection); it does not interfere with sexual functioning. The procedure does not take an hour; it takes only a few minutes.

22. (2) The first few ejaculations contain sperm that are already in the tubes. Before he is considered sterile, he should have two ejaculates a month apart that test sperm-free. It is usually at least 6–8 weeks before a man is considered sterile following a vasectomy. The surgeon does not flush the sperm from the man's tubes.

23. (1) A vasectomy does not prevent ejaculation. The ejaculate does not contain sperm. The man's sexual functioning is not affected. The client asks for information. The most appropriate response is to give the information. There is no evidence in the question that the man is concerned about his sexual identity. The nurse should answer the client's question, not interject her own experience in answering this question.

24. (3) Most urinary calculi that form as a result of prolonged immobility are alkaline. Cranberry juice leaves an acid ash, which keeps the urine acidic. The other liquids leave an alkaline ash, which could lead to the development of calculi.

25. (2) A diuretic causes increased urine output. Monitoring daily weights is the best way to assess changes in hydration status. Testing urine for sugar and acetone is not indicated for

this client. There is no data stating that the client is a diabetic. Intake and output may be indicated, but daily weights will give a more reliable indication of actual fluid loss. It is not wrong to assess for pedal edema, but daily weights will give a better indicator of fluid loss. Edema can be in places other than the feet.

26. (2) The irrigating solution goes in through the catheter, bathes the bladder, and flows out through the tubing into the collection bag. The nurse should measure the total amount of drainage and subtract the amount of irrigating solution infused, because this is not urine output. Choice number 1 makes no sense because the drainage is larger than the amount of irrigating solution used. The question asked how the nurse calculates total urine output. Answer 3 does not address the issue of calculating the total urine output. Recording total fluid intake will most likely be done for this client, but subtracting it from the drainage does not tell us the client's urine output.

27. (1) Total drainage from the bag is 2,550 ml. The amount of irrigant infused is 1,825 ml. Subtract 1,825 ml from 2,250 ml and the answer is 725 ml of urine.

28. (1) When obtaining a history of the present illness, the nurse questions the client about precipitating factors. Acute glomerulonephritis (AGN) usually occurs 10–14 days after a streptococcal infection. Strep throat or strep-related otitis media is the most common precipitating event. Chicken pox is caused by herpes zoster virus and is not usually associated with AGN. A bladder infection is not usually associated with AGN. AGN follows a streptococcal infection and is not specifically an inherited condition.

29. (4) It is important to tell the client that his urine will be red during the post-surgical period so that he is not frightened. The client will have an indwelling urinary catheter after surgery. He may even have a continuous, normal saline irrigation. There is no need to give instructions regarding voiding until after the catheter has been removed. Walking does not usually relieve bladder spasms. Coughing and deep-breathing are important post-operative interventions, but they do not prevent clot formation.

30. (4) Renal colic is severe pain associated with ureteral spasms when the ureter is irritated by a stone. A stone may occlude the ureter and block urine flow from the kidney. This can also result in hydronephrosis, a complication that can lead to kidney necrosis. Anemia and hypertension are complications of renal failure. Polyuria is not associated with renal colic.

31. (4) Bacteria may enter the urethra during intercourse. Voiding soon after intercourse helps flush organisms from the urinary tract. Daily fluid intake should be at least 2,500 to 3,000 ml to prevent recurring cystitis. Showers, not baths, are recommended. Sitting in a tub may cause a reflux of bacteria into the bladder. Finishing all medication is an appropriate response to a current infection, but does not prevent recurring infections.

32. (3) Lung sounds should be assessed to monitor for pulmonary edema, which is a complication of chronic renal failure. Inserting a catheter does not increase kidney function. The client will be oliguric in late-stage chronic renal failure. Elevating the feet increases fluid flow to the heart, making the heart work harder. This should not be done, because congestive heart failure is associated with chronic renal failure. Protein intake is restricted in chronic renal failure.

33. (3) All males past the age of puberty should perform self-testicular examination every month. The man should do this on the same day every month; such as the 1st or the 15th. The exam should be done in the shower, followed by a visual inspection looking in the mirror. There is no relation to sexual intercourse. Self-testicular examination is performed by the man himself. A physician will examine the testicles when a physical is done. This may not be yearly for young men.

Testicular cancer is primarily a disease of young men.

34. (4) A puffy face (moon face) and swollen feet may be side effects of steroid medications. A person who has had an organ transplant will receive immunosuppressant drugs including a steroid for the rest of his/her life. A person who has had a kidney transplant should be able to return to work once strength has been regained. If the client's work involved excessive exposure to infectious agents, the client might have to change jobs. Wearing gloves is an excellent way to reduce the chance of contracting an infection. The client will be taking a number of anti-rejection drugs life-long.

35. (2) Shortness of breath when eating crab meat suggests an allergy to iodine. Iodine dye is used to visualize the kidney during an IVP. This should be reported immediately to the physician. The client will have an intravenous needle, but fear of needles is not the greatest concern. Feeling nauseated or a feeling of warmth along the vein are normal sensations when receiving iodine dye. Tetanus allergy does not indicate an allergy to iodine.

Chapter 9

The Musculoskeletal System

Sample Questions

1. A plaster cast has just been applied to a client's left forearm, and he is in 10 lbs Russell traction on his left leg. Which of the following nursing concerns takes priority in the care of this client?

   1. The casted extremity may swell and the cast will become a tourniquet.
   2. Heat conduction from the wet cast can cause burning to the skin below.
   3. Muscle atrophy of the areas involved can lead to decreased muscle tone.
   4. Skin irritation from the cast edges can cause abrasions.

2. The nurse is caring for a client with a newly applied plaster cast. How should the nurse touch and move the wet cast?

   1. Use the palms of the hands.
   2. Use the fingertips only.
   3. Use a towel sling.
   4. Touch the cast only on the petals at the edges.

3. The nurse is caring for a client who has just had a cast applied. Which statement best describes the expected client outcome relative to the circulatory system for a client with a cast?

   1. There will be no increase in pain in the extremity.
   2. The client will have no circulatory impairment.
   3. The integrity of the cast will be maintained.
   4. The client will report any feelings of skin irritation.

4. The nurse gently elevates the client's newly casted arm on a pillow and explains that this is necessary for the first 24–48 hours after casting. What is the chief purpose of this action?

   1. It helps a damp cast to dry more evenly.
   2. It reduces the amount of pain medication needed.
   3. Venous return is enhanced, and edema is decreased.
   4. It is more comfortable than keeping the arm dependent.

5. An adolescent male was in an accident and is hospitalized with multiple fractures. The nurse enters the room and observes that he has his back to the door and is staring at the wall with a sad expression on his face. What is the best response for the nurse to make at this time?

    1. "You seem sad."
    2. "Don't be too down on yourself."
    3. "I know it is hard to be out of school."
    4. "Do you miss your family and friends?"

6. The client is in Russell's traction. Which statement best describes how Russell's traction works?

    1. The legs are suspended vertically with the hip flexed at 90° and knees extended.
    2. A straight pull on the affected leg is assured.
    3. A belt is applied just above and surrounding the iliac crests. The belt is then attached to a pulley system.
    4. Vertical traction is used at the knee at the same time a horizontal force is exerted on the tibia and fibula.

7. The nurse is assessing the leg of a client in Russell's traction. Which area is it essential to assess?

    1. Brachial area
    2. Femoral area
    3. Popliteal area
    4. Inner aspect of the thigh

8. It is necessary to pull the client, who is in Russell's traction, up in bed. Which action should the nurse take?

    1. Leave the weights in place.
    2. Remove the weights completely.
    3. Reduce the weight of the traction by one half.
    4. Have one nurse lift the weights while the others pull the client.

9. The client has been flat in bed in traction for two weeks and she is to be allowed out of bed for the first time today. What must the nurse be particularly alert for when getting the client out of bed?

    1. Renal complications
    2. Depression
    3. Orthostatic hypotension
    4. Skin breakdown

10. The client is a 73-year-old woman who fell in her home and suffered a right hip fracture. She tells the nurse that she was walking across the kitchen and felt something "snap" in her hip and this made her fall. What type of fracture is the client most likely to have had?

    1. Comminuted fracture
    2. Greenstick fracture
    3. Open fracture
    4. Pathological fracture

11. The nurse knows that elderly women have a high incidence of hip fracture for which reason?

    1. Decreased progesterone secretion
    2. Decreased mobility due to arthritic conditions
    3. Increased calcium absorption
    4. Osteoporosis in the skeletal structure

12. The nurse is caring for a person prior to surgery to repair a broken right hip. Which nursing care measure is essential?

    1. Get the client out of bed twice a day to maintain mobility.
    2. Use pillows to maintain the right hip in a state of abduction.
    3. Elevate the foot of the bed to 25 degrees.
    4. Feed the client to conserve her energy.

13. A femoral head replacement was performed on an elderly client. Post-operatively the nurse

positions the client with an abductor pillow between the client's legs. What is the primary reason for this?

1. This position will promote greater comfort.
2. Abduction promotes greater circulation to the hip joint.
3. Abduction will prevent the prosthesis from snapping out of the socket.
4. This position will help to prevent pressure on the sciatic nerve.

14. The client with rheumatoid arthritis has been taking 15 or 20 extra-strength aspirin a day. Which additional statement the client makes would be of greatest concern to the nurse?

1. "I sometimes have ringing in my ears."
2. "I have a rash under my arms."
3. "My fingers are swollen sometimes."
4. "I don't have very much energy."

15. The physician orders prednisone for a client with rheumatoid arthritis for painful wrists and joints. Which instruction is it essential for the nurse to give the client?

1. "Take the pills with milk or food."
2. "Be sure to take the medication between meals."
3. "Stop the pills at once if your face begins to get puffy."
4. "Your urine may turn pinkish while taking this."

16. The client is a 64-year-old male admitted to the hospital with gout and has severe pain in his right big toe, which is red and swollen. Which nursing care measure is most essential for the nurse to perform at this time?

1. Use a bed cradle on the bed.
2. Put a bed board on the bed.
3. Obtain a heat lamp.
4. Prepare to catheterize the client.

17. The nurse is to give the client with gout one tablet of colchicine every hour until relief or toxicity occurs. Which of the following is an indication for stopping the colchicine?

1. Ringing in the ears
2. Nausea and vomiting
3. A rash on the client's hips
4. A temperature of 101°F

18. The nurse is teaching the client with gout about a diet low in purines. Which of the following is lowest in purine?

1. Roast chicken
2. Beef liver
3. Fried shrimp
4. Scrambled eggs

19. The client is now over an acute episode of gout. He is to be discharged on allopurinol (Zyloprim). What instruction must the nurse give to this client?

1. "Take your medicine on an empty stomach."
2. "Report any nausea to your physician at once."
3. "Drink two to three quarts of fluids daily."
4. "Do not take over-the-counter cold medicine."

20. The client with arthritis is receiving sodium salicylate and asks the nurse what the drug will do for her. The nurse's reply should include information that the drug is given for which of these effects?

1. Antipyretic
2. Antibiotic
3. Anticoagulant
4. Anti-inflammatory

21. The client with newly diagnosed rheumatoid arthritis asks what can happen if no treatment is done. The nurse knows that if rheumatoid arthritis is left untreated, which of the following would be most apt to develop?

    1. Bony ankylosis
    2. Chronic osteomyelitis
    3. Pathological fractures
    4. Joint hypermobility

22. The client with rheumatoid arthritis is to receive prednisone 2.5 mg P.O. a.c. and h.s. What is the primary expected action of the drug?

    1. Maintenance of sodium and potassium balance
    2. Improvement of carbohydrate metabolism
    3. Production of androgen-like effects
    4. Interference with inflammatory reactions

23. The client is admitted to the hospital for a diagnostic workup. The client has vague symptoms of malaise, coughing, chest discomfort, low-grade fever, diffuse rashes, and musculoskeletal aches and pains. A diagnosis of probable lupus erythematosus has been made. The night nurse finds the client crying and saying, "I would rather die than suffer with this disease for the rest of my life." Which response by the nurse would be most therapeutic at this time?

    1. Telling the client there are support groups to join after discharge
    2. Offering to stay with the client to discuss concerns and questions
    3. Advising the client to write concerns on paper to discuss with the doctors and nurses tomorrow
    4. Offer the client a back rub and a warm cup of milk

24. The client is an elderly man who has had diabetes and peripheral vascular disease for several years. He now has had a right below-the-knee amputation. Which pre-operative nursing action will do most to help the client adjust to having an amputation?

    1. Encouraging deep-breathing
    2. Asking him if he understands the full effects of the planned surgery
    3. Discussing the effects of diabetes on the vascular system
    4. Having a recovered amputee visit him

25. The client has returned to the nursing unit following a right below-the-knee amputation. How should the nurse position the client?

    1. Supine with head turned to the side
    2. Place shock blocks under the foot of the bed
    3. Semi-Fowler's position with knees bent
    4. Left lateral with pillows between the knees

26. The day after an amputation, the client begins to hemorrhage from his stump. What action should the nurse take first?

    1. Apply a pressure dressing to the stump.
    2. Place a tourniquet above the stump.
    3. Notify the physician.
    4. Apply an ice pack to the stump.

27. The client continues to recover following a below-the-knee amputation. What nursing action should the nurse take to help prevent the most common complication following leg amputation?

    1. Clean the wound with hydrogen peroxide three times a day.
    2. Have the client lie prone several times a day.
    3. Ask the client to flex and extend the toes on the remaining leg.
    4. Encourage the client to completely empty his/her bladder.

28. A young adult is discharged to home with crutches. Which exercise should the nurse teach the client in order to strengthen the triceps muscles for crutch-walking?

    1. Pushing the buttocks up off the mattress

    2. Pulling the body up, using an overhead trapeze

    3. Raising the legs straight up and down

    4. Squeezing a rubber ball in each hand

29. The client is ordered to be positioned flat following a myelogram. The nurse understands the primary reason for this is which of the following?

    1. To prevent infection

    2. To prevent spinal headache

    3. To prevent seizures

    4. To promote excretion of dye

30. The client has a fractured right ankle that has just been casted. The nurse is instructing the client in crutch-walking techniques. Which method is most appropriate?

    1. Move the right crutch, then the left foot, then the left crutch, and finally the right foot.

    2. Balance weight on the left foot and move right foot and both crutches forward, then bear weight on both crutches and move the left foot forward.

    3. Move the right crutch and left foot forward together; then the left crutch and right foot.

    4. Move the right crutch and right foot together and then the left crutch and the left foot.

Answers and Rationales

1. (1) The nurse must elevate the extremity to prevent swelling, which could cut off circulation. The wet plaster cast gives a sensation of heat to the client but will not burn the skin. There will be muscle atrophy to both the arm and the leg. However, this is a long-term problem and will best be addressed after the cast and traction are removed. Abrasions are a cause for concern after the cast has dried but not at this time.

2. (1) The nurse should touch the cast using only the palms of the hands to prevent making indentations in a wet cast. Indentations could cause irritation of the skin. Fingertips would cause indentations in the wet cast. A towel sling is not appropriate. The cast is not petalled until it has dried. It would be impossible to move the casted extremity just by touching the petalled area at the edge of the cast.

3. (2) The cast should not be so tight as to cause circulatory impairment, which would be evidenced by swelling and changes in color or temperature. Pain is usually evidence of neurological impairment. The integrity of the cast should be maintained, but that does not describe an outcome relative to the circulatory system. Skin irritation is not an indicator of circulatory impairment.

4. (3) Elevation of the extremity increases venous return and reduces swelling. Elevation does not help a damp cast to dry more evenly. Changing the position of the pillow beneath the cast and not covering the cast will help it dry more evenly. Elevating a casted extremity does not directly reduce the amount of pain medication needed. A casted extremity that is elevated usually is more comfortable than one that is dependent; the chief purpose of elevation is to prevent edema formation. The prevention of edema is what makes the extremity more comfortable.

5. (1) The nurse should open communication. The nurse is sharing with the client the nurse's perception of the client's behavior. This is therapeutic and should open communication. Answer 2 tells him what not to do and will probably block communication. Answers 3 and 4 assume that the nurse knows what is causing

his sadness and do not allow him to discuss his feelings.

6. (4) This best describes Russell's traction. Answer 1 describes Bryant's traction. Answer 2 is Buck's extension traction. Answer 3 is pelvic traction.

7. (3) The popliteal area should be assessed for adequacy of circulation. In Russell's traction, there is a vertical pull at the popliteal area that could obstruct circulation. The brachial area is in the arm.

8. (1) The weights should remain in place at all times. They should not be removed or reduced or lifted up while the client is moved.

9. (3) The client has been flat for two weeks. Orthostatic hypotension is likely. The nurse should let the client dangle on the side of the bed before ambulating. While the client would have an increased possibility of kidney stones after being immobilized, this is not related to getting the client out of bed. Depression and skin breakdown can also occur in clients who have been immobilized. However, they are not apt to cause problems when the client gets out of bed for the first time.

10. (4) The description fits that of a pathological fracture in which the bone fractured first and then she fell. This is usually related to a decrease of calcium in the bone. With a comminuted fracture, the bone is broken into several pieces. A greenstick fracture occurs in children. One side of the bone is broken and the other side is splintered, like breaking a green stick. An open or compound fracture is one in which a wound through the soft tissue communicates with the site of the break.

11. (4) Osteoporosis or the loss of calcium is caused by a number of factors and is often related to the decrease in estrogen following menopause. Osteoporosis is thought to be related to decreased estrogen after menopause, not decreased progesterone. Elderly women do not all have decreased mobility due to arthritis. The cause is usually related to decreased

calcium absorption rather than increased calcium absorption.

12. (2) The hip should be maintained in abduction to keep the hip in the best alignment. She cannot get out of bed. The foot is not elevated. There is no data indicating a need to feed the client.

13. (3) Abduction is necessary to keep the hip from coming out of the socket. This position may or may not be most comfortable. Comfort, while important, is not of highest priority. Abduction does not necessarily promote greater circulation to the hip joint. Abduction does not prevent pressure on the sciatic nerve.

14. (1) Tinnitus is a sign of aspirin toxicity. Swollen fingers and decrease in energy are typical of rheumatoid arthritis. A rash under the arms is not likely to be related to aspirin ingestion.

15. (1) Corticosteroids are very irritating to the stomach and are taken with food or milk to reduce the chance of ulcer development. The client will develop a puffy face from the steroid. This is not an indication to discontinue the drug. Steroids should not be stopped abruptly. They should always be tapered. Answer 4 is not true; the urine does not turn pinkish. Dilantin, an anti-seizure drug, may turn the urine pinkish.

16. (1) The pain of gout is very severe. A bed cradle will keep the bed linens off his toe. There is no indication for a bed board. Bed boards are indicated for back problems. A heat lamp is not part of the therapy for gout. There is no indication of a need to catheterize the client.

17. (2) Nausea, vomiting, and diarrhea indicate toxicity to colchicine. Tinnitus indicates aspirin toxicity. Rash and fever are not usual signs of colchicine toxicity.

18. (4) Eggs are lowest in purine. Chicken, organ meats such as liver, and shrimp are high in purines.

19. (3) It is essential to force fluids when taking allopurinol, a uricosuric drug. This will help the

uric acid crystals to be excreted in the urine and not collect in the kidneys and form stones. The medicine should be taken with food. Nausea can be a side effect of the allopurinol. However, the priority instruction is to drink large amounts of fluid. There is no contraindication with over-the-counter cold medicine.

20. (4) Sodium salicylate has all of the effects except antibiotic. However, it is given to a person with arthritis primarily for its anti-inflammatory effect. The anticoagulant action can be an adverse effect for this client.

21. (1) Bony ankylosis occurs in untreated rheumatoid arthritis. Osteomyelitis is a bone infection and is not related to rheumatoid arthritis. Pathological fractures are usually the result of severe osteoporosis, not arthritis. Joints lose mobility and become ankylosed; they do not have hypermobility.

22. (4) Prednisone is a corticosteroid and has an anti-inflammatory effect. It does affect sodium and potassium balance, carbohydrate metabolism, and causes androgen-like effects; however, these are seen as bothersome side effects when given to a client who has arthritis.

23. (2) Offering help and letting the client express feelings is most therapeutic at this time. Telling the client about support groups may be appropriate later. Advising the client to write her concerns on paper to discuss tomorrow could be appropriate after the nurse had listened to the client's concerns and feelings. At this time, that response closes communication. Giving the client a back rub and a warm cup of milk could be done after listening to the client.

24. (4) Seeing an amputee who is living successfully will do the most to help him adjust to having an amputation. All of the others might be done but do not help him to adjust to an amputation.

25. (2) The foot of the bed should be raised to prevent edema formation in the stump. Shock blocks are the best way to accomplish this.

Pillows can be used for the first 24–28 hours only. Note that the client has returned to the nursing unit. The client will be awake before returning to the nursing unit, and so turning the head to the side is not needed. Positioning the client in semi-Fowler's position with knees bent would cause swelling of the surgical site and is contraindicated. Positioning the client on the side with pillows between the knees is not the most appropriate position.

26. (2) Applying a tourniquet is the best action because the bleeders are usually too large to be controlled by pressure. This is one of the very few times when applying a tourniquet is indicated. An ice pack will be ineffective in controlling hemorrhage from the stump. The nurse should notify the physician but should attempt to stop the bleeding before leaving the client to call the physician.

27. (2) The most common complication is flexion contracture of the hip or knee. Having the client lie prone will help to prevent flexion contractures of the hip and knee. The wound should be kept clean, but not usually with hydrogen peroxide three times a day. Asking the client to flex and extend the toes on the remaining leg will help to prevent thrombophlebitis in the remaining leg and is certainly appropriate. However, thrombophlebitis is not the most common complication following leg amputation. It is appropriate to encourage the client to empty the bladder. However, a bladder infection is not the most common complication following leg amputation.

28. (1) Pushing one's buttocks up off the mattress is a resistive exercise that improves the strength and tone of the triceps muscles. Pull-ups strengthen the biceps muscles. Straight leg raises strengthen the hip flexor and quadriceps. Squeezing a rubber ball strengthens finger flexors.

29. (2) When a client is ordered to be flat following a myelogram, the nurse knows the physician used an oil-based dye. The reason for the flat

position is to prevent development of spinal headache. If the client had been ordered to be in a low-Fowler's position, the nurse would know that a water-based dye had been used. The water-based dye is not removed, and the client is in low-Fowler's position to prevent irritation of the meninges and seizures. With a water-based dye, fluids are encouraged to promote excretion of the dye. Positioning does not prevent development of infection.

30. (2) A three-point gait is indicated when the client can bear no weight on one foot. This correctly describes a three-point gait for someone with a right foot problem. Answer 1 describes a four-point gait. The client must be able to bear weight on both feet for this gait. Answer 3 correctly describes a two-point gait. The client must be able to bear weight on both feet for this gait. Answer 4 does not correctly describe any gait.

Chapter 10

The Endocrine System

Sample Questions

1. What should be included in the nursing care plan for a client with diabetes insipidus?

   1. Blood pressure every hour
   2. Strict intake and output
   3. Urine for ketone bodies
   4. Glucose monitoring qid

2. What must the nurse do when preparing a client for a CT scan?

   1. Administer a laxative prep.
   2. Encourage fluids.
   3. Explain the procedure.
   4. Administer a radioisotope.

3. Antibiotics are ordered for a client who has had a transphenoidal hypophysectomy. He asks why he is receiving an antibiotic when he does not have an infection. The nurse's response is based on the knowledge that:

   1. Antibiotics will help to prevent respiratory complications following surgery.
   2. Meningitis is a complication following transphenoidal hypophysectomy.
   3. Fluid retention can cause dangerously high cerebral spinal fluid pressure.
   4. Hormone replacement is essential after hypophysectomy.

4. Twelve hours after a transphenoidal hypophysectomy, the client keeps clearing his throat and complains of a drip in his mouth. In order to accurately assess this, the nurse should test the fluid for:

   1. Sugar
   2. Protein
   3. Bacteria
   4. Blood

5. The client is ready for discharge following an adrenalectomy. Which statement that the client makes indicates the best understanding of the client's condition?

   1. "I will continue on a low-sodium, low-potassium diet."
   2. "My husband has arranged for a marriage counselor because of our fights."
   3. "I will stay out of the sun so I will not turn splotchy brown."
   4. "I will take all of those pills every day."

6. What is the nursing priority when administering care to a client with severe hyperthyroidism?

   1. Assess for recent emotional trauma.
   2. Provide a calm, non-stimulating environment.
   3. Provide diversionary activity.
   4. Encourage range-of-motion exercises.

7. Which problem is most likely to develop if hyperthyroidism remains untreated?

   1. Pulmonary embolism
   2. Respiratory acidosis
   3. Cerebral vascular accident
   4. Heart failure

8. Which nursing care measure is essential because a client has exophthalmos?

   1. Administer artificial tears.
   2. Encourage the client to wear her glasses.
   3. Promote bed rest.
   4. Monitor her pulse rate every four hours.

9. A client who has just had a thyroidectomy returns to the unit in stable condition. What equipment is it essential for the nurse to have readily available?

   1. Tracheostomy set
   2. Thoracotomy tray
   3. Dressing set
   4. Ice collar

10. What is the best way to assess for hemorrhage in a client who has had a thyroidectomy?

   1. Check the pulse and blood pressure hourly.
   2. Roll the client to the side and check for evidence of bleeding.
   3. Ask the client if he/she feels blood trickling down the back of the throat.
   4. Place a hand under the client's neck and shoulders to feel bed linens.

11. Which finding would be the greatest cause for concern to the nurse during the early post-operative period following a thyroidectomy?

   1. Temperature of 100°F
   2. A sore throat
   3. Carpal spasm when the blood pressure is taken
   4. Complaints of pain in the area of the surgical incision

12. An adult is admitted to the hospital with a diagnosis of hypothyroidism. Which findings would the nurse most likely elicit during the nursing assessment?

   1. Elevated blood pressure and temperature
   2. Tachycardia and weight gain
   3. Hypothermia and constipation
   4. Moist skin and coarse hair

13. Which diet would most likely be ordered for the client with hypothyroidism?

   1. High protein, high calorie
   2. Restricted fluids, low protein
   3. High roughage, low calorie
   4. High carbohydrate, low roughage

14. An adult with myxedema is started on thyroid replacement therapy and is discharged. The client returns to the doctor's office one week later. Which statement that the client makes is most indicative of an adverse reaction to the medication?

   1. "My chest hurt when I was sweeping the floor this morning."
   2. "I had severe cramps last night."
   3. "I am losing weight."
   4. "My pulse rate has been more rapid lately."

15. The nurse's next door neighbor calls. He says he cannot awaken his 21-year-old wife. The nurse notes that the client is unconscious and is having deep respirations. Her breath has a

fruity smell to it. The husband says that his wife has been eating and drinking a lot recently and that last night she vomited before lying down. What is the most appropriate action for the nurse to take?

1. Start cardiopulmonary resuscitation.

2. Get her to a hospital immediately.

3. Try to rouse her by giving her coffee.

4. Give her sweetened orange juice.

16. The client is diagnosed as having insulin-dependent diabetes mellitus (IDDM). She received regular insulin at 7:30 A.M. When is she most apt to develop a hypoglycemic reaction?

1. Mid-morning

2. Mid-afternoon

3. Early evening

4. During the night

17. The nurse is teaching a client to administer insulin. The instructions should include teaching the client to

1. Inject the needle at a 90-degree angle into the muscle.

2. Vigorously massage the area after injecting the insulin.

3. Rotate injection sites.

4. Keep the open bottle of insulin in the refrigerator.

18. An adolescent with IDDM is learning about a diabetic diet. He asks the nurse if he will ever be able to go out to eat with his friends again.

1. "You can go out with them, but you should take your own snack with you."

2. "Yes. You will learn what foods are allowed so you can eat with your friends."

3. "When you get food out in a restaurant, be sure to order diet soft drinks."

4. "Eating out will not be possible on a diabetic diet. Why don't you plan to invite your friends to your house?"

19. At 10 A.M., a client with IDDM becomes very irritable and starts to yell at the nurse. Which initial nursing assessment should take priority?

1. Blood pressure and pulse

2. Color and temperature of skin

3. Reflexes and muscle tone

4. Serum electrolytes and glucose

20. An elderly woman has been recently diagnosed as having non-insulin-dependent diabetes mellitus (NIDDM). Which of the following complaints she has is most likely to be related to the diagnosis of diabetes mellitus?

1. Pruritus vulvae

2. Cough

3. Eructation

4. Singultus

21. A client has a transphenoidal hypophysectomy to remove a pituitary tumor. When the client returns to the nursing unit following surgery, the head of the bed is elevated 30 degrees. What is the primary purpose for placing the client in this position?

1. To promote respiratory effort

2. To reduce pressure on the sella turcica

3. To prevent acidosis

4. To promote oxygenation

22. The nurse is discussing discharge plans with a client who had a transphenoidal hypophysectomy. Which statement made by the client indicates a need for more teaching?

1. "I won't brush my teeth until the doctor removes the stitches."

2. "I will wear loafers instead of tie shoes."

3. "Where can I get a Medic Alert bracelet?"

4. "I will take all these new medicines until I feel better."

23. A woman with a tumor of the adrenal cortex says to the nurse, "Will I always look this ugly? I hate having a beard." What is the best response for the nurse to make?

1. "After surgery you will not develop any more symptoms, but the changes you now have will linger."

2. "That varies from person to person. You should ask your physician."

3. "After surgery, your appearance should gradually return to normal."

4. "Electrolysis and plastic surgery should make your appearance normal."

24. The client develops hypoparathyroidism after a total thyroidectomy. What treatment should the nurse anticipate?

1. Emergency tracheostomy

2. Administration of calcium

3. Oxygen administration

4. Administration of potassium

25. A woman with newly diagnosed IDDM says she wants to have children. She asks if she will be able to have children and if they will be normal. What is the best answer for the nurse to give?

1. "Women with diabetes should not get pregnant because it is very difficult to control diabetes during pregnancy."

2. "Babies born to diabetic mothers are very apt to have severe and non-correctable birth defects."

3. "You should be able to safely have a baby if you go to your doctor regularly during pregnancy."

4. "You should consult carefully with a geneticist before getting pregnant to determine how to prevent your baby from developing diabetes."

26. A client is admitted to the hospital with recently diagnosed diabetes mellitus and is to have fasting blood work drawn this morning. At 7:00 A.M., the lab has not arrived to draw the blood. The client's dose of regular insulin is scheduled for 7:30 A.M. What is the best action for the nurse to take?

1. Give the insulin as ordered.

2. Withhold the insulin until the lab comes and the client will be eating within 15–30 minutes.

3. Withhold the insulin until the blood has been drawn and the client has eaten.

4. Do not administer insulin until the blood work has been drawn and the results have been called back to the unit.

27. An adolescent with newly diagnosed IDDM asks the nurse if he can continue to play football. What is the best answer for the nurse to give?

1. "Now that you have diabetes, you should not play football because you may get a cut that will not heal."

2. "If you work with your physician to regulate the insulin dosage and your diet, you should be able to play football."

3. "It would be better for you to work as equipment manager so you will not be under as much stress."

4. "You can probably continue to play football if you can regulate it so that you have the same amount of exercise each day."

28. The client is a 62-year-old woman who is 30 pounds overweight. She comes to the doctor's office complaining of headaches, frequent hunger, excessive thirst, and urination. The presenting complaints suggest that the nurse should assess for other signs of which condition?

1. Hypothyroidism

2. Acute pyelonephritis

3. Addison's disease

4. Diabetes mellitus

29. An elderly client with NIDDM develops an ingrown toenail. What is the best action for the nurse?

    1. Put cotton under the nail and clip the nail straight across.
    2. Elevate the foot immediately.
    3. Apply warm, moist soaks.
    4. Notify the physician.

30. A woman with hypothyroidism asks the nurse why the doctor told her she cannot have a sedative. The nurse's response is based on which of the following facts?

    1. Sedatives potentiate thyroid replacement medication.
    2. Clients with hypothyroidism have increased susceptibility to all sedative drugs.
    3. Sedatives will have a paradoxical affect on clients with hypothyroidism.
    4. Sedatives would cause fluid retention and hypernatremia.

Answers and Rationales

1. (2) Diabetes insipidus is excessive urine output due to decreased amounts of antidiuretic hormone. Because of the excessive urine output, it is necessary to monitor intake and output.

2. (3) Explanation is all that is necessary. The client is not given a radioisotope. Fluids are not pushed prior to the procedure. The client frequently is given an iodine dye, so the nurse should ask about allergies to shellfish.

3. (2) A transphenoidal approach goes through the roof of the mouth, which has many organisms. Meningitis can occur. Answer 1 is a true statement but not the primary reason in this case. Antibiotics do not lower spinal fluid pressure. Answer 4 is a true statement, but antibiotics are not hormones.

4. (1) Dripping in the back of the throat after a transphenoidal hypophysectomy may be cerebrospinal fluid (CSF). CSF contains glucose. Saliva and mucus do not.

5. (4) The client must take steroid replacements every day for the rest of his/her life. Answer 1 is not an appropriate diet. The fights should decrease as mood swings decrease after surgery.

6. (2) A calm environment is important to reduce activity. Hyperthyroidism makes a person hyperactive and easily distractible. There is no reason to assess for emotional trauma. The hyperthyroid client is usually hyperactive, so there would be no need for range of motion exercises.

7. (4) Hyperthyroidism causes tachycardia, which can be severe enough to cause heart failure. Pulse rates can be 100 to 150/minute.

8. (1) Exophthalmos (protrusion of the eyes) may be so severe that the eyelids cannot close. Artificial tears will keep the eyes moist so that abrasions do not occur.

9. (1) Swelling in the operative site could cause airway obstruction. The nurse should have a tracheostomy set and oxygen readily available for 48 hours after thyroidectomy. A thoracotomy tray is not indicated. This client is not likely to need intervention in the thoracic cavity. A dressing set is unlikely to be needed. An ice collar might be indicated, but is not critical to have at the bedside.

10. (4) Following a thyroidectomy, the client is in semi-Fowler's position so drainage would go to the back of the neck. Because of the neck incision, the client should not be rolled to the side. The bleeding is unlikely to be inside the throat. Blood trickling down the throat might be seen in a client who has had a tonsillectomy.

11. (3) Carpal spasm is a sign of tetany and is known as Chovstek's sign. Tetany may occur if the parathyroids have been inadvertently removed. The parathyroids regulate calcium

phosphorus balance. Hypocalcemia causes tetany. Most clients who have been intubated during surgery have a sore throat. Pain in the incision area is normal in the immediate post-operative period.

12. (3) Hypothyroidism causes decreased metabolic rate, which will cause lowered body temperature and pulse and decreased digestion of food. The skin is dry and the hair thins.

13. (3) Hypothyroidism causes constipation and obesity. A diet high in roughage and low in calories is appropriate. The client should not be given a high-calorie diet. There is no need for fluid restriction or alteration in protein.

14. (1) Chest pain on exertion suggests angina. In addition to a slow heart rate, the client with hypothyroidism frequently has atherosclerosis. Thyroxin will increase the heart rate, and the heart will require more oxygen. Angina is a likely and serious complication that can occur. She will also probably lose weight and have an increased pulse. These are expected when taking thyroxin. Cramps are not likely to be related to taking thyroxin.

15. (2) Her symptoms suggest ketoacidosis. She must receive medical treatment at once. Coffee will not help her. She is unresponsive. Sweetened orange juice is not indicated for ketoacidosis. It would be appropriate for hypoglycemia. There is no data to suggest the need for CPR.

16. (1) Hypoglycemic reactions occur at peak action time. Peak action time for regular insulin is two to four hours after injection.

17. (3) Injection sites should be rotated to prevent tissue damage. Insulin is injected at a 90-degree angle into the deep subcutaneous tissue, not the muscle. Insulin does not need to be refrigerated. The open vial should be kept in the box to protect it from light. Insulin should not be kept at temperature extremes, such as the glove compartment of the car on a hot day.

18. (2) Eating out with friends is very important to an adolescent. Snacks will be allowed on his diet. He should be taught how to use the exchange lists in managing his diet.

19. (2) The nurse should immediately assess the skin. Behavior change and irritability suggest hypoglycemia. If the client is hypoglycemic, the client will have pale, cold, clammy skin, and needs treatment (ingestion of a rapid acting carbohydrate) at once.

20. (1) Pruritus vulvae (itching of the vulva) frequently accompanies diabetes. Monilial infections are common due to the change in pH. Eructation is belching or burping, and singultus is hiccups. Neither of these is particularly related to diabetes.

21. (2) Slight head elevation will reduce pressure on the sella turcica, where the pituitary gland is located, and edema formation in the area. This position may help promote respiratory effort. However, that is not the primary reason in this client. This position does not prevent acidosis or promote oxygenation.

22. (4) Because the pituitary or master gland was removed, the client will need to take life-long medications, not just until the client feels better. All of the other actions are appropriate. The client should not bend over to tie shoes, because this increases intracranial pressure. Answer 1 is correct. Remember, the client had a transphenoidal procedure in which the incision is in the mouth above the gum line. The client must take medications daily for the rest of his/her life so a Medic Alert bracelet is appropriate.

23. (3) A gradual return to normal will occur after adrenalectomy, when there are no longer abnormal amounts of steroids being produced.

24. (2) Hypoparathyroidism causes a decrease in calcium, which is manifested by tetany. Calcium will be administered.

25. (3) Most diabetic women can safely have babies if they receive good medical supervision during

pregnancy. There is a slightly higher incidence of fetal loss and malformations in babies of diabetic mothers, but not enough to preclude the chance of a normal baby. There is no way to prevent the child from later developing diabetes. Diabetes is an inherited condition.

26. (2) Regular insulin onsets within 30 minutes. It should not be given until he can eat within 15–30 minutes so that he will not develop hypoglycemia.

27. (2) Diabetes is not a contraindication for sports. Changes in activity level will alter the utilization of glucose, so he will need to work closely with his physician to regulate exercise, insulin, and diet control.

28. (4) The symptoms are the cardinal symptoms of diabetes mellitus: polydipsia, polyphagia, and polyuria. The client with hypothyroidism would have fatigue, weight gain, and complain of being cold all the time. The person with acute pyelonephritis would probably complain of frequent urination and flank pain and might have a fever. The person with Addison's disease would have polyuria, low blood sugar, and might go into hypovolemic shock.

29. (4) An ingrown toenail may cause infection, which can be very serious for the diabetic client. The physician should be notified. It is not appropriate for the practical nurse to initiate treatment.

30. (2) In hypothyroidism, the metabolic rate is decreased. This causes an increased susceptibility to sedative drugs.

Chapter 11

The Integumentary System

Sample Questions

1. Burns of what part of the body have the highest mortality rate?

    1. Lower torso
    2. Upper part of the body
    3. Hands and feet
    4. Perineum

2. Which of the following persons with burns has the poorest prognosis?

    1. A 20-year-old with second- and third-degree burns over 60% of the body
    2. An 80-year-old with second- and third-degree burns over 50% of the body
    3. A 35-year-old with second- and third-degree burns over 60% of the body
    4. A 2-year-old with second- and third-degree burns over 30% of the body

3. Which of these clients should have his clothing removed immediately?

    1. A 32-year-old man who was burned while working on high tension wires
    2. A 14-year-old who suffered severe smoke inhalation during a fire at school
    3. A 78-year-old who was burned during a fire that started when the client fell asleep while smoking
    4. A 19-year-old who spilled chemicals on himself in the chemistry lab at school

4. A 28-year-old man received severe burns of the chest, abdomen, back, legs, and hands when the house caught fire. In the emergency room, a nasogastric tube was inserted and the client was ordered NPO. What is the primary reason for maintaining NPO on this client?

    1. To prevent the deadly complication of aspiration
    2. To make the client more comfortable
    3. To help prevent paralytic ileus
    4. To help prevent excessive fluid loss

5. An indwelling catheter was inserted in a severely burned client for which reason?

   1. To prevent contamination of burned areas
   2. To measure hourly urine output
   3. To prevent urinary tract infection
   4. To detect internal injuries quickly

6. A severely burned man had his last tetanus shot when he started work at his job two years ago. What should the nurse expect to administer now?

   1. Tetanus toxoid booster
   2. Tetanus antitoxin
   3. Hyperimmune human tetanus globulin
   4. DPT booster

7. A severely burned client is to be admitted from the emergency department. What type of room should the nurse prepare for the client?

   1. A semi-private room with a non-infectious client
   2. A room with a post-operative client
   3. An isolation room
   4. A private room with a private bath

8. The nurse is planning care for a newly burned client. What is the priority nursing observation to be made during the first 48 hours after the burn?

   1. Hourly blood pressure
   2. Assessment of skin color and capillary refill
   3. Hourly urine measurement
   4. Frequent assessment for pain

9. Cimetidine (Tagamet) is ordered IV every six hours for a person with severe burns. What is the primary reason for administering Tagamet?

   1. To prevent infection
   2. To restore electrolyte balance
   3. To promote renal function
   4. To prevent Curling's ulcers

10. A client who was severely burned goes to the Hubbard tank daily. Tanking sessions are limited to a half hour for which reason?

    1. A longer period of time is too tiring.
    2. Eschar becomes difficult to remove with longer soaking.
    3. Prolonged soaking causes electrolyte dilution.
    4. The water becomes too cool and may cause chilling.

11. Silver nitrate dressings are applied to burns on an adult. What should be included in the nursing care plan?

    1. Change the dressings every two hours.
    2. Keep the dressings moist.
    3. Carefully monitor fluid intake.
    4. Observe for black discoloration.

12. Which assessment is essential when the client is having silver nitrate dressings applied?

    1. BUN
    2. Blood gases
    3. CBC
    4. Serum electrolytes

13. A young man has extensive burns on the front and back of the chest. His treatment includes the use of sulfamylon to the burned areas. What is the best method for applying topical antimicrobials?

    1. With the sterile, gloved hand
    2. With a sterile applicator
    3. With sterile 4 × 4's
    4. By aerosol spray

14. An electrician was wearing a glove that had a hole in it when he grabbed a "hot" wire. His coworkers came to him immediately and called the rescue squad. When the industrial nurse reached him, the electric current had been shut off. What action should the nurse take initially?

1. Dress the entrance and exit wounds.

2. Check respirations and pulse rate.

3. Remove clothing from the burned area.

4. Roll him in a blanket.

15. A client who has just been diagnosed with psoriasis asks the nurse what should be done to prevent family members from getting the condition. What should the nurse include when responding to this question?

   1. Showering daily with antiseptic soap should be sufficient.

   2. Wearing clothing over the affected part and washing clothes separately from the rest of the family is all that is necessary.

   3. Psoriasis is not contagious, so no special precautions are necessary.

   4. Psoriasis is transmitted primarily by direct contact with the skin.

16. The nurse is teaching a class on the prevention of cancer. Which information should be included regarding how to reduce the risk of skin cancer?

   1. Avoid prolonged exposure to the sun.

   2. Shower immediately after being out-of-doors.

   3. Avoid strong perfumes, hand creams, and body lotions.

   4. After being in the woods or in tall grass, check for ticks.

17. The client mentions all of the following to the nurse. Which should the client be encouraged to report to the physician immediately?

   1. A small mole on the right thigh that has looked the same ever since the client can remember

   2. A pigmented area that is pink-red in color and has been present since birth

   3. Three small warts on the right hand that have been present for some time

4. A black and purple mole that is growing larger and has a funny shape

18. The nurse is caring for an adult who has herpes zoster. What medication is most likely to be administered to this client?

   1. Penicillin

   2. Acyclovir

   3. Tetracycline

   4. Benadryl

19. The nurse is caring for a person who has severe poison ivy. Soaks with Burrow's solution are ordered. What is the primary reason for using Burrow's solution soaks?

   1. To disinfect the wound

   2. To prevent pain from the lesions

   3. To stop the pruritus associated with the condition

   4. To help dry the oozing lesions

20. A woman who has herpes simplex I around the mouth and nose asks the nurse if she can give the sores to her husband. What should the nurse include when answering this client?

   1. Herpes simplex I is a fever blister and is not contagious.

   2. She should not kiss her husband or anyone else because it can be transmitted to susceptible persons.

   3. Fever blisters are seen only in persons who have fevers.

   4. The virus is transmitted through coughing and sneezing.

Answers and Rationales

1. (2) Persons with burns of the upper part of the body frequently have respiratory involvement. Airway problems increase the mortality rate.

2. (2) The very old and the very young are at the highest risk and have the highest mortality rate. The very old are half-dehydrated before the burn occurred and have greater difficulty with the fluid shifts. The very young have a greater percent of their body weight that is supposed to be water. They have more difficulty with the fluid shifts that occur following a burn.

3. (4) Clothing should be removed from persons with chemical burns so that they will not be further contaminated. A flame burn should be smothered. If necessary soak the area with water but do not remove the clothing until the person is in the emergency room. A person who suffered from smoke inhalation does not have an immediate need to remove clothing. A person who received an electrical burn does not have an immediate need to have his clothes removed.

4. (3) Burn victims are very prone to paralytic ileus. The client will remain NPO until bowel sounds have returned.

5. (2) Measurement of urine output is a high priority. Fluid replacement is based on output. The goal is to prevent the client from going into shock by maintaining a urine output of 50–100 ml/hr.

6. (1) Tetanus toxoid is given when the client has had prior tetanus inoculations. Hyperimmune tetanus globulin is given when the person has not had prior tetanus immunization. DTP is not given past the age of six years. Tetanus antitoxin is given when a person has not been immunized and considerable time has elapsed from the time of the injury. Tetanus antitoxin helps to fight a tetanus infection that is developing. Tetanus toxoid and immune globulin help to prevent tetanus infection from developing.

7. (3) Burn victims should be placed in isolation because they are very susceptible to infection.

8. (3) Fluid replacement is based on hourly measurement of urine output. The other observations are important and should be done, but they are not the highest priority.

9. (4) Curling's (stress) ulcers occur frequently in burn victims. Tagamet is a histamine blocker that reduces gastric acid and helps to prevent the development of ulcers.

10. (3) The water in the Hubbard tank is hypotonic, and sodium loss occurs through the open wounds. The bath may be painful and fatiguing for the patient. The primary reason is the physiologic problem of sodium loss.

11. (2) Silver nitrate dressings must always be kept wet or the silver nitrate is not effective. Silver nitrate does cause black discoloration, but this is incidental and not a major nursing consideration.

12. (4) Silver nitrate can cause depletion of potassium, sodium, and chloride; therefore, serum electrolytes are essential.

13. (1) The sterile, gloved hand is the preferred way to apply topical antimicrobials.

14. (2) Electric burns cause cardiac arrhythmias. Checking respiration and the pulse rate is highest priority. There is no need to remove clothing or roll a victim of an electric burn in a blanket because there are no flames. Dressing wounds is of lesser priority than assessing cardiac and respiratory functioning.

15. (3) Psoriasis is not contagious.

16. (1) Prolonged exposure to ultraviolet rays is the major risk factor for skin cancer. Showering immediately after being outdoors will not reduce the risk of skin cancer. Skin cancer is not caused by perfumes, hand creams, or body lotions. Checking for ticks after being outdoors is helpful in preventing Rocky Mountain Spotted Fever and Lyme Disease but will not prevent skin cancer.

17. (4) A mole that changes shape and has multiple colors and irregular borders is suggestive of malignant melanoma. This should be reported immediately. A mole that has not changed in appearance is of no particular concern. The pigmented area that has been present since birth sounds like a nevus or a birthmark and is not of particular concern. The client may want

to report the three small warts and have them removed for cosmetic reasons. They are not an immediate threat to health and do not need to be reported immediately.

18. (2) Acyclovir, an antiviral agent, is most likely to be given to the person who has herpes zoster, a infection with the chicken pox virus that affects the nerves. Penicillin and tetracycline are given for bacterial infections. Benadryl is an antihistamine and will help with itching. The person who has herpes zoster or shingles is likely to need pain medication, not antihistamines.

19. (4) Burrow's solution is used to help dry up oozing lesions such as poison ivy. It does not disinfect, prevent pain, or stop itching.

20. (2) Herpes simplex I can be transmitted through direct contact if the other person has any breaks in the skin or mucous membrane. She should not kiss anyone until after the lesions have disappeared. While blisters do sometimes occur when a person has a fever, a fever is not necessary for a herpes simplex infection. Herpes simplex virus is transmitted by direct contact, not coughing and sneezing.

Unit III

Maternity and Pediatrics

UNIT OUTLINE

Chapter 12

The Female Reproductive System, Maternity, and Newborns

Sample Questions

1. A 45-year-old woman has been having menorrhagia and metrorrhagia for several months. She is also feeling very tired and run down. Which is the most likely explanation for her fatigue?

   1. Hormonal changes related to menopause
   2. Psychological exhaustion produced by continuous worry about her illness
   3. Interference with digestion due to pressure on the small bowel
   4. Decreased oxygen-carrying capacity of the blood due to chronic loss of iron stores

2. A 45-year-old woman was found to have several large fibroid tumors. She is to have an abdominal panhysterectomy. She asks what a panhysterectomy includes. The nurse knows that a panhysterectomy consists of the removal of:

   1. Uterine fundus and body
   2. Uterine fundus and body and uterine cervix
   3. Uterine fundus and body, uterine cervix, fallopian tubes, and ovaries
   4. Uterine fundus and body, uterine cervix, fallopian tubes, ovaries, and vagina

3. The nurse is caring for a woman who had a hysterectomy. Which vascular complication should the nurse be especially alert for because of the location of the surgery?

   1. Thrombophlebitis
   2. Varicose veins
   3. Cerebral embolism
   4. Aortic aneurysm

4. The nurse is caring for an adult woman who had a vaginal hysterectomy today. The client is now returned to the nursing care unit following an uneventful stay in the post-anesthesia care unit. What is the priority nursing action for this client?

   1. Offer her the bedpan.
   2. Encourage coughing and deep breathing.
   3. Immediately administer pain medication.
   4. Assess chest tubes for patency.

5. A young woman has been having lower abdominal pain and amenorrhea. She is diagnosed as having an ovarian cyst. She asks the nurse what the usual treatment is for an ovarian cyst. What is the best response for the nurse to make?

   1. "Most women with your condition are placed on estrogen therapy for 6 to 12 months until the symptoms disappear."
   2. "The most effective treatment for ovarian cysts is to shrink the cyst with radiation therapy."
   3. "Ovarian cysts are usually surgically removed."
   4. "Steroid therapy is often given. The cyst usually resolves in three months."

6. A 39-year-old woman is seen in the gynecology clinic and asks the nurse about menopause. What is the best explanation for the nurse to give her?

   1. "It usually occurs about the age of 40. You can expect severe hot flashes."
   2. "It usually occurs after the age of 45 and frequently marks the end of a woman's sex life."
   3. "You can expect to have symptoms for about three years while your body adjusts to additional hormones."
   4. "No more ovarian hormones are produced, so you will stop menstruating."

7. A 42-year-old woman sees her physician because of painless spotting between periods that is worse after intercourse. A pap smear is done. The results come back as Stage III. The client is undergoing further testing and treatment. She asks the nurse what a Stage III pap smear means. The nurse's response is based on the knowledge that a Stage III pap smear indicates that

   1. Only normal cells are present.
   2. Atypical cells are present.
   3. Cells suggestive but not diagnostic of malignancy are present.
   4. Many malignant cells are present.

8. A woman is to have internal radiation as part of her treatment for cancer of the cervix. In teaching her about the pre-operative preparation for this procedure, the nurse should include which information?

   1. A high-residue diet will be ordered.
   2. An indwelling catheter will be inserted.
   3. A nasogastric tube will be inserted.
   4. Several units of blood will be ready for transfusion if needed.

9. The nurse is caring for a woman after insertion of radium rods for treatment of cancer of the cervix. The nurse positions her in a supine position with legs extended for which reason?

   1. To keep the rods in the correct position
   2. To prevent the urinary bladder from becoming over-distended
   3. To reduce pressure on the pelvic and back areas
   4. To limit the amount of radiation exposure

10. The nurse is caring for a woman after the insertion of radium rods for treatment of cancer of the cervix. Which discomfort

should the nurse anticipate that the client may have while the rods are in place?

1. Headache
2. Urinary retention
3. Constipation
4. Uterine cramps

11. The nurse is caring for a woman the day after the insertion of radium rods for treatment of cancer of the cervix. The woman calls the nurse and says, "There is something between my legs. It fell out of me." What is the most appropriate initial action for the nurse to take?

1. Call the radiation safety officer.
2. Put on rubber gloves and put the radiation rod in the bathroom until help arrives.
3. Using long forceps, place the radium needle in a lead-lined container.
4. Calmly reinsert the rod in the vagina.

12. A 14-year-old female comes to the clinic for contraceptive advice. She says she wants to take the pill. Vital signs are within normal limits. What question is it most important for the nurse to ask her?

1. How much exercise do you get each day?
2. What do you usually eat each day?
3. How many cigarettes do you smoke each day?
4. Are you under stress?

13. A young woman asks the nurse if oral contraceptives have any side effects. What is the best response for the nurse to make?

1. "Nausea, fluid retention, and weight gain."
2. "Why do you ask? Look at the benefits."
3. "Are you concerned about something?"

4. "Increased libido, decreased breast size, and diarrhea."

14. A client asks the nurse the difference between an IUD (intrauterine device) and the diaphragm. The nurse's response should be based on which information?

1. The diaphragm is inserted into the uterine cavity, and the IUD covers the cervix.
2. The IUD is 97% effective, and the diaphragm is 50% effective.
3. The IUD is placed into the uterine cavity by the doctor, and the diaphragm is placed into the vagina each time by the user.
4. The IUD must be used with contraceptive jelly, and the diaphragm does not require contraceptive jelly.

15. A young woman tells the nurse that her boyfriend used a "rubber" once. What is the most important information about condoms for the nurse to provide the client?

1. Always use Vaseline as a lubricant.
2. Apply the condom to the penis right before ejaculation.
3. You don't need a medical prescription.
4. It must be applied before any penile-vaginal contact.

16. A woman is to have a routine gynecological examination tomorrow. What instructions should the nurse give this client?

1. "Bring a urine sample with you."
2 "Be sure to drink plenty of fluids in the morning before you come so that your bladder will be full."
3. "Be sure not to douche today or tomorrow."
4. "Don't eat breakfast. You will be able to eat right after the exam."

17. A 46-year-old woman visits her gynecologist because she has been spotting. She is to be evaluated for carcinoma of the cervix. If she has cancer of the cervix, she is most likely to report that vaginal spotting occurred at what time?

    1. On arising
    2. While sitting
    3. After intercourse
    4. On stair climbing

18. The nurse is discussing self breast examination with a group of women in a clinic. One woman asks, "When should I do this examination?" What is the best response for the nurse?

    1. "You should perform self breast examination early in the morning for most accurate results."
    2. "Self breast examination should be done a few days after your period every month."
    3. "Self breast examination should be done by women after the age of 40 on the first of every month."
    4. "Self breast examination is best done just before you expect your menstrual period."

19. The physician prescribes clomiphene (Clomid) for a woman who has been having difficulty getting pregnant. When discussing this drug with the woman, the nurse should know that which of the following is known to be a side effect of clomiphene?

    1. Infertility
    2. Multiple births
    3. Vaginal bleeding
    4. Painful intercourse

20. A newly married couple asks the nurse which method of contraception is the best and the one that they should use. Which response is most helpful to the couple?

    1. "The pill is the best because it is 100% effective with few side effects."
    2. "The best method is the one that you both agree upon and will use consistently."
    3. "The condom is the best because it prevents diseases as well as pregnancy."
    4. "No method is completely effective; you should practice abstinence until you are ready to have children."

21. A woman is being treated for trichomonas vaginalis with metronidazole (Flagyl). Which statement the woman makes indicates a need for further teaching?

    1. "My husband is also taking the medication."
    2. "I will take Flagyl with meals."
    3. "The doctor said I might get a metallic taste in my mouth while I am taking Flagyl."
    4. "I will drink only one glass of wine per meal while I am taking Flagyl."

22. A client who is being treated for syphilis says to the nurse, "Why does the doctor want to know who I have had sex with?" What should the nurse include when responding to this question?

    1. It really is not any of the physician's concern.
    2. The physician wants to help her make better decisions about her lifestyle.
    3. Reporting of sexual contacts is mandatory so that the contacts can receive testing and treatment.
    4. Studies need to be done on sexual activities to learn how to reduce the spread of the disease.

23. During the early period following a right modified radical mastectomy, which nursing

action would be appropriate to include in the client's plan of care?

1. Position the patient in the right lateral position.
2. Encourage a high fluid intake.
3. Ambulate as soon as sensation and motion have returned.
4. Elevate the right arm on pillows.

24. The nurse is caring for a client who has had a right modified radical mastectomy this morning. Which exercise should the nurse encourage the client to perform this evening?

1. Hair combing exercises with the right arm
2. Wall climbing exercises with the right arm
3. Movement of the fingers and wrists of the right arm
4. Exercises of the left arm only

25. The client is being discharged following a left simple mastectomy. Which statement the client makes indicates an understanding of discharge teaching?

1. "I won't let anyone take blood pressures on my left arm."
2. "I understand that I should not have sexual relations for at least three months."
3. "I won't move my arm any more than necessary."
4. "I will not lift my arm above my head for the next two weeks."

26. A 21-year-old woman thinks she may be pregnant. She goes to her physician and tells the nurse that the drugstore test was positive for pregnancy. She asks the nurse if the test is reliable. What is the best response for the nurse to make?

1. "The tests are quite reliable. In order to be sure you are pregnant, I need to get some more information from you."
2. "The tests are less reliable than the one the doctor does. We will have to repeat it."
3. "Those kits are not very reliable. Your doctor should make the diagnosis."
4. "They are very reliable. You can be sure you are pregnant."

27. The nurse is assessing a woman who thinks she may be pregnant. Which information from the client is most significant in confirming the diagnosis of pregnancy?

1. She is experiencing nausea before bedtime and after meals.
2. The client says she has gained six pounds and her slacks are tight.
3. She has noticed it is difficult to sleep on her "stomach" because her breasts are tender.
4. The client has a history of regular menstrual periods since age 13, and she has missed her second period.

28. After her examination by the physician, the antepartal client tells the nurse the doctor said she had positive Chadwick's and Goodell's signs. She asks the nurse what this means. What is the best response for the nurse to make?

1. "Chadwick's sign is a dark blue coloring of the vagina and cervix. Goodell's sign is softening of the cervix of the uterus."
2. "These help to confirm pregnancy. They refer to color changes and changes in the uterus caused by increased hormones of pregnancy."
3. "Those are medical terms. You don't need to be concerned about them."
4. "It refers to changes that occasionally happen in pregnancy but are unlikely to cause problems."

29. An antepartal client asks when her baby is due. Her last menstrual period was August 28. Using Naegele's rule, calculate the EDC (estimated date of confinement).

    1. May 21
    2. May 28
    3. June 4
    4. June 28

30. In establishing a teaching plan for a client who is in the first trimester of pregnancy, the nurse identifies a long list of topics to discuss. Which is most appropriate for the first visit?

    1. Preparation for labor and delivery
    2. Asking the woman what questions and concerns she has about parenting
    3. Nutrition and activity during pregnancy
    4. Dealing with heartburn and abdominal discomfort

31. When a woman in early pregnancy is leaving the clinic, she blushes and asks the nurse if it is true that sex during pregnancy is bad for the baby. What is the best response for the nurse to make?

    1. "The baby is protected by his sac. Sex is perfectly alright."
    2. "It is unlikely to harm the baby. What you do with your personal life is your concern."
    3. "In a normal pregnancy, intercourse will not harm the baby. However, many women experience a change in desire. How are you feeling?"
    4. "Intercourse during pregnancy is usually alright, but you need to ask the doctor if it is acceptable for you."

32. The doctor told a pregnant woman to eat a well-balanced diet and increase her iron intake. She says, "I hate liver. How can I increase my iron?" What is the best response for the nurse to make?

    1. "Although liver is a good source of iron, beets, poultry, and milk are also good sources."
    2. "Many people dislike liver. Red meats, dark green vegetables, and dried fruits are also good sources of iron."
    3. "You should eat liver as it is the best source of iron. There are lots of ways to disguise the taste."
    4. "You can eat almost anything you like because your prenatal vitamins have all the vitamins and minerals needed for a healthy pregnancy."

33. The nurse is teaching a prenatal class. A woman in the class who is eight months pregnant asks why her feet swell. The nurse includes which of the following information in the answer?

    1. Swollen feet during pregnancy can indicate a serious problem.
    2. The enlarging baby reduces venous return, causing retention of fluid in the feet and ankles.
    3. Swelling of the feet during pregnancy is usually related to pregnancy-induced hypertension.
    4. Swelling of the feet during pregnancy is due to the increased blood volume and will disappear after delivery.

34. A woman who is at about six weeks gestation asks if she can listen to the baby's heart beat today. What should be included in the nurse's reply?

    1. The heart is not beating at six weeks.
    2. The heart is formed and beating but is too weak to be heard with a stethoscope.
    3. The heart beat can be heard with an electronic fetoscope.
    4. The heart does not start beating until 20 weeks gestation.

35. A woman who is in early pregnancy asks the nurse what to do about her "morning sickness." What should the nurse include in the reply?

1. Eating a heavy bedtime snack containing fat helps to keep nausea from developing in the morning.
2. Eating dry crackers before getting out of bed may help.
3. Drinking liquids before getting up in the morning helps relieve nausea.
4. The doctor can prescribe an antiemetic if she has had three or more vomiting episodes.

36. A woman who is 38 weeks gestation tells the nurse that she sometimes gets dizzy when she lies down. Which information is it important for the nurse to give the client?

1. This is a sign of a serious complication and should be reported to the physician whenever it occurs.
2. Try to sleep in an upright position on your back to prevent the dizziness.
3. Try lying on your left side rather than on your back.
4. Sleeping on your back with several pillows should help.

37. The nurse asks the newly pregnant woman if she has a cat for which of the following reasons?

1. Cats may suffocate new babies and should not be in the home when a baby arrives.
2. Cat feces may cause toxoplasmosis, which can lead to blindness, brain defects, and stillbirth.
3. If the mother gets scratched by a cat, the baby may develop heart defects.
4. Cats are jealous of babies and may try to kill them during infancy.

38. The nurse is caring for a woman who is 30 weeks gestation and has gained 17 pounds during the pregnancy, has a blood pressure of 110/70, and she states that she feels warmer than everyone around her. Which interpretation of these findings is most correct?

1. All of these findings are normal.
2. Her weight gain is excessive for this point in pregnancy.
3. The blood pressure is abnormal.
4. She should be evaluated for a serious infection, because pregnant women are usually cooler than other people.

39. What should the nurse do to assess for a positive sign of pregnancy?

1. Perform a pregnancy test on the woman's urine.
2. Auscultate for fetal heart sounds.
3. Ask the woman when she had her last menstrual period.
4. Ask the woman if her breasts are tender.

40. An oxytocin challenge test is ordered for a woman who is 42 weeks pregnant. What should the nurse plan for in the care of this client?

1. Place her in the supine position during the test.
2. Keep her NPO before the test.
3. Have her empty her bladder before the test.
4. Prepare the client for the insertion of internal monitors.

41. A woman comes to the doctor's office for her routine checkup. She is 34 weeks gestation. The nurse notes all of the following. Which would be of greatest concern to the nurse?

1. Weight gain of two pounds in two weeks
2. Small amount of dependent edema
3. Fetal heart rate of 155/minute
4. Blood pressure of 150/94

42. A pregnant woman is admitted to the hospital. Her initial admitting vital signs are blood pressure 160/94; pulse 88; respirations 24; and temperature 98°F. She complains of epigastric pain and headache. What should the nurse do initially?

1. Insert an indwelling catheter.
2. Give Maalox 30 cc now.
3. Contact the doctor stat with findings.
4. Supportive care for impending convulsion

43. Magnesium sulfate is ordered for a client who is hospitalized for PIH. What effects would the nurse expect to see as a result of this medication?

1. Central nervous system depression
2. Decreased gastric acidity
3. Onset of contractions
4. Decrease in number of bowel movements

44. A client with PIH asks the nurse, "When will I get over this?" What is the best response for the nurse to make?

1. "Your disease can be controlled with medication."
2. "After your baby is born."
3. "After delivery, you will need further testing."
4. "You could have this condition for years."

45. A 40-year-old who is 28 weeks gestation comes to the emergency room with painless, bright-red bleeding of 1½ hours duration. What condition does the nurse suspect this client has?

1. Abruptio placenta
2. Placenta previa
3. Hydatidiform mole
4. Prolapsed cord

46. A woman who is 28 weeks gestation comes to the emergency room with painless, bright-red bleeding of 1½ hours duration. Which of the following would the nurse expect during assessment of this woman?

1. Alterations in fetal heart rate
2. Board-like uterus
3. Severe abdominal pain
4. Elevated temperature

47. A woman is admitted with suspected placenta previa. What test will be done to confirm the diagnosis?

1. Internal exam
2. Non-stress test
3. Oxytocin challenge test
4. Ultrasound

48. A pregnant 16-year-old asks the nurse if she should have an abortion. How should the nurse respond initially?

1. "You should ask your parents for advice."
2. "Abortion is the deliberate killing of a human being."
3. "An abortion would let you finish growing up before you have children."
4. "What are your feelings about abortion?"

49. A 25-year-old is four months pregnant. She had rheumatic fever at age 15 and developed a systolic murmur. She reports exertional dyspnea. What instruction should the nurse give her?

1. "Try to keep as active as possible, but eliminate any activity that you find tiring."
2. "Carry on all your usual activities, but learn to work at a slower pace."
3. "Avoid heavy housework, shopping, stair climbing, and all unnecessary physical effort."
4. "Get someone to do your housework and stay in bed or in a wheelchair."

50. A pregnant woman comes for her six-month checkup and mentions to the nurse that she is gaining so much weight that even her shoes and rings are getting tight. What should the nurse plan to include in her care?

1. Teaching about the food pyramid and the importance of a well-balanced diet

2. Further assessment of her weight, blood pressure, and urine

3. Encouraging the use of a comfortable walking shoe with a medium heel

4. Reassurance that weight gain is normal as long as it does not exceed 25 pounds

51. A 23-year-old woman, G1 P0, is admitted to the labor room with contractions every 5 minutes lasting 45 seconds. Upon vaginal exam, she is noted to be completely effaced and 5 cm. dilated. Station is 0. She asks the nurse for pain medication. What is the best response for the nurse to make?

1. "I'll ask your doctor for medication."

2. "Can you hold out for a few more minutes? It's too soon for you to have medication."

3. "Pain medication will hurt your baby. We would rather not give you any unless absolutely necessary."

4. "Can your husband help you with your breathing techniques?"

52. After several hours of active labor, a woman says to the nurse, "I have to push. I have to push." What is the best initial response for the nurse to make?

1. "Pull your knees up to your chest and hold on to them. Take a deep breath and push down as though you are having a bowel movement."

2. "Let me have the RN examine you before you start to push."

3. "That means the baby is coming. I'll take you into the delivery room now."

4. "Women often feel that way during labor. Turn on your left side and you will be more comfortable."

53. A laboring woman is to be transferred to the delivery room. The nurse is positioning her on the table when she has a very strong contraction and starts to bear down. What should the nurse tell her to do?

1. Pant

2. Bear down strongly

3. Put her legs up in the stirrups

4. Ignore the contraction

54. A 32-year-old, G2 P1 is admitted to the labor room. Her previous delivery was a normal, spontaneous vaginal delivery without complications. She has been having contractions for four hours at home. The registered nurse examines her and determines that she is 4 cm. dilated and 70% effaced. The fetus is in the breech position. She calls for the nurse saying, "My water just broke!" What should the practical nurse do initially?

1. Notify the physician.

2. Do a vaginal exam.

3. Check the fetal heart rate.

4. Prepare for delivery.

55. The fetus is in the breech position. Inspection of the amniotic fluid after the membranes rupture shows a greenish-black cast to the fluid. What is the best interpretation of this finding?

1. The baby is in acute distress.

2. The fluid is contaminated with feces from the mother.

3. The mother has diabetes mellitus.

4. It may be normal since the baby is presenting breech.

56. A woman in labor does not continue to dilate. The physician decides to perform a cesarean section. A healthy 7 lb, 12 oz baby boy is delivered. What is the most essential nursing intervention in the immediate postpartum period?

   1. Check the fundus for firmness.

   2. Assess the episiotomy for bleeding.

   3. Assist the woman with accepting the necessity of having had a c-section.

   4. Encourage fluid intake.

57. A woman, G2 P2, who has just had an unexpected cesarean delivery asks the nurse if having a cesarean means that she cannot have any more children. What is the best response for the nurse to give this mother?

   1. "Most women are able to have another child after having had a cesarean delivery."

   2. "Since you have two healthy children, it would be better not to attempt another delivery."

   3. "Is it important for you to have more children?"

   4. "That is a question you will have to discuss with your physician."

58. A 26-year-old, gravida 3, para 0, in early labor is admitted to labor and delivery. She is not sure if her membranes have ruptured. She has had some leakage of fluid. How should the nurse begin the assessment?

   1. "Tell me about your other labor experiences."

   2. "How old are your other children?"

   3. "Did you bring an example of the fluid that was leaking with you?"

   4. "Describe your contractions to me."

59. A woman, 38 weeks pregnant, arrives in the labor and delivery suite and tells the nurse that she thinks her membranes have ruptured. The nurse uses phenaphthazine (Nitrazine) paper to test the leaking fluid. The nurse expects the Nitrazine paper to turn which color if amniotic fluid is present?

   1. Red

   2. Orange

   3. Blue

   4. Purple

60. A 29-year-old gravida 1, para 0 woman is admitted to labor and delivery. She is three centimeters dilated, 80% effaced, and head at 0 station. She and her husband have been to prepared childbirth classes and are eager to give birth naturally. During her first contraction in the hospital, which lasts 30 seconds, the nurse observes the client using rapid pant-blow breathing. What is the most appropriate response for the nurse to make at this time?

   1. "Don't pant. It's too early in labor for panting."

   2. "Continue using pant-blow breathing until the RN checks to see if you are fully dilated."

   3. "Good. You are using your breathing from class. Keep it up."

   4. "What kinds of breathing techniques did you learn in childbirth class?"

61. The physician is performing an amniotomy on a woman in labor. What is the most important nursing action during this procedure?

   1. Assist the physician.

   2. Keep the mother informed.

   3. Monitor fetal heart tones.

   4. Encourage slow chest breathing.

62. The nurse is caring for a woman in labor who is having contractions every 5–7 minutes that last 45–50 seconds. Her husband asks if this is transition because his

wife is getting restless and irritable and feels pressure. What is the best response for the nurse to make?

1. "Transition is still a long way off. Don't you remember this from your classes?"
2. "Her contractions are not typical of transition, but I'll have the RN check her."
3. "The contractions are typical of transition. You are very observant."
4. "It's impossible to tell where she is without doing an exam."

63. As labor progresses, a client becomes increasingly irritable with her husband, complaining of lower back pain and fatigue. What is the most appropriate response for the nurse to make?

1. Have the client turn on her side and give her a back rub.
2. Ask the client if she would like the doctor to give her something for the discomfort.
3. Reassure the husband that irritability is normal now and teach him to apply pressure to his wife's lower back.
4. Encourage the client to try and get some rest and ask her husband if he would like to take a coffee break.

64. An epidural block is ordered for a woman in labor. Which nursing action is essential because the client has epidural anesthesia?

1. Monitoring the uterus for uterine tetany
2. Giving oxytocin to counteract the effect of the epidural in slowing contractions
3. Having the woman lie flat in bed to avoid post-anesthesia headache
4. Monitoring blood pressure for possible hypotension

65. The nurse is positioning a laboring woman who has not reached the transition phase. The nurse should avoid placing her in the supine position because the supine position has which effect?

1. It increases gravitational forces and prolongs labor.
2. It causes decreased perfusion of the placenta.
3. It may impede free movement of the symphysis pubis.
4. It frequently leads to transient episodes of hypertension.

66. A woman in labor is experiencing very strong contractions every 2–3 minutes, lasting 60–75 seconds. She complains of a severe backache and is irritable. The best interpretation of these data is that the woman is in which stage/phase of labor?

1. Early first stage of labor
2. Transition phase of labor
3. Late second stage of labor
4. Early third stage of labor

67. A woman who is completely dilated is pushing with contractions. After 30 minutes of pushing, the baby is still at 0 station. What is the most appropriate nursing action at this time?

1. Assess for a full bladder.
2. Prepare for a cesarean delivery.
3. Monitor fetal heart tones.
4. Turn the mother to her left side.

68. Which nursing action has the highest priority for a client in the second stage of labor?

1. Help the mother push effectively.
2. Prepare the mother to breastfeed on the delivery table.
3. Check the fetal position.
4. Administer medication for pain.

69. A woman, gravida 5 para 4, is unable to get to the hospital since labor has progressed very rapidly. The nurse, who lives upstairs, comes down to assist her with the emergency home delivery. The nurse examines the woman and assesses that the perineum is bulging. What is the priority nursing measure at this time?

    1. Encourage the woman to push during the contraction.
    2. Place a clean sheet under the perineal area.
    3. Accurately time the contractions.
    4. Contact the physician by phone for instructions.

70. During an emergency home delivery, the head is beginning to crown. What is the most appropriate action for the nurse to take at this time?

    1. Instruct the mother to push down vigorously.
    2. Press down on the fundus to expel the baby.
    3. Apply gentle perineal pressure to prevent rapid expulsion of the head.
    4. Direct the mother to take prolonged deep breaths to improve fetal oxygenation.

71. What is the most common complication associated with too rapid delivery in precipitate labor?

    1. Pitting edema of the baby's scalp
    2. Dural or subdural tears in fetal brain tissue
    3. Premature separation of the placenta
    4. Prolonged retention of the placenta

72. The nurse has just completed emergency delivery of a term infant. What is the priority nursing concern at this time?

    1. Controlling hemorrhage in the mother

    2. Removing the afterbirth
    3. Keeping the infant warm
    4. Cutting the umbilical cord

73. What should the nurse do to stimulate the separation of the placenta after emergency home delivery of a baby?

    1. Ask the mother to push down vigorously.
    2. Push the fundus down vigorously.
    3. Encourage the baby to breastfeed.
    4. Place gentle tension on the umbilical cord.

74. A woman delivered a baby in the car on the way to the hospital. In the emergency room, the physician examined the mother. What is the priority action for the nurse at this time?

    1. Gently tug on the cord and massage the uterus to see if the placenta is ready to be delivered.
    2. Clamp and cut the cord with sterile scissors.
    3. Note and record the Apgar score.
    4. Clear the mucus from the baby's mouth and nose.

75. A woman who is giving birth at home wonders if her baby will need drops in the eyes because she knows that neither she nor her husband have gonorrhea. The best answer for the nurse to give should include which of the following?

    1. It is desirable for the baby to receive the eye drops, but it is not essential.
    2. If you do not want your baby to have the eye drops, you must sign a waiver stating that you refuse them.
    3. The baby needs the drops but does not have to receive them for up to two hours after birth.
    4. The drops are needed to prevent the eye condition known as retrolental fibroplasia.

76. The nurse is caring for a laboring woman who has a history of rheumatic heart disease. How should the nurse position her during labor?

    1. Supine
    2. Semirecumbent
    3. Side-lying
    4. Sitting

77. The nurse is caring for a laboring woman who has a history of rheumatic heart disease. Which instruction should the nurse give to her during the second stage of labor?

    1. Avoid prolonged bearing down.
    2. Breathe shallowly and rapidly.
    3. Sit on the side of the bed.
    4. Sleep between contractions.

78. A woman spontaneously delivers a baby girl who is immediately handed to the nurse. Which action is of highest priority for the nurse?

    1. Do an Apgar assessment.
    2. Check neonatal heart rate.
    3. Apply identification bracelets.
    4. Clean the nasopharynx.

79. At one minute after birth, an infant is crying, has a heart rate of 140, has acrocyanosis, resists the suction catheter, and keeps his arms extended and his legs flexed. What is the Apgar score?

    1. 4
    2. 6
    3. 8
    4. 10

80. The delivery room nurse is explaining Apgar scoring to new parents. Which information pertaining to the purpose of a five-minute Apgar score should be included in the explanation?

    1. It evaluates the effectiveness of the labor and delivery.
    2. It measures the adequacy of transition to extrauterine life.
    3. It assesses the possibility of respiratory distress syndrome.
    4. It gives an estimate of the gestational age of the infant.

81. The nurse is caring for a woman who has had a spinal anesthetic. Which of the following would be most likely to occur after spinal anesthesia?

    1. The client states that she is dizzy and light-headed.
    2. The temperature is 101°F.
    3. The nurse observes the client shivering.
    4. The client develops a red, itchy rash on her back and chest.

82. What action is essential for the nurse during the fourth stage of labor?

    1. Firmly massage the fundus every 15 minutes.
    2. Take the vital signs q 1 h.
    3. Turn the client on her side during a lochia check.
    4. Assist the client to the bathroom to void.

83. Which of the following is the most important nursing assessment during the fourth stage of labor?

    1. Bonding behaviors
    2. Distention of the bladder
    3. Ability to relax
    4. Knowledge of newborn behavior

84. A woman who is 32 weeks gestation is admitted with contractions every four minutes. Ritodrine is given for which of the following purposes?

    1. To suppress uterine activity
    2. To make her more comfortable
    3. To enhance contractions
    4. To increase fetal oxygenation

85. The nursing care plan for a woman who has placenta abruptio should include careful assessment for signs and symptoms of:

    1. Jaundice
    2. Hypovolemic shock
    3. Impending convulsions
    4. Hypertension

86. A woman who had a normal vaginal delivery two hours ago has just arrived on the postpartum floor. Vital signs are normal. When assessing her uterus, the nurse notes that it is boggy. What should be the nurse's initial intervention?

    1. Massage the uterus.
    2. Report to the charge nurse.
    3. Contact the doctor stat.
    4. Continue to assess it frequently.

87. The nurse is caring for a woman who had a normal vaginal delivery two hours ago and has just arrived on the postpartum floor. Two hours later her uterus is displaced to the right. What is the most likely explanation for this?

    1. A fibroid tumor
    2. A full bladder
    3. An increase in interstitial fluid
    4. Retained placental fragments

88. The day after delivery, a new mother asks why her milk is so creamy and yellow. What is the best response for the nurse to make?

    1. "I wouldn't worry about it."
    2. "This is normal. It will soon turn to real milk."
    3. "You're coming along fine."
    4. "You haven't gotten your milk in yet."

89. A new mother is in the first period of adjustment following birth called the taking-in phase. What type of maternal behavior would the nurse expect her to exhibit?

    1. Passivity and dependence
    2. Preoccupation with baby's needs
    3. Independence
    4. Resuming control of life

90. A new mother has decided not to breastfeed her baby. Which statement indicates the best understanding of the management of engorgement?

    1. "I will stand with my back to the shower."
    2. "I will take a sitz bath every day."
    3. "I will apply a warm compress to my breasts three times a day."
    4. "I will drink a lot of liquids for the next few days."

91. A new mother is about to be discharged from the hospital. Which statement made by a new mother indicates a need for more instruction?

    1. "I will use my old diaphragm for contraception."
    2. "I have an appointment for my six-week check up."
    3. "My mother will be helping me with the children for the next two weeks."
    4. "I plan to go back to my job as a secretary in six weeks."

92. A woman who delivered today by cesarean delivery asks the nurse, "How come my baby has such a round head? My other baby's head was not so round, and she was more red." What is the best response for the nurse to make?

1. "Each baby is different. It is not a good idea to compare your children."
2. "Were forceps used when your older child was delivered?"
3. "Babies born by cesarean have rounder heads because they do not go through the birth canal."
4. "A round head is a sign the baby is very intelligent. Your child should do very well in school."

93. A new mother is checking the list of supplies she will need at home for care of the newborn. She asks the nurse why she needs rubbing alcohol. What is the best response for the nurse to make?

1. "Rubbing alcohol is good for the baby's skin. You should apply it to his body three times a day."
2. "Apply the rubbing alcohol to the baby's circumcision to speed healing."
3. "Wipe his bottom off with alcohol after each bowel movement."
4. "Clean his cord stump with alcohol each time you change his diaper."

94. A woman is admitted to the postpartum unit two hours after delivery of a baby. What action is especially important because the membranes were ruptured for 28 hours before delivery?

1. Monitor her temperature every two hours.
2. Provide perineal care with zephiran every four hours.
3. Maintain a strict perineal pad count.

4. Have the mother take a sitz bath four times a day.

95. The nurse is caring for a woman who delivered a baby three hours ago. The woman pulls the emergency call light and says she is bleeding all over the bed. The nurse enters the room and sees the blood-soaked bed. What is the best initial action for the nurse to take?

1. Assess and massage the fundus if soft.
2. Take vital signs.
3. Place the client in sharp Trendelenburg position.
4. Notify the physician immediately.

96. Methergine 5 mg qid is ordered for a postpartum client. An hour after taking the drug, the woman complains of uterine cramping. What is the best explanation for the nurse to give her?

1. "This is an unfortunate side effect, but you need the medicine."
2. "The cramping is uncomfortable, but it is a sign that the drug is keeping your uterus contracted so you won't bleed too much."
3. "Since you are experiencing cramps, I'll ask the doctor to discontinue the drug."
4. "The cramping should decrease soon. If it does not, let me know. I'll see if the doctor will decrease the dosage."

97. The nurse is caring for a woman who had a postpartum hemorrhage. Which of the following facts about her delivery most likely contributed to her hemorrhage?

1. The baby weighed 10 lb 6 oz.
2. She received pitocin after delivery of the placenta.
3. She delivered 10 days after her due date.
4. Her second stage of labor lasted an hour.

98. A woman who has just delivered has chosen to bottle feed. What should the nurse teach her about breast care?

    1. "Take long warm showers, allowing the shower to hit your breasts."
    2. "Massage your breasts every three hours to increase circulation."
    3. "Wear a supportive bra, and do not handle your breasts."
    4. "Hold the baby away from your chest so he will not smell the breast milk."

99. The nurse is observing a new mother for good maternal infant attachment. Which observation would be a sign of inappropriate attachment?

    1. Calling the baby "little bit."
    2. Holding the baby in "en face" position.
    3. Telling the baby "You look just like your Daddy."
    4. Continually saying, "I'm too tired to hold the baby."

100. A woman who had a cesarean section tells the nurse, "I guess I flunked natural childbirth because I had to have a cesarean." This statement is most indicative of which phase of postpartum adjustment?

    1. Taking in
    2. Working through
    3. Taking hold
    4. Letting go

101. Six hours after delivery, the nurse notes that a woman's fundus is two finger breadths above the umbilicus and deviated to the right of the midline. What is the most likely cause of this finding?

    1. Retained placental fragments
    2. Bladder distention
    3. Normal involution
    4. Second degree uterine atony

102. Which area of health teaching will a new mother be most responsive to during the taking-in phase of the postpartum period?

    1. Family planning
    2. Newborn care
    3. Community support groups
    4. Perineal care

103. On the first day after a cesarean section, the client is ambulating. She is uncomfortable and asks the nurse, "Why am I being made to walk so soon after surgery?" What is the nurse's best response?

    1. "You can get to hold your baby more quickly if you walk around."
    2. "Early walking keeps the blood from pooling in your legs and prevents blood clots."
    3. "Walking early will prevent your wound from opening."
    4. "Early walking helps lower the incidence of wound infection."

104. A pregnant woman tells the nurse that she is planning to breastfeed because "You don't have to take contraceptives until you wean the baby." What is the best response for the nurse?

    1. "Lactation does suppress ovulation, so you are not likely to get pregnant."
    2. "You will not get pregnant until you start to menstruate again."
    3. "When a woman is breastfeeding, she may not menstruate although she may ovulate. It is best to use some type of birth control."
    4. "You will find that you won't be interested in resuming sexual activity until after you wean the baby."

105. A new mother who has been breastfeeding her infant for six weeks calls the nurse at the doctor's office and says her right nipple is

cracked and sore, she has a temperature, and feels as though she has the flu. How should the nurse respond to the woman?

1. "Try putting warm compresses over your right breast."

2. "Immediately stop nursing and apply cold compresses to your breasts."

3. "Come to see the physician. You may need medication to help."

4. "Reduce the time the baby nurses on your right breast, and call again if the breast is not better in two days."

106. At three hours of age, a term newborn seems jittery and has a weak and high-pitched cry and irregular respirations. The nurse suspects that the infant may have which of the following?

1. Hypoglycemia

2. Hypercalcemia

3. Hypervolemia

4. Hypothyroidism

107. The mother of a newborn is breastfeeding her infant on the delivery table. How can the nurse best assist her?

1. Touch the infant's cheek adjacent to the nipple to elicit the rooting reflex.

2. Leave the mother and baby alone and allow the infant to nurse as long as desired.

3. Position the infant to grasp the nipple so as to express milk.

4. Give the infant a bottle first to evaluate the baby's ability to suck.

108. Parents of a newborn note petechiae on the newborn's face and neck. The nurse should tell them that this is a result of which of the following?

1. Increased intravascular pressure during delivery

2. Decreased Vitamin K level in the newborn infant

3. A rash called erythema toxicum

4. Excessive superficial capillaries

109. A newborn has a total body response to noise or movement that is distressing to her parents. What should the nurse tell the parents about this response?

1. It is a reflexive response that indicates normal development.

2. It is a voluntary response that indicates insecurity in a new environment.

3. It is an automatic response that may indicate that the baby is hungry.

4. It is an involuntary response that will remain for the first year of life.

110. When changing her newborn infant, a mother notices a reddened area on the infant's buttocks. How should the nurse respond?

1. Have staff nurses instead of the mother change the infant.

2. Use both lotion and powder to protect the area.

3. Encourage the mother to cleanse and change the infant more frequently.

4. Notify the physician and request an order for a topical ointment.

111. A woman, 32 weeks gestation, delivers a 3-pound, 8-ounce baby boy two hours after arriving at the hospital. What is the baby at risk for because of his gestational age?

1. Mental retardation and seizures

2. Hypothermia and respiratory distress

3. Acrocyanosis and decreased lanugo

4. Patent ductus arteriosus and pneumonia

112. Orders for a premature infant are for nipple feedings or gavage. What assessment findings are necessary before nipple feedings are given?

1. The baby must have a respiratory rate of 20–30 and heart rate of 110–130.
2. The baby must be alert and rooting.
3. Sucking and gag reflexes must be present.
4. Weight and temperature must be stable.

113. The mother of a 3-pound preterm infant has expressed a desire to breastfeed her baby. Because of his prematurity, she expresses fear that she can't. What is the best response for the nurse to make?

1. "The baby won't be able to nurse for several weeks, but you can try at that time."
2. "Breast milk does not have enough calories for premature babies."
3. "You must be very disappointed that he is so small. Special formula is necessary. Perhaps you can nurse your next baby."
4. "Breast milk is very good for premature babies. Even if he is not strong enough to nurse now, we will help you pump your breasts and give him the milk."

114. The mother of a term newborn born two hours ago asks the nurse why the baby's hands and feet are blue. What information should the nurse include when responding?

1. Blue hands and feet can indicate possible heart defects.
2. This is normal in newborns for the first 24 hours.
3. This pattern of coloration is more common in infants who will eventually have darker skin color.
4. Once the baby's temperature is stabilized, the hands and feet will warm up and be less blue.

115. A newborn is thought to have toxoplasmosis. The nurse explains to the family that toxoplasmosis is most likely to have been transmitted to the infant in which manner?

1. Through a blood transfusion given to the mother
2. Through breast milk during breastfeeding
3. By contact with the maternal genitals during birth
4. It crosses the placenta during pregnancy.

116. A newborn infant is with his mother, who is a diabetic. He appeared pink and alert and his temperature was stable when he left the nursery 15 minutes ago. His mother calls the nurse and says, "Look at his legs." The nurse observes spontaneous jerky movements. What is the best INITIAL action for the nurse to take?

1. Tell his mother that this is normal behavior for a newborn.
2. Tell the mother to feed him his glucose water now.
3. Do a Dextrostix test on the infant.
4. Take the baby back to the nursery and observe him for other behaviors and neurologic symptoms.

117. The nurse is caring for a premature infant. Immediately after arrival in the nursery, which nursing action is essential?

1. Take the rectal temperature.
2. Examine for anomalies.
3. Check the airway for patency.
4. Cleanse the skin of vernix.

118. A baby boy was born at 2:45 A.M. after a 35-week gestation. He weighed 1,170 grams. Upon admission to the premature nursery, he had slight respiratory distress, nasal flaring, grunting, intercostal retractions,

and slight cyanosis. Apgar score at 1 minute was 4 and at 5 minutes was 6. Apical pulse 164, respirations 44, axillary temperature 96°F. What was the most likely cause of the baby's cyanosis?

1. Increased serum concentration of bilirubin
2. Inadequate oxygenation of arterial blood
3. Excessive number of red blood cells
4. Lack of subcutaneous fatty tissue

119. When assessing a newborn's need for oxygen, which should the nurse assess because it is the best indicator?

1. Respiratory rate
2. Skin color
3. Pulse rate
4. Arterial pO$_2$

120. On the evening of the second day after birth, the nurse notes that an infant appears icteric. What is the most likely cause?

1. Rupture of a great number of fragile red cells in a short period of time
2. Inflammatory obstruction of hepatic bile ducts and resorption of pigments
3. Extravasation of blood from ruptured capillaries into subcutaneous tissue
4. Faulty melanin metabolism due to absence of enzymes for normal protein synthesis

121. On the evening of the second day after birth, an infant was observed to be icteric, so he was exposed to blue light. What is the purpose of the blue light?

1. To stimulate increased formation of Vitamin K in the skin
2. To enhance pigment breakdown by increasing body temperature

3. To convert indirect bilirubin to a less toxic compound
4. To increase brain electrical activity by stimulating the optic nerve

122. A young woman delivered her first baby this morning. She asks the nurse why the top of the baby's head is so soft and doesn't seem to have any bone. What should the nurse include when responding to the mother?

1. This soft spot is called a fontanel and is normal; it makes delivery easier.
2. It is a condition that occurs in some babies and will disappear within a few days.
3. The physician is monitoring the infant for any problems which might occur with this common defect.
4. It is called caput succadaneum and is caused by bleeding under the scalp during birth.

123. Which finding, if present, would suggest to the nurse that the infant was not at term when born?

1. The scrotum has rugae.
2. Testicles are not descended.
3. Scanty vernix
4. Sparse lanugo

124. The nurse is preparing a three-day-old infant for discharge from the hospital. When checking the record for completeness, the nurse checks to see that the infant has had which of the following?

1. DTP and polio immunizations
2. MMR immunization and tuberculin test
3. Pneumococcal vaccine and HIV test
4. Hepatitis B vaccine and PKU test

125. The physician has told the parents that their child probably has phenylketonuria. The parents ask the nurse what special needs the child will have. What should the nurse include in the response?

1. The baby will most likely not develop normally for longer than six months and will die in a few years.
2. The baby will have a special formula and cannot eat protein foods during childhood.
3. Special feeding techniques are necessary until the child has surgery.
4. The baby will not be able to void normally and will need to be catheterized frequently.

Answers and Rationales

1. (4) Menorrhagia means heavy menstrual flow, and metrorrhagia means bleeding between periods. Such increased loss of blood results in fatigue due to the chronic loss of blood (iron stores). Hormonal changes may cause fatigue, but the data in this question do not support that reason. Excessive worry can cause fatigue, but the data in this question do not support that. There is no data to support interference with digestion due to pressure on the small bowel. If the woman has fibroid tumors, there may be pressure on the bowel-but that would not cause interference with digestion and fatigue.

2. (3) A panhysterectomy consists of the removal of the entire uterus, including the cervix and the tubes and ovaries. The vagina is left intact.

3. (1) Persons who have had surgery in the pelvic area are apt to develop thrombophlebitis. Varicose veins are a complication of pregnancy.

4. (2) Coughing and deep-breathing are very important in the immediate post-operative period. She will have an indwelling catheter after a vaginal hysterectomy. Pain medication is given for pain. There is no indication of pain. She will not have chest tubes after pelvic surgery.

5. (3) Large ovarian cysts are usually surgically removed. Women who have small ovarian cysts may be given birth control pills (progesterone) to suppress ovarian activity and resolve the cyst. Radiation therapy, estrogen, and steroids are not appropriate for persons with ovarian cysts.

6. (4) Menopause is the cessation of production of ovarian hormones. Amenorrhea will occur. Not all women have hot flashes. It is not the end of a woman's sex life. It is the end of her capacity to reproduce. It occurs when a woman is in her 40s or 50s.

7. (3) Stage III is characterized by cells suggestive but not diagnostic of malignancy. Stage I contains normal cells. Stage II contains atypical cells. Stage IV contains malignant cells.

8. (2) During the time the radium rods are in place, the client should have as little movement as possible to prevent dislodgment of the radium. She will have an indwelling catheter in place so her bladder will not become full and also to prevent damage to the bladder from the radiation. She will have an enema before the procedure and a low-residue or clear liquid diet before surgery and while the rods are in place. There is no need for a nasogastric tube or blood transfusions.

9. (1) The client is kept flat to prevent the rods from becoming dislodged. She will have an indwelling catheter in place. Positioning does not reduce radiation exposure.

10. (4) Uterine cramping occurs frequently. She will be on a clear liquid or low-residue diet so that she is not likely to be constipated. She will have a catheter in place so she will not have urinary retention.

11. (3) There should always be long forceps and a lead-lined container readily available whenever a person has radium inserted. The

nurse should pick up the rod with the long forceps and immediately place it in a lead-lined container. The radiation safety officer should then be notified. Leaving the rod between the client's legs exposes her and others to unnecessary radiation. Rubber gloves offer no protection from radiation. The nurse does not reinsert the radium.

12. (3) Cigarette smoking is a contraindication for the use of the pill. There is a higher incidence of thromboembolic problems when a person smokes.

13. (1) These are side effects of the pill. Answer 2 and answer 3 do not answer the question asked. Answer 4 is not correct.

14. (3) The IUD must be inserted into the uterus by the physician. The woman inserts the diaphragm before each act of intercourse. Both types are very effective when used as directed. The diaphragm requires contraceptive jelly; the IUD does not.

15. (4) Pre-ejaculatory secretions may contain sperm. It must be applied before there is any penile-vaginal contact. Vaseline should never be used as a lubricant. Lubricants should always be water soluble, such as K-Y jelly or Surgilube. Answer 3 is a true statement but not the most important information to give the client.

16. (3) There is no special preparation for a gynecological exam. The patient should not douche, however. There is no need to bring a urine specimen. The client may be asked to give a specimen prior to the examination. Drinking plenty of fluids would be appropriate prior to a pelvic ultrasound examination. There is no need to fast before a gynecological exam.

17. (3) Post-coital (after intercourse) spotting is often seen with cancer of the cervix. The other responses are not correct.

18. (2) The best time to perform self breast examination is a few days after your period begins because the breasts are least tender at this time. It should be done every month. Answer 1 is incorrect. It does not matter what time of day the exam is performed. Self breast examination should be done monthly, starting right after puberty. The incidence of breast cancer does increase in age, but it can occur in teenagers. The breasts are most tender just before the period starts; this is the least desirable time to do a self breast examination.

19. (2) One of the major side effects of fertility drugs such as clomiphene, which increases ovulation, is multiple births. Clomiphene is used to treat infertility; it does not cause infertility. Clomiphene does not cause vaginal bleeding or painful intercourse.

20. (2) The best method for any couple is one they will use consistently. The only 100% effective method is abstinence, which is not a realistic choice for most couples. To be effective, contraception must be used consistently and correctly. Answer 1 is not correct. If the pill is not taken exactly as directed, pregnancies can and do occur. The pill has several side effects, including nausea, weight gain, and enlarged breasts. Answer 3 contains correct information in that the condom does help to prevent disease transmission. However, with a married couple this is not likely to be an issue. Answer 4 is an unrealistic answer for a married couple and therefore is not very helpful.

21. (4) Alcohol taken with Flagyl causes an Antabuse-like reaction, nausea, and vomiting. The client should drink no alcoholic beverages. The husband (partner) should also be treated, even if he has no symptoms, to prevent reinfection. Flagyl, unless it is extended release, should be taken with food to decrease GI side effects. People commonly get a metallic taste when taking Flagyl.

22. (3) Sexual contacts must be reported so that they can be contacted, tested, and treated to avoid the serious complications of untreated syphilis. Answer 1 is not correct. It is possible that there might be some truth to answer 2. However, the information regarding contacts

is usually obtained in a nonjudgmental manner for the reasons described. Answer 4 is not correct.

23. (4) The arm on the affected side should be elevated on pillows to help prevent the development of lymphedema. The client should not be positioned on the affected side. Once the client is awake following anesthesia, the head of the bed will be elevated. The client may have liquids following surgery, but there is no particular need to encourage a high fluid intake. The client will begin to ambulate fairly quickly. However, the client will not have had an epidural anesthetic for a mastectomy, so the return of sensation and motion is not an issue. A mastectomy is too high for an epidural. Epidurals are not given for surgery above the waist.

24. (3) The day of surgery, the client should be encouraged to move the fingers and wrists of the affected arm. Hair combing and wall climbing exercises will be performed later, not the day of surgery. The client should be encouraged to exercise the fingers and wrists of the affected extremity the day of surgery as well as exercising the unaffected arm.

25. (1) The person who has had a mastectomy should not have blood drawn or blood pressures taken on that arm. There is no reason why she should not have sexual relations for three months. As soon as she feels well enough, sexual relations can resume. She should use a position that does not put pressure on her left side. Answer 3 and answer 4 are incorrect. A woman who has had a mastectomy will need to perform arm exercises regularly. These will include lifting the arm above the head in exercises like hair combing and wall climbing.

26. (1) The tests are quite reliable. They are based on the presence of HCG (human chorionic gonadotropin), which is secreted during pregnancy. Physician tests use the same principle. The nurse should take a history to confirm the results of the tests. The physician will examine the woman to help confirm the test results.

27. (4) Amenorrhea in an otherwise healthy woman of childbearing age is strongly suggestive of pregnancy. Nausea, weight gain, and tender breasts are all presumptive signs but are not as significant as amenorrhea.

28. (2) This answer is most appropriate to give the client. Answer 1 is a true statement but uses vocabulary that is inappropriate for the client. These changes are normal changes and occur in most pregnancies. Answer 3 is a real put-down to the client. Answer 4 is not correct. These are normal findings that help to confirm the diagnosis of pregnancy.

29. (3) Add nine months or take away three months and then add seven days. August 28 minus three months is May 28. Adding seven days would make it May 35. Since there are only 31 days in May, the days are carried into June—making June 4 the EDC. Answer 1 subtracts seven days instead of adding seven days. Answer 2 does not add seven days. Answers 3 and 4 subtract only 2 months instead of 3 months and do not add seven days.

30. (3) Nutrition and activity are important concerns from the first trimester onward. Labor and delivery is a third trimester concern, and parenting is of most concern in either the third trimester or post delivery. Heartburn and abdominal discomfort do not usually occur until the third trimester.

31. (3) Intercourse is not harmful during a normal pregnancy. This response recognizes the changes in libido which may occur during pregnancy and allows for the expression of feelings. Answer 1 is factual information but answer 3 allows the woman to express her feelings. The questions says "she blushes." This may indicate that the woman has concerns about sex. Answer 2 gives factual information but does not allow the woman to express her concerns. Answer 4 again does

not give the woman a chance to discuss this with the nurse. The nurse should be able to answer this question.

32. (2) This answer recognizes that a dislike of liver is common and suggests good sources of iron. Answer 1 includes information that is not correct; milk contains no iron. Answer 3 has some correct information; liver is high in iron. It is also high in cholesterol. There are many other sources of iron. It is not necessary to eat liver to get iron in the diet. At one time, eating liver regularly was thought to be the best way to get iron. Answers 3 and 4 are not the best answers. Prenatal vitamins do contain iron. However, they should not be considered a substitute for a proper diet.

33. (2) The enlarging fetus presses on the veins returning fluid from the lower extremities, causing fluid retention. Swelling of the upper extremities or face may indicate pregnancy-induced hypertension. There is an increased blood volume during pregnancy, but this does not by itself cause swelling in the lower extremities.

34. (2) The heart chambers are formed and the' heart is beating by four weeks gestation. However, it can not be heard even with a fetoscope. Answer 1 is incorrect. The heart is beating by four weeks. Answer 3 is not correct. It cannot be heard at this time. Answer 4 is incorrect. The heart rate will be audible with a standard fetoscope by 20 weeks, but it has been beating since about four weeks.

35. (2) Eating dry carbohydrates in the morning before rising often helps. The woman should avoid fatty foods and those with strong odors. Drinking liquids in the morning usually makes morning sickness worse, not better. Antiemetics are not prescribed because of the possible teratogenic effect on the developing embryo.

36. (3) Dizziness when lying on the back suggests that she may have vena caval syndrome—pressure on the vena cava from the enlarged

uterus and fetus that decreases venous return and causes the blood pressure to drop. Lying on the left side usually reduces pressure on the vena cava and prevents the drop in blood pressure and dizziness. Sleeping in an upright position on her back will cause vena caval syndrome. Sleeping on the back with several pillows is similar to answer 2, which was incorrect.

37. (2) Cats may become infected with toxoplasmosis, which if ingested by the mother can cause toxoplasmosis and can lead to neurological lesions causing blindness, brain defects, and death. Parents should be alert for safety with any pet, but cats do not suffocate new babies or try to kill them. It is not being scratched by a cat that is the biggest danger during pregnancy; it is the possibility of developing toxoplasmosis from the feces. Raw meat can also carry toxoplasmosis.

38. (1) All of these findings are within normal limits. Weight gain during the first trimester is usually 3–5 pounds. After that, the normal weight gain is around 12 ounces (¾ of a pound) a week. Using these guidelines, her weight gain should be 16–18 lbs. Her blood pressure is well within normal limits, even though we are not given a baseline. Pregnant women have a high metabolic rate and usually feel warmer than everyone else.

39. (2) Fetal heart sounds, sonograms, and X-rays are positive signs of pregnancy. A positive pregnancy test is a probable sign of pregnancy. Amenorrhea and breast tenderness are presumptive signs of pregnancy.

40. (3) The mother should empty her bladder before oxytocin is given and contractions begin. It is not necessary to be supine; the head will be elevated. NPO is not essential. The monitor with an oxytocin challenge test is external, not internal.

41. (4) A B.P. of 150/94 is indicative of pregnancy-induced hypertension. Weight gain of a

pound a week, slight dependent edema, and a fetal heart beat of 155 are all normal.

42. (4) Epigastric pain and headache suggest that a seizure is imminent. Supportive care to protect the client from injury is essential. An indwelling catheter may be inserted but only after the nurse assures that the client is safe should a seizure occur. The epigastric pain is most likely related to preeclampsia, not gastritis. The doctor should be notified, but the client should be made safe first.

43. (1) Magnesium sulfate is a central nervous system depressant. It is given to prevent seizures. Magnesium hydroxide gel is an antacid. Oxytocin is given to initiate contractions. Magnesium sulfate may decrease contractions. Magnesium sulfate does not cause constipation. Some laxatives contain magnesium.

44. (2) Preeclampsia is pregnancy-induced hypertension and disappears shortly after the birth of the baby.

45. (2) Placenta previa is characterized by painless bleeding in the third trimester. Abruptio is characterized by abdominal pain and a rigid abdomen with or without obvious bleeding. Shock develops rapidly in placenta abruptio. Hydatidiform mole is characterized by severe nausea and vomiting and the passage of grapelike vesicles. Prolapsed cord often occurs when the membranes rupture and is not characterized by bleeding.

46. (1) The history suggests placenta previa. The baby may well develop fetal distress. A boardlike abdomen and severe pain are characteristic of abruptio placenta. Elevated temperature is not characteristic of placenta previa.

47. (4) A sonogram will show the position of the placenta in the uterus. An internal exam will probably not be done because it can cause severe bleeding when there is a placenta previa. The non-stress test and the oxytocin challenge test are done to see how the fetus responds to contractions.

48. (4) The nurse should initially encourage the client to formulate and express her thoughts and concerns. The nurse should not try to impose her/his values on the client as answers 2 and 3 do. Answer 1 tells the client what to do and is not appropriate for an initial response, although discussing the issue with her parents should be encouraged.

49. (3) The client reports exertional dyspnea. The answer relates to avoiding exertion or things requiring extra effort. The data do not suggest that it is necessary at this point to stay in bed or in a wheelchair. Answers 1 and 2 do not relate to the data, which includes exertional dyspnea.

50. (2) Her symptoms suggest pregnancy-induced hypertension; particularly significant is the fact that her rings are getting tight. Upper body edema is highly suggestive of PIH. The nurse should record her weight and note how much weight has been gained in the last month. Monitoring blood pressure for elevation and checking urine for protein will help to determine if this woman has PIH. Dietary teaching as described in answer 1 is important, but the action relating to the data in the question is assessment for PIH. The advice in answer 3 regarding a comfortable walking shoe is also appropriate for a pregnant woman but does not relate to the data in this question. More important than total weight gain is the pattern of weight gain. A sudden increase in weight gain may indicate fluid retention accompanying PIH, even if the total is not yet 25 or 30 lbs.

51. (1) Analgesia can usually be safely given after 5 cm of dilation and until one to two hours before delivery. Answer 2 is not appropriate, because according to the data given, the mother is a good candidate for some type of analgesia. Answer 3 is not true. Pain medication too early may slow labor, and pain medication too late may depress the baby's respirations and heart beat. Pain medication given appropriately is often very helpful during labor. Answer 4 is not appropriate. It

does not address the question that the client asked about pain medication.

52. (2) Before encouraging the mother to push, the nurse should determine that the mother has completed transition and is fully dilated. She should not push before she is fully dilated. Answer 1 is a good description of pushing. However, the woman should not push until she is fully dilated. Most women need to push for a while before the baby is born. Answer 4 is a true statement; however, it is not the best response for the nurse to make.

53. (1) When it is not desirable for a woman to push, such as when moving from bed to table, she should be instructed to pant. It is not possible for a woman to pant and push at the same time. The mother will probably be unable to put her legs up in stirrups during a contraction. At this stage of labor, she will be unable to ignore contractions.

54. (3) The practical nurse should initially check the fetal heart rate, and then the registered nurse should perform a vaginal exam. A breech fetus is at high risk for a prolapsed cord when the membranes rupture. Following assessment of the fetal heart rate, the RN will perform a vaginal exam. A woman with a breech presentation may need a cesarean delivery. After the initial assessments, the physician will be notified because this baby is in a breech position. The physician is not automatically notified when the membranes rupture.

55. (4) Breech presentations frequently have amniotic-stained fluid. Amniotic-stained fluid in a vertex presentation is a sign of fetal distress. Maternal diabetes does not cause amniotic-stained fluid unless the fetus happens to be in distress.

56. (1) Checking the fundus for hemorrhage is of highest priority. The placenta has separated from the uterus in a woman who has had a cesarean delivery just as it does in a vaginal delivery. Both types of deliveries have a risk of postpartum hemorrhage. It is essential to keep the fundus firm for both types of deliveries. The woman who had a cesarean delivery has no episiotomy. Assisting with emotional adjustment will be a part of nursing care but is not the highest priority. Encouraging fluid intake is important but is not the highest priority.

57. (1) A cesarean delivery is not in itself a contraindication for another pregnancy. Many women can have a vaginal delivery after a cesarean. The old rule of only two cesarean deliveries is no longer true. Remember this client had one vaginal delivery and one cesarean. Answer 2 does not give accurate information. Choice 3 does not answer the question. Answer 4 contains some truth, but the nurse should be able to give general information to this mother.

58. (4) This is the appropriate assessment in early labor. Because she is para 0, the nurse knows that she has not carried a pregnancy at least 20 weeks. She has not had labor and has not given birth, so answers 1 and 2 are not appropriate. It is not reasonable to expect the woman to bring a sample of the fluid with her.

59. (3) Amniotic fluid is alkaline and turns Nitrazine paper blue. Urine is acidic and turns Nitrazine paper red.

60. (4) Panting is not the appropriate breathing pattern at this time. Panting is important when the woman has the desire to push but she should not push. Further assessment is needed to help her alter her breathing to a more appropriate pace. If she continues panting at this time, she will be at risk for developing respiratory alkalosis and exhausting herself. Answer 1 is a true statement but is a put-down to the client. Answer 2 is not correct. Her contractions are not compatible with late first stage labor (transition), when the pant-blow breathing pattern is appropriate. Answer 3 is not correct. She is using an inappropriate breathing technique.

61. (3) Amniotomy can be stressful for the fetus. Assessing the fetal heart rate is the priority nursing measure during amniotomy. Keeping the mother informed is not as important as fetal safety. The procedure is painless, so breathing techniques are not necessary.

62. (2) Contractions during transition usually occur every 2–3 minutes and last 60–90 seconds. Her contractions are not typical of transition, but the only way to be sure is to have the RN do a vaginal exam. Answer 1 ignores the symptoms and puts the client down. Answer 3 is incorrect information; her contractions are not typical of transition. Irritability and restlessness can be signs of transition. Answer 4 is not a useful response. It is not completely true, and it is certainly not a therapeutic response.

63. (3) Rubbing the lower back usually helps the husband deal with his feelings of helplessness and fosters the couple's sense of mutual experience. Answer 1 is not appropriate, because it is better for the mate to give the back rub if he is able and willing than for the nurse to do it. Answer 2 is not appropriate because she has said that she wants to have a natural childbirth. Answer 4 is not realistic. It is not realistic to encourage a woman in active labor to rest. Sending the husband away is not appropriate.

64. (4) Hypotension is a frequent side effect of regional anesthesia. Maternal hypotension causes fetal bradycardia and hypoxia. Answer 1 is not correct, because epidural anesthesia does not cause uterine tetany. Answer 2 is not correct. Even though contractions are sometimes slowed after administering an epidural, oxytocin is not routinely administered. Answer 4 is not correct. The woman who has had an epidural anesthesia will have her head elevated to prevent respiratory depression. Post-anesthesia headache occurs after spinal or saddle block anesthesia, not after epidural anesthesia.

65. (2) Pressure of the uterus against major blood vessels reduces circulation, causing decreased perfusion of the placenta. Answer 1 is not correct; the supine position does not prolong labor. Choice 3 is not correct; the supine position does not impede free movement of the symphysis pubis. Answer 4 is not correct; the supine position does not cause transient episodes of hypertension in the laboring woman.

66. (2) Contractions during the transition phase typically occur every 2–3 minutes and last 60–90 seconds. The woman is often irritable and has a backache. Answer 1 is not correct. Early first stage labor contractions are usually several minutes apart, lasting only a few seconds. Backache and irritability are not common in early first stage labor. Answer 3 is not correct. Late second stage labor is the "pushing stage" just before delivery. Early third stage labor is after delivery of the baby, just before the placenta is expelled. Third stage labor is usually only a few minutes.

67. (1) Lack of descent is often related to a full bladder. Answer 2 is not correct. Until a full bladder has been ruled out as a cause of failure to descend, cesarean delivery would not be considered. Answer 3 is not correct. Routine fetal assessment will of course be done. However, there is no specific data suggesting a fetal problem and no need for additional fetal monitoring. Answer 4 is not correct. Position is not the most likely cause for failure to descend. Turning the mother to the left side would be an appropriate intervention for a sudden drop in blood pressure resulting from vena caval syndrome.

68. (1) The second stage of labor is the pushing stage. The nurse should help the mother push effectively. Answer 2 is not correct. The mother cannot breastfeed the infant until it is born. Breastfeeding on the delivery table might be an appropriate action in the third stage of labor. Answer 3 is not correct. Checking the fetal position is not the highest priority action during second stage labor. Answer 4 is not correct. Pain medication should not be administered in the second stage because it will cause a sleepy baby.

69. (2) The woman is a G5 P4, and the perineum is bulging. Delivery is imminent. Contamination will be minimized by catching the infant on a clean surface. Answer 1 is not correct. The woman will not need to be encouraged to push; she will be doing it on her own. Secondly, it will be more appropriate to have her pant so that the delivery can be controlled. Answer 3 is not correct. Delivery is imminent. There is no time or need to time the contractions. Answer 4 is not correct. Delivery is imminent. There is no time to contact the physician for instructions. The nurse should be able to handle this emergency delivery.

70. (3) Applying gentle counter pressure to the perineum prevents too rapid expulsion of the head, which can lead to increased intracranial pressure in the infant and laceration in the mother. Answer 1 is not correct. The mother will be encouraged to pant so that the delivery can be controlled. Answer 2 is not correct. The nurse does not press down on the fundus to expel the baby. Answer 4 is not correct. There is no need to tell the mother to take prolonged deep breaths. Applying gentle perineal pressure is by far the most appropriate action for the nurse at this time.

71. (2) The sudden change of pressure tends to tear away dural linings. The mother can also get perineal tears. Answer 1 is not correct. Edema of the scalp is not a complication with precipitate labor. Sometimes prolonged labor can cause caput succadaneum, where the baby has bleeding under the scalp. Answers 3 and 4 are not correct. Rapid delivery is not particularly associated with placental problems.

72. (3) Newborns have immature temperature regulating mechanisms. The nurse should dry the infant and place it in a blanket or towel on the mother's abdomen. Answer 1 is not correct. The first concern is clearing the infant's airway and keeping the infant warm. The mother is not likely to hemorrhage at this time. Maternal hemorrhage would be more likely after delivery of the placenta. Answer 2

is not correct. The afterbirth or placenta should separate and deliver itself within 5 to 15 minutes after the baby is born. The nurse should care for the baby until this happens. Answer 4 is not correct. There is no hurry to cut the cord. The cord should never be cut with anything that is not sterile because the baby could develop a fatal infection.

73. (3) Breastfeeding stimulates uterine contractions, which will help the placenta to separate. Answer 1 is not correct. Having the mother push down vigorously will not stimulate the placenta to separate. Answer 2 is not correct. The nurse should not push down on the fundus. This is not necessary for the placenta to separate. Answer 4 is not correct. The nurse should never pull on the cord. This could cause inversion of the uterus.

74. (4) A clear airway for the infant is first priority. Answer 1 is not correct. Tugging on the cord before the placenta is expelled could cause inversion of the uterus. Answer 2 is not correct. The cord does not need to be cut immediately. Clearing the infant's airway is a much higher priority. Answer 3 is not correct. The nurse may assess the infant and get an Apgar score. However, the airway is a much higher priority than the Apgar.

75. (3) Antibiotic eye drops have to be instilled into the neonate's conjunctival sacs to prevent infection, not just from gonorrhea and chlamydia but also from pathogens in the birth canal such as pneumococcus and streptococcus. It is safe to wait up to two hours to instill the drops. This allows time for maternal-child eye contact and interaction, which facilitates attachment. Answers 1 and 2 are not correct. There is a legal requirement to give the baby eye prophylaxis. Answer 4 is not correct. Retrolental fibroplasia results from too much oxygen concentration in immature retinal vessels during oxygen therapy for the compromised neonate.

76. (2) Semirecumbent or semi-Fowler's position would be the most appropriate position to reduce the cardiac work load and ease

breathing. The laboring woman who has a history of rheumatic heart disease is at risk for congestive heart failure. The supine and side-lying positions would increase the cardiac work load. Sitting upright is not the best choice.

77. (1) The woman with cardiac disease should not bear down excessively. She will be given an epidural anesthesia, and outlet forceps may be indicated to shorten the second stage of labor. Answer 2 is not correct. Breathing shallowly and rapidly will cause respiratory alkalosis. Answer 3 is not correct. Sitting on the side of the bed is not an appropriate action during second stage labor. Second stage labor is the expulsion stage. Answer 4 is not correct. Sometimes mothers do dose between contractions in second stage. However, answer 1 is the priority instruction that the nurse should give this mother.

78. (4) Always make sure the airway is clear first. Apgar scoring is not the LPN's responsibility, and it is not the highest priority. Checking heart rate and applying identification bracelets are secondary to clearing the airway.

79. (3) He receives two points for respiratory effort because he is crying. He receives two points for his heartbeat because it is over 100. He receives one point for acrocyanosis (blue extremities). He receives two points for reflexes because he resists the suction catheters. He receives one point instead of two because his arms are extended instead of flexed. He receives 8 points out of the maximum score of 10 points.

80. (2) The Apgar score assesses the infant on respiratory effort, heart rate, color, reflexes, and muscle tone. These indicate his adaptation to extrauterine life. The purpose of the Apgar score is not to evaluate the effectiveness of labor and delivery, assess respiratory distress syndrome, or give an estimate of gestational age of the infant.

81. (3) Chills occur frequently after the administration of a regional anesthetic such

as Carbocaine. A spinal anesthesia does not usually cause the client to be dizzy and light-headed. Fever and rash are not likely to occur after spinal anesthesia.

82. (3) Lochia can accumulate under the buttocks. It cannot be accurately observed in a supine position. The nurse assesses the fundus every 15 minutes and massages it only when it is soft. Vital signs will be q 15 minutes, not every hour. The client will not get up to void this soon after delivery.

83. (2) A distended bladder may interfere with involution of the uterus and cause excessive bleeding. The nurse will observe for appropriate bonding behaviors and maternal relaxation and maternal knowledge of newborn behavior but the most important is assessment for bladder distention (because that could cause uterine relaxation and hemorrhage).

84. (1) This woman is in premature labor. Ritodrine is used to suppress uterine activity. Note that answers 1 and 3 are opposites. Usually when there are opposites, one of the opposites is the correct answer. It would not be logical to enhance contractions in a woman who is not at term. Ritodrine is not an analgesic and does not increase fetal oxygenation.

85. (2) Abruptio placenta causes hemorrhage, either apparent or concealed. The nurse must observe for hypovolemic shock. Jaundice is not seen with placenta abruptio. Convulsions occur with eclampsia or pregnancy-induced hypertension. The client who is hemorrhaging will develop shock, not hypertension. Note the opposites; shock is low blood pressure and hypertension is high blood pressure. The answer is likely to be one of the opposites.

86. (1) The initial response is to massage the uterus. Most of the time, massaging the uterus will cause it to firm up immediately. If it does not respond to massage by becoming firm, then the practical nurse should report it

to the charge nurse or contact the physician. The nurse will continue to assess frequently after massaging the fundus. Note that the question asked for the initial intervention.

87. (2) A full bladder causes the uterus to be elevated above the umbilicus and displaced to the right. A fibroid tumor, if present, would not cause a change in position of the uterus in a two-hour time period. Interstitial fluid does not accumulate in the uterus and could not cause the uterine position change. Retained placental fragments would cause an increase in vaginal bleeding or a boggy fundus, but not displacement of the fundus.

88. (2) The client is describing colostrum. Milk comes in about 72 hours after delivery. Answers 1 and 3 do not address the question asked by the mother. Answer 4 is technically accurate but does not give as much information and reassurance as Answer 2.

89. (1) The taking-in period is characterized by passivity and dependence. The mother relives her labor and integrates it into her being. Preoccupation with the baby's needs and reasserting independence are characteristic of the taking-hold phase, which follows the taking-in phase. Resuming control of life is characteristic of the letting-go phase.

90. (1) Standing with her back to the shower will keep the warm water from stimulating milk production. Cool compresses will help with engorgement; warm compresses stimulate milk flow. A sitz bath is indicated for an episiotomy. It is not related to the care of the breasts. Pushing fluids will encourage milk production.

91. (1) A woman should be resized for a diaphragm after the birth of a baby. The old one may no longer be the correct size. The resizing will occur after involution is completed, usually at her six-week checkup. If sexual activity is resumed before that time, another means of contraception (such as the condom) should be used if she does not wish

to get pregnant. All of the other responses are good responses.

92. (3) Babies born by cesarean delivery do not have molded heads because they have not passed through the pelvis and the birth canal. The other responses are not helpful. Answer 1 does not address the questions. Forceps can cause distinctive marks on the head. A round head is not a sign of intelligence.

93. (4) Alcohol is used to dry the cord. The other answers are not correct and are contraindicated. Alcohol is too drying to apply to the skin. Alcohol is not applied to the circumcision; it would cause great pain. Petrolatum (Vaseline) gauze is applied to the circumcision. The baby's bottom should not be wiped with alcohol because it will cause drying of the skin.

94. (1) Temperature over 100.4°F after the second day usually indicates infection. Infection is the most frequent maternal complication after prolonged rupture of the membranes. Zephiran perineal care is not a current practice and is not related to prolonged rupture of the membranes. A strict perineal pad count is not necessary. Sitz baths are a comfort measure for a sore perineum and are not related to prolonged rupture of the membranes.

95. (1) The biggest cause of postpartum hemorrhage is uterine atony. Always assess and massage the fundus first. Taking vital signs and notifying the physician will be done after the nurse massages the fundus. The client will not be placed in the Trendelenburg position.

96. (2) This response explains the drug's action to the client. Methergine is an oxytocic drug that helps the uterus to contract and prevents postpartum bleeding. Answer 1 is not correct because it does not give the mother the information she needs to understand why she is cramping. Answers 3 and 4 are not accurate.

97. (1) An over-stretched uterus is subject to hemorrhage. A large baby causes additional

stretching of the uterus. Answer 2 is not correct. Pitocin contracts the uterus and decreases hemorrhage. It is also standard procedure following delivery. Answer 3 is not correct. Delivering after the due date itself does not increase postpartum hemorrhage. However, the large baby does. Answer 4 is not correct. An hour second stage is normal.

98. (3) Decreasing stimulation will decrease milk production. Hot showers and massaging breasts stimulates milk production. The baby should be held close to the chest regardless of the feeding method.

99. (4) This may mean she is rejecting the baby. Nicknames, holding the baby in "en face" position (so the mother can look at the baby's face) and seeing family resemblance are positive signs of attachment.

100. (1) By discussing her experience, she is bringing it into reality. This is characteristic of the taking-in phase. The taking-hold phase is when the mother tries to reassert her control of the family, and letting-go is when the baby is integrated into the family. Working through is not one of the phases of postpartum adjustment.

101. (2) Bladder distention causes uterine displacement, which interferes with involution and may lead to postpartum hemorrhage. With normal involution, the fundus would be at or slightly above the umbilicus and in the midline. Retained placental fragments and uterine atony would cause excessive bleeding.

102. (4) During the taking-in phase, the mother is more self-centered. She will be most responsive to perineal care. She will be most responsive to family planning and newborn care during the taking-hold phase. Awareness of community support groups would be in the taking-hold or letting-go phase.

103. (2) Early walking helps to prevent thrombophlebitis. She does not have to walk in order to hold her baby. Walking does not prevent dehiscence or wound infection.

104. (3) The bottle-feeding mother's ovulation and menstrual cycle has been noted to occur as early as 36 days; the breastfeeding mother's, as early as 39 days. Lactation sometimes, but not always, suppresses ovulation. A nursing mother may ovulate and not menstruate, so another method of contraception is recommended. Lactation does not have an effect on sexual desire. Breastfeeding is not a reliable method of contraception.

105. (3) The data suggest that the mother has mastitis. Antibiotics may be a part of the treatment. She should be seen by the physician. Warm compresses might be helpful, but the woman needs to be seen by the physician. Cold compresses are not indicated for infection. She will probably not need to stop nursing or reduce feeding on that breast.

106. (1) Being jittery and having a weak and high-pitched cry and irregular respirations are classic symptoms of hypoglycemia.

107. (1) The rooting reflex is stimulated when the cheek next to the breast is gently stroked. Answer 2 is not correct. The nurse should not leave the mother and baby alone until the nurse is confident that mother and baby are doing well. The infant should not nurse long enough to cause sore nipples. Answer 3 is not correct. The infant should grasp the areola, not the nipple. Answer 4 is not correct. Giving a bottle first would serve no purpose and might interfere with nursing.

108. (1) Increased intravascular pressure during delivery can cause petechiae. These will quickly disappear. Decreased Vitamin K level in the infant might predispose the infant to bleeding from the umbilical cord but does not cause petechiae on the face and neck. Erythema toxicum is a generalized rash sometimes seen in newborns. It is not limited to the face and neck. Petechiae are not a result of excessive superficial capillaries.

109. (1) The response described is the startle reflex and is normal in newborns. It lasts only a few months.

110. (3) More frequent changing and cleaning of the area should help to prevent diaper rash. The mother should learn how to care for her baby and should be encouraged to change the infant. Using both lotion and powder would create a caked mess. The description in the question suggests a diaper rash. There is no need to contact the physician. The nurse will, of course, record the observation on the client's record.

111. (2) A premature infant lacks fat cells and is not able to alter body temperature. He has decreased surfactant and is apt to develop respiratory distress. Mental retardation and seizures are possible later complications of prematurity. Acrocyanosis is normal. Decreased lanugo is seen at term; a premature infant has more lanugo. Patent ductus arteriosus is not specifically related to prematurity. Pneumonia is not specifically related to prematurity.

112. (3) Before an infant can be given nipple feedings, he/she must have sucking and gag reflexes to prevent aspiration. The respiratory rate and heart rate given in answer 1 are below those of term infants and are totally unrealistic. A baby who is alert and rooting but does not have sucking and gag reflexes should not be given nipple feedings. Stable weight and temperature are not requirements for nipple feeding.

113. (4) This response helps to reinforce the mother's positive feelings as well as giving correct information. Answer 1 denies the mother's feelings and does not give correct information. Answers 2 and 3 are not correct. Breast milk is the best food for premature babies.

114. (2) Acrocyanosis or blue hands and feet is normal for the first 24 hours of life and is thought to be related to the establishment of circulation after delivery. Acrocyanosis in the first 24 hours does not suggest heart defects. Continuing acrocyanosis might. Bluish discoloration over the lower back and buttocks are called Mongolian spots and are typical in infants with more pigment in their skin. Acrocyanosis is not related to the regulation of temperature as much as it is related to the establishment of nonfetal circulatory patterns.

115. (4) Toxoplasmosis is transmitted from the mother to the baby through the placenta. The mother most likely acquired it from cat feces or eating raw meat. The mother could contract HIV or hepatitis from a blood transfusion. HIV could then affect the fetus. HIV can probably be transmitted through breast milk. Gonorrhea, chlamydia, and herpes can all be picked up by the infant during the birth process.

116. (3) The nurse needs more data on which to make an assessment. Dextrostix will test for blood sugar. The baby of a diabetic mother is apt to develop hypoglycemia. If the blood sugar is 35 mg/dl or less, he will be given glucose water and the physician will be notified. Jerky movements of the extremities are not normal and suggest hypoglycemia.

117. (3) The airway should be checked for patency immediately. Removing vernix is not a high priority. The temperature will be monitored, but this is not the highest priority. The nurse will check for anomalies, but this is not the highest priority. When the infant is stable, it will be bathed, and bloody material will be removed. Vernix is good for the skin.

118. (2) Cyanosis is indicative of inadequate oxygenation. Increased bilirubin would be evidenced by jaundice. It is normal for newborns to have excessive red blood cells. This does not cause cyanosis. Lack of subcutaneous fatty tissue is common in premature infants and causes poor temperature regulation.

119. (4) Arterial pO_2 is the best indicator of oxygen levels. Respiratory rate, skin color, and pulse

rate can be affected by factors other than oxygenation. They are indicators but are not the most reliable.

120. (1) Red blood cells of premature infants are fragile and break down rapidly, causing an increase in bilirubin, which causes icterus or jaundice. The timing is key. Jaundice occurring after 48 hours is usually physiologic jaundice. Jaundice presenting at birth or within the first 24 hours is usually pathologic in nature. Obstruction of hepatic bile ducts would be a pathologic cause of jaundice and would occur earlier. Answer 3 is not realistic. This might cause a bruising appearance but not jaundice. Answer 4 makes no sense.

121. (3) The bili light or blue light enhances the breakdown of indirect bilirubin to a less-toxic compound. Vitamin K is not made in the skin, it is made in the intestines. Vitamin D is absorbed by the skin. Increasing temperature does not enhance pigment breakdown. The eyes are covered when the blue light is used to protect the eyes against damage.

122. (1) The mother appears to be describing the anterior fontanel, or soft spot, which occurs in all babies. The skull bones are not completely fused, allowing molding of the head during the birth process. This should close between 12 and 18 months. It is a normal condition occurring in all babies and is not a defect. Caput succadaneum is a

swelling that may occur on the head following delivery. It crosses suture lines and is due to bleeding under the scalp during birth. It is normal and disappears in a few days. This is not what is described in the question.

123. (2) Testicles normally descend into the scrotum at eight months gestation. An infant born prior to that time will have undescended testicles. A term infant will have rugae on the scrotum. Vernix and lanugo are less with a term infant than with a premature infant.

124. (4) Hepatitis B vaccine is given within the first 12 hours after birth. A PKU test is done when the infant has had milk feedings for 24 hours. DTP and polio immunizations are usually started at two months of age. MMR is given at 15 months. A tuberculin test is usually done at one year. Pneumococcal vaccine is not routinely given to infants. Newborns are not routinely tested for HIV.

125. (2) Phenylketonuria is a disorder of purine metabolism in which phenylalanine is not metabolized properly and builds up in the blood and brain and causes severe mental retardation if not treated promptly. The treatment is to avoid foods containing phenylalanine. The child will have a special formula (Lofenalac) and cannot eat protein-containing foods. If diagnosed early and if the proper diet is followed, the child should do well.

Chapter 13

Pediatrics

Sample Questions

1. A three-month-old infant is admitted. Upon admission, the nurse assesses her developmental status as appropriate for age. Which of the following would the client be least likely able to do?

    1. Smile in response to mother's face
    2. Reach for shiny objects but miss them
    3. Hold head erect and steady
    4. Sit with slight support

2. A three-month-old infant is doing well after the repair of a cleft lip. The nurse wants to provide the client with appropriate stimulation. What is the best toy for the nurse to provide?

    1. Colorful rattle
    2. String of large beads
    3. Mobile with a music box
    4. Teddy bear with button eyes

3. Which toys would be best for a five-month-old infant who has infantile eczema?

    1. Soft, washable toys
    2. Stuffed toys
    3. Puzzles and games
    4. Toy cars

4. Which diversion would be appropriate for the nurse to plan to use with an eight-month-old infant?

    1. A colorful mobile
    2. Large blocks to stack
    3. A colorful rattle
    4. A game of peek-a-boo

5. Which activity would best occupy a 12-month-old child while the nurse is interviewing the parents?

    1. String of large snap beads and a large plastic bowl
    2. Riding toy
    3. Several small puzzles
    4. Paste, paper, and scissors

6. An 18-month-old is admitted for a repeat cardiac catheterization. The parents are continuously present and do everything for the child: dress him, feed him, even play for him. The nurse wants to prepare the child and the parents for the procedure. Which should be included in the care plan?

    1. Give the child simple explanations.
    2. Talk with the parents to assess their knowledge and how they can help with the child's care.
    3. No specific action will be necessary because the child and family have been through a cardiac catheterization previously.
    4. Ask the parents to stay away as much as possible because they upset the child.

7. In planning care for an 18-month-old, the nurse would expect him to be able to do which of the following?

   1. Button his shirt and tie his shoes
   2. Feed himself and drink from a cup
   3. Cut with scissors
   4. Walk up and down stairs

8. The mother of a two-year-old child asks the nurse how to cope with the child's frequent temper tantrums when he does not get what he wants immediately. What information should the nurse include when responding?

   1. As long as the child is safe, ignore him during the tantrum.
   2. If the child's demands are reasonable, give him part of what he wants.
   3. Spank the child if the tantrum continues for more than five minutes.
   4. Explain to the child why he cannot have what he wants and promise him a reward when he stops crying.

9. A three-year-old is admitted to the pediatric unit for diagnostic tests. His mother is discussing the child's hospitalization with the nurse. She is concerned about staying with this child and caring for her other two children at home. Which suggestion to the mother will most help the child adjust to being in the hospital?

   1. Do not visit the child until discharge so that your child won't cry when you leave.
   2. Spend the night in the hospital with your child.
   3. Bring your child's favorite teddy bear and security blanket to the hospital.
   4. Buy your child a gift to let the child know you care deeply.

10. The parents of a three-year-old are leaving for the evening. Which behavior would the nurse expect the child to exhibit?

    1. Wave good-bye to the parents
    2. Cry when the parents leave
    3. Hide his/her head under the covers
    4. Ask to go to the playroom

11. When planning outdoor play activities for a normal four-year-old child, which activity is most appropriate?

    1. Two-wheeled bike
    2. Sandbox
    3. Climbing trees
    4. Push toy lawn mower

12. A five-year-old had major surgery several days ago and is allowed to be up. When planning diversion activity, which action by the nurse is most appropriate?

    1. Give the child a book to read.
    2. Play a board game with the child.
    3. Encourage the child to play house with other children.
    4. Turn on the television so the child can watch cartoons.

13. A six-year-old is admitted for a tonsillectomy. Considering the child's age, which of the following would be the most important to include in a pre-operative physical assessment?

    1. Characteristics of tongue, gum, or lip sores
    2. Any sign of tonsilar inflammation
    3. The number and location of any loose teeth
    4. The location and presence of tenderness in any swollen lymph nodes

14. A six-year-old child is in the terminal stage of leukemia. The child appears helpless and afraid. How can the nurse best help the child?

    1. Allow the child to make the major decisions for her care.

2. Make all decisions for the child.

3. Discuss with the child the fears that dying children usually have.

4. Discuss with the child the reasons for her fears.

15. The nurse is preparing a six-year-old for cardiac surgery. Which pre-operative teaching technique is most appropriate?

1. Have the child practice procedures that will be performed post-operatively, such as coughing and deep breathing.

2. Arrange for the child to tour the operating room and surgical ICU.

3. Encourage the child to draw pictures illustrating the operation.

4. Arrange for the child to discuss heart surgery and post-operative events with a group of children who have undergone heart surgery.

16. A 10-year-old girl is being treated for rheumatic fever. Which would be an appropriate activity while she is on bed rest?

1. Stringing large wooden beads

2. Engaging in a pillow fight

3. Making craft items from felt

4. Watching television

17. A 10-year-old who is immobilized in a cast following an accident has been squirting other children and the staff with a syringe filled with water. The nurse wants to provide other activities to help him express his aggression. Which activity would be most appropriate?

1. Cranking a wind-up toy

2. Pounding clay

3. Putting charts together

4. Writing a story

18. An 11-year-old boy is admitted to the pediatric unit in traction with a fractured femur sustained in a motorcycle accident. His uncle, who was driving the cycle when the accident occurred, received only minor injuries. The child tells the nurse that his uncle was not to blame for the accident. He is "the best motorcycle rider in the world." The nurse interprets this to mean that the child is exhibiting which defense mechanism?

1. Denial

2. Repression

3. Hero worship

4. Fantasy

19. The nurse is planning care for an 11-year-old who has a fractured femur and is in traction. Which activity would be most appropriate?

1. Dramatizing with puppets

2. Building with popsicle sticks

3. Watching television

4. Coloring with crayons or colored pencils

20. A two-year-old is hospitalized for a fractured femur. During his first two days in the hospital, he lies quietly, sucks his thumb, and does not cry. Which is the best interpretation of his behavior?

1. He has made a good adjustment to being in the hospital.

2. He is comfortable with the nurses caring for him.

3. He is experiencing anxiety.

4. He does not have a good relationship with his parents.

21. A hospitalized two-and-a-half-year-old has a temper tantrum while her mother is bathing her. Her mother asks the nurse how she should handle this behavior. Which information should be included in the nurse's reply?

1. Temper tantrums in a hospitalized child indicate regression.

2. Tantrums suggest a poorly developed sense of trust.

3. Discipline is necessary when a child has a temper tantrum.

4. This behavior is a normal response to limit setting in a child of this age.

22. A three-year-old resists going to bed at night. Her mother asks the nurse what she should say to her. Which response should the nurse suggest to the mother as most appropriate?

1. "I don't love you anymore because you don't know how to listen."

2. "All good children go to bed on time."

3. "If you go to sleep now, I'll take you to the zoo tomorrow."

4. "Here is your blanket. It's time to go to sleep."

23. An eight-year-old is terminally ill. Considering the child's age, which statement would you most expect the child to make?

1. "After I'm dead, will you come visit me?"

2. "Who will take care of me when I am dead?"

3. "Will it hurt me when I die?"

4. "Can you help me do a videotape about dying from leukemia?"

24. A father has brought his four-month-old daughter to the well-baby clinic. Which statement he makes is greatest cause for concern to the nurse?

1. "She cannot sit up by herself."

2. "She does not hold the rattle as well as she did at first."

3. "She does not follow objects with her eyes."

4. "She spits up after a feeding."

25. A three-year-old has all of the following abilities. Which did he acquire most recently?

1. Walking

2. Throwing a large ball

3. Riding a tricycle

4. Stating his name

26. The mother of a two-year-old calls the doctor's office because her child swallowed "the rest of the bottle of adult aspirin" about a half hour ago. The nurse determines that there were about 15 tablets left in the bottle. What initial assessment findings are consistent with aspirin ingestion?

1. Bradypnea and pallor

2. Hyperventilation and hyperpyrexia

3. Subnormal temperature and bleeding

4. Melena and bradycardia

27. A toddler who has swallowed several adult aspirin is admitted to the emergency room. When admitted, the child is breathing but is difficult to arouse. What is the immediate priority of care?

1. Administration of syrup of ipecac

2. Cardiopulmonary resuscitation

3. Ventilatory support

4. Gastric lavage

28. A six-month-old is being seen for a well-baby visit. The child has received all immunizations as recommended so far. What immunizations does the nurse expect to give at this visit?

1. DTP, MMR, IPV
2. DTP, hepatitis B, HIB
3. HIB, IPV, varicella
4. MMR, hepatitis B, HIB

29. The mother of a six-year-old who has chicken pox asks the nurse when the child can go back to school. What information should be included in the nurse's response? The child is contagious

    1. Until all signs of the disease are gone.
    2. As long as the child has scabs.
    3. As long as there are fluid-filled vesicles.
    4. Until the rash and fever are gone.

30. A two-year-old child is in for an annual examination. Which comment by the mother alerts the nurse to a risk for lead poisoning?

    1. "Why does he eat paint off the window sills?"
    2. "Will his temper tantrums ever stop?"
    3. "I haven't been able to toilet train him yet."
    4. "He is such a messy eater."

31. A six-year-old has Tetralogy of Fallot. He is being admitted for surgery. The nurse knows that which problem is not associated with Tetralogy of Fallot?

    1. Severe atrial septal defect
    2. Pulmonary stenosis
    3. Right ventricular hypertrophy
    4. Overriding aorta

32. A six-year-old with Tetralogy of Fallot is being admitted for surgery. While the nurse is orienting the child to the unit, the child suddenly squats with the arms thrown over the knees and knees drawn up to the chest. What is the best immediate nursing action?

    1. Observe and assist if needed.
    2. Place the child in a lying position.
    3. Call for help and return the child to the room.
    4. Assist the child to a standing position.

33. A six-year-old with Tetralogy of Fallot is being admitted for surgery. What is most important to teach the child during the pre-operative period?

    1. Strict hand washing technique
    2. How to cough and deep-breathe
    3. The importance of drinking plenty of fluids
    4. Positions of comfort

34. A six-year-old with Tetralogy of Fallot has open heart surgery. The septal defect was closed, and the pulmonic valve was replaced. When the child returns to the unit, he has oxygen, IVs, and closed chest drainage. How should the nurse position the chest drainage system?

    1. Above the level of the bed
    2. At the level of the heart
    3. Below the level of the bed
    4. Alternating above and below the bed level every two hours

35. A parent brings a three-week-old infant to the clinic. The parent states that the baby does not eat very well. She takes 45 cc of formula in 45 minutes and gets "tired and sweaty" when eating. The nurse observes the baby sleeping in the parent's arms. Her color is pink, and the child is breathing without difficulty. What is the best response for the nurse to make?

   1. "It's normal for an infant to get tired while feeding. That will go away as the child gets older."
   2. "It's normal for an infant to get tired while feeding. You could try feeding the baby smaller amounts of formula more frequently."
   3. "This could be a sign of a health problem. Does your baby's skin color change while eating?"
   4. "This could be a sign of a health problem. How does your baby's behavior compare with your other children when they were that age?"

36. The nurse is explaining cardiac catheterization to the parents of a child. The nurse explains to the parents that information about which of the following can be obtained during cardiac catheterization?

   1. Oxygen levels in the chambers of the heart
   2. Pulmonary vascularization
   3. Presence of abdominal aortic aneurysm
   4. Activity tolerance

37. The nurse is caring for a toddler who is six hours post cardiac catheterization. The nurse is administering antibiotics. The child's mother asks why the child needs to have antibiotics. The nurse's response should indicate that antibiotics are given to the client to prevent which type of infection?

   1. Urinary tract infection
   2. Pneumonia
   3. Otitis media

   4. Endocarditis

38. The nurse is caring for a toddler with a cardiac defect who has had several episodes of congestive heart failure in the past few months. Which data would be the most useful to the nurse in assessing the child's current congestive heart failure?

   1. The degree of clubbing of the child's fingers and toes
   2. Amount of fluid and food intake
   3. Recent fluctuations in weight
   4. The degree of sacral edema

39. A child with a cyanotic heart defect has an elevated hematocrit. What is the most likely cause of the elevated hematocrit?

   1. Chronic infection
   2. Recent dehydration
   3. Increased cardiac output
   4. Chronic oxygen deficiency

40. The nurse is administering the daily digoxin dose of .035 mg to a 10-month-old child. Before administering the dose, the nurse takes the child's apical pulse and it is 85. Which of the following interpretations of these data is most accurate?

   1. The child has just awakened, and the heart action is slowest in the morning.
   2. This is a normal rate for a 10-month-old child.
   3. The child may be going into heart block due to digoxin toxicity.
   4. The child's potassium level needs to be evaluated.

41. The nurse is discussing dietary needs of a child with a serious heart defect. The child is being treated with digoxin and hydrochlorothiazide (Hydrodiuril). The nurse

should stress the importance of giving the child which of these foods?

1. Cheese and ice cream
2. Finger foods such as hot dogs
3. Apricots and bananas
4. Four glasses of whole milk per day

42. A child with a cyanotic heart defect has a hypoxic episode. What should the nurse do for the child at this time?

1. Administer prn oxygen and position the child in the squat position.
2. Position the child side-lying and give the ordered morphine.
3. Ask the parents to leave and start oxygen.
4. Give oxygen and notify the physician.

43. The nurse notes that a child who has had a serious heart condition since birth does not do the expected activities for that age. The child's mother says, "I worry constantly about my child. I don't let the older children or the neighbor kids play with my child very much. I try to make things as easy for my child as I can." What is the best interpretation of this data?

1. The child is physically incapable due to his cardiac defect.
2. The child's mother is overprotective and allows the child few challenges to develop skills.
3. The child is probably mentally retarded from the effects of continual hypoxia.
4. The child has regressed due to the effects of hospitalization.

44. Ten days after cardiac surgery an 18-month-old is recovering well. The child is alert and fairly active and is playing well with the parents. Discharge is planned soon. The nurse notes that the parents are still very reluctant to allow the child to do anything without help.

What is the best initial action for the nurse to take?

1. Re-emphasize the need for autonomy in toddlers.
2. Provide opportunities for autonomy when the parents are not present.
3. Reassess the parent's needs and concerns.
4. Discuss the success of the surgery and how well the child is doing.

45. The nurse makes an initial assessment of a four-year-old admitted with possible epiglottitis. Which observation is most suggestive of epiglottitis?

1. Low-grade fever
2. Retching
3. Excessive drooling
4. Substernal retractions

46. Which nursing action could be life-threatening for a child with epiglottitis?

1. Examining the child's throat with a tongue blade
2. Placing the child in a semi-Fowler's position
3. Maintaining high humidity
4. Obtaining a nasopharyngeal culture

47. Which factor would most likely be a cause of epiglottitis?

1. Acquiring the child's first puppy, the day before the onset of symptoms
2. Exposure to the parainfluenza virus
3. Exposure to Hemophilus influenza, type B
4. Frequent upper respiratory infections as an infant

48. The nurse is caring for a child who has epiglottitis. What position would the child be most likely to assume?

1. Squatting
2. Sitting upright and leaning forward, supporting self with hands
3. Crouching on hands and knees and rocking back and forth
4. Knee-chest position

49. The nurse is assessing a child who has epiglottitis and is having respiratory difficulty. Which is the nurse most likely to assess in the child?

1. Flaring of the nares; cyanosis; lethargy
2. Diminished breath sounds bilaterally; easily agitated
3. Scattered rales throughout lung fields; anxious and frightened
4. Mouth open with a protruding tongue; inspiratory stridor

50. Which is the most important goal of nursing care in the management of a child with epiglottitis?

1. Preventing the spread of infection from the epiglottis throughout the respiratory tract
2. Reduction of high fever and prevention of hyperthermia
3. Maintaining a patent airway
4. Maintaining him in an atmosphere of high humidity with oxygen

51. Which is the most important nursing action when caring for a child with epiglottitis?

1. Cardiac monitoring
2. Blood pressure monitoring
3. Temperature monitoring
4. Monitoring intravenous infusion

52. A five-year-old is admitted with his first asthma attack. Which would have been least likely to have precipitated his asthma attack?

1. A new puppy in the house
2. A visit from his uncle who smokes cigars
3. An unusually early snowstorm
4. Eating fresh fruit salad

53. During aminophylline infusion, a child becomes restless, nauseated, and his blood pressure drops. What is the appropriate nursing response to these findings?

1. Because these are common side effects of the drug, which will pass when the infusion is completed, simply chart the response.
2. Stop the infusion immediately and notify the physician or charge nurse, because the symptoms are suggestive of an adverse response to aminophylline.
3. Continue to monitor the child, because the symptoms are probably related to the child's illness because they are not commonly associated with aminophylline.
4. Continue to monitor the child, because these are expected responses to aminophylline.

54. The nurse is teaching a child with asthma to blow cotton balls across a table. Which is the best explanation for this play technique?

1. It decreases expiratory pressure.
2. It provides for an extended expiratory phase of respiration.
3. It promotes a fuller expansion of the thoracic cavity during inspiration.
4. It develops the accessory muscles of respiration.

55. After having chronic sore throats and repeated absences from school over the past year, a six-year-old has been admitted to the pediatric unit for a tonsillectomy. Which

would be the most important information to obtain in a pre-operative health history?

1. Evidence of bleeding tendencies
2. Parent's responses to anesthesia, especially adverse reactions
3. Child's perception of the surgical procedure
4. Frequency and type of bacterial tonsilar infections

56. A six-year-old has just returned from having a tonsillectomy. The child's condition is stable but the child remains quite drowsy. How should the nurse position this child?

1. On her back with head elevated 30 degrees
2. High-Fowler's
3. Semi-prone
4. Trendelenburg

57. The nurse is caring for a child who had a tonsillectomy this morning. The child is observed to be swallowing continuously. What is the most appropriate initial nursing action?

1. Administer acetaminophen for pain.
2. Place an ice collar around her throat.
3. Call the surgeon immediately.
4. Encourage the child to suck on ice chips.

58. The nurse is caring for a six-year-old who had a tonsillectomy this morning. Once the child is fully awake and alert, which liquid is the best to offer her?

1. A cherry popsicle
2. Apple juice
3. Orange juice
4. Cranberry juice

59. A 10-year-old has had diagnosed bronchial asthma for three years. The child has been admitted to the pediatric unit in acute respiratory distress. Which would be most characteristic of the child's asthmatic attack upon admission?

1. Expiratory wheezing
2. Inspiratory stridor
3. Cyanotic nail beds
4. Prolonged inspiratory phase

60. A child is admitted with asthma. Which aspects of the health history would be most closely associated with asthma?

1. The child's grandfather died of emphysema at age 76.
2. The child's grandmother died of lung cancer.
3. The child had respiratory distress syndrome following premature birth.
4. The child had eczema as an infant and toddler.

61. A stat dose of epinephrine is ordered for a child with asthma. How should the nurse administer the epinephrine?

1. Intramuscular
2. Sublingual
3. Subcutaneous
4. Nebulization

62. A child with an asthma attack has received epinephrine. The child is also to receive isoproteronol (Isuprel) via intermittent positive pressure breathing. When should the isoproteronol be given in relation to the epinephrine?

1. Isoproteronol should be given 30 minutes prior to the administration of epinephrine.

2. Isoproteronol should never be given in conjunction with epinephrine. Check with the physician.

3. Isoproteronol should not be given within one hour after the administration of epinephrine.

4. Isoproteronol should be given at the same time as epinephrine for maximum benefit.

63. A child is having an asthma attack. The nurse places the child in high-Fowler's position for which of the following reasons?

1. To prevent the aspiration of mucous

2. To visualize abnormal inspiratory excursion

3. To prevent atelectasis

4. To relieve dyspnea

64. A thirteen-month-old is diagnosed with croup and placed in a croup tent. Which toy is most appropriate for the nurse to give the child?

1. A doll made of cotton

2. A music box

3. A soft fuzzy toy made of synthetic materials

4. A wind-up bunny

65. The nurse is caring for a five-year-old who has cystic fibrosis. What should the nurse do to help the child manage secretions and avoid respiratory distress?

1. Administer continuous oxygen therapy.

2. Perform chest physiotherapy every four hours.

3. Administer pancreatic enzymes as ordered.

4. Encourage a diet high in calories.

66. The nurse is to administer pancreatic enzymes to an eight-month-old who has cystic fibrosis. When should this medication be administered?

1. A half hour before meals

2. With meals

3. An hour after meals

4. Between meals

67. A ten-month-old is being treated for otitis media. What is the most important nursing action to prevent recurrence of the infection?

1. Administer acetaminophen as ordered.

2. Encourage the parents to maintain a smoke-free home environment.

3. Explain to the parents that they must give the child all of the prescribed antibiotic therapy.

4. Encourage the parents to bottle-feed the child in an upright position.

68. The nurse is caring for a six-month-old infant who is in a croup tent. The child's mother calls and tells the nurse that the child's clothes are all wet. What is the best action for the nurse to take?

1. Explain to the mother that this is normal because the croup tent has high humidity.

2. Change the child's clothing.

3. Cover the child with a dry blanket.

4. Remove the child from the croup tent until his clothes are dry.

69. A five-year-old has cystic fibrosis. What is best to offer the child on a hot summer day?

1. Kool-aid

2. Ice cream

3. Lemonade

4. Broth

70. Which assessment finding in a 10-month-old indicates a need for further neurologic evaluation?

1. Inability to crawl

2. Speaking only 2–4 words

3. Inability to sit up without support

4. Presence of crude pincer grasp

71. What should the nurse do to protect a child from injury during a seizure?

1. Restrain the child's arms and legs.

2. Place a tongue blade in the child's mouth.

3. Place a pillow under the child's head.

4. Provide a waterproof pad for the bed.

72. The nurse is teaching the parents of a child who has cerebral palsy to feed a child. What position is best to recommend?

1. A normal eating position and provide stabilization of the jaw

2. A semi-reclining position

3. Upright while using a nasogastric or gastrostomy tube

4. Hyperextension of the neck

73. A one-year-old child is admitted to the pediatric unit with the diagnosis of bacterial meningitis. Which room should the nurse assign to this child?

1. A room with a two-year-old who had surgery for a hernia repair

2. A room with a one-year-old child who has pneumonia

3. A room with a two-year-old who has cerebral palsy

4. A private room with no roommates

74. The nurse is caring for an infant who is admitted with bacterial meningitis. What is the first priority when providing nursing care for this child?

1. Administer ordered antibiotics as soon as possible.

2. Keep the room quiet and dim.

3. Explain all procedures to the parents.

4. Begin low-flow oxygen via mask.

75. A newborn has a myelomeningocele. What is the most important nursing action prior to surgery?

1. Turn the infant every two hours.

2. Encourage holding and cuddling by the parents.

3. Apply sterile, moist, nonadherent dressings over the lesion.

4. Administer pain medication every 3–4 hours.

76. A three-year-old is being seen in the neurology clinic for a routine visit. The child had a repair of a myelomeningocele shortly after birth. The child's mother asks the nurse when she can accomplish bladder training. What is the best reply?

1. "You need to take your child to the bathroom every two hours."

2. "We will teach you how to do intermittent, clean catheterization."

3. "Continue to diaper the child until school age."

4. "Your child needs to learn how to do self-catheterization."

77. Which assessment regularly performed on newborns and infants will do most to help with early identification of infants who might have hydrocephalus?

    1. Head circumference
    2. Weight measurement
    3. Length measurement
    4. Presence of reflexes

78. How should the nurse position a four-month-old infant who has hydrocephalus?

    1. Side lying
    2. Sitting up in an infant seat
    3. Alternating prone and supine
    4. Left Sims

79. The parents of a child who has otitis media ask the nurse why the doctor told them to give the child acetaminophen instead of aspirin. What should the nurse include when answering?

    1. Acetaminophen is more effective against ear pain than aspirin.
    2. Acetaminophen is better at reducing temperature than aspirin.
    3. Aspirin may cause gastritis in children.
    4. Aspirin is thought to cause Reye's syndrome, a very serious disease.

80. The parents of a child who is newly diagnosed with Tay-Sachs disease ask the nurse if they have more children could they be affected. Which information should be included when responding to the parents?

    1. Boys are more likely to inherit the disease than girls.
    2. Tay-Sachs is not inherited, so there is little chance other children will have it.
    3. There is a one-in-four chance that each pregnancy will result in a child who has the disease.

    4. Fifty percent of the girls will have the disease.

81. When planning care for an infant who has Tay-Sachs, the nurse knows that the care is aimed at which of the following?

    1. Providing supportive care until the child dies
    2. Preventing spread of the disease to others
    3. Curing the underlying problem so the child will grow normally
    4. Providing for maximum development of the child

82. An infant is born with a meningomyelocele. How should the nurse position the infant before surgery?

    1. Prone with a pillow under the legs
    2. Supine with head elevated
    3. Sidelying with a pillow at the back
    4. Semi-Fowler's with a small pillow

83. The parents of a two-year-old who has meningitis ask the nurse why the lights are dim in the child's room even in the day time. What information should the nurse include in the answer?

    1. Rest is essential, and a dimly lit room promotes rest.
    2. The child is sensitive to light and may develop seizures.
    3. The IV medications are very sensitive to light.
    4. Light could cause severe damage to the eyes and possible blindness.

84. A six-year-old child is brought to the doctor's office with crusts on the eyelid and a very red conjunctiva. The doctor prescribes antibiotic eye drops. The child's mother asks the nurse if the child can go

back to school this afternoon. How should the nurse respond?

1. Teach the child not to touch his eyes, and take him back to school.

2. He should stay out of school today but can go back tomorrow.

3. He should stay out of school for a week because it usually takes a week for the condition to clear.

4. This condition is very contagious. The child should stay out of school for the next two days.

85. The nurse is administering eye drops to a child who has conjunctivitis. Where should the eye drops be placed?

1. On the pupil

2. In the conjunctival sac

3. By the inner canthus

4. On the sclera

86. The nurse is caring for a five-month-old infant who had a craniotomy following a head injury. Which observation the LPN/LVN makes should be reported to the charge nurse?

1. Respirations of 38

2. Difficulty arousing the baby from a nap

3. Pulse rate of 120

4. The baby cannot sit up by herself.

87. The nurse is caring for a child who has cerebral palsy. The nurse notes that the child does not writhe when sleeping but is in constant motion when awake. How should the nurse interpret this observation?

1. The child should be encouraged to do something productive so she will not think about writhing.

2. This indicates that the child could control the movements if she wanted to. A behavior modification program may be effective.

3. This is typical of cerebral palsy. The nurse should assist the child with ADL as needed.

4. The child should be sedated much of the time to prevent the dangerous writhing that occurs during waking.

88. A ten-year-old tells his neighbor, a nurse, that his eyes were "stuck together" this morning when he woke up. The nurse notes that his eyes are red and the conjunctiva is inflamed. What should the nurse neighbor recommend to the boy's mother?

1. Tell his mother that he may have a contagious disease and should be seen by his doctor today.

2. Encourage the mother to make an appointment to see the eye doctor.

3. Suggest to the mother that the boy go to school today but make an appointment with the doctor if the condition does not clear up soon.

4. Explain to the boy that he should wash his face and eyes with a wash cloth as soon as he wakes up.

89. The nurse is caring for an infant who has had surgery for a meningomyelocele. When thinking of long-term care needs, which understanding is most accurate?

   1. The surgery corrects the defect, and the infant should develop normally.
   2. The infant will probably have lower body paralysis and bowel and bladder dysfunction.
   3. The infant should develop normally physically but is likely to have some degree of mental retardation.
   4. The surgery may need to be repeated if the condition recurs.

90. The nurse is teaching the mother of a newborn who has a cleft lip and palate to feed the infant. Which would be least appropriate to include?

   1. Place the tip of the asepto at the front of the baby's mouth so that the baby can suck.
   2. Rinse the mouth with sterile water after each feeding to minimize infections.
   3. Feed the baby in an upright position and bubble frequently to reduce air in the stomach.
   4. Apply lanolin to lips to reduce dryness associated with mouth breathing.

91. The mother of a two-month-old infant with a cleft lip and palate calls the clinic. She tells the nurse that the baby has a temperature of 102°, has been turning her head from side to side, and has been eating poorly. What should the nurse advise?

   1. Clean the baby's ears with warm water.
   2. Give the baby infant Tylenol 0.3 cc and call back in four hours after taking her temperature.
   3. Bring the baby into the clinic for evaluation.
   4. Give the baby 4 ounces of water and retake her temperature in one hour.

92. A three-month-old infant is hospitalized for repair of a cleft lip. Following surgery, the baby returns to the unit with a Logan bow in place. The baby is awake and beginning to whimper. The baby's color is pink and pulse is 120 with respirations of 38. An IV is ordered in the baby's right hand at 15 cc per hour. The fluid is not infusing well. Her right hand is edematous. The jacket restraint has loosened, and one arm has partially come out. What is the priority nursing action?

   1. Recheck the baby's vital signs.
   2. Check the baby's IV site for infiltration.
   3. Check to see if the baby has voided.
   4. Replace the restraints securely.

93. Following surgery for repair of a cleft lip, it is important to prevent excessive crying by the infant. What should the nurse do to accomplish this?

   1. Give the baby a pacifier to meet his/her sucking needs.
   2. Place the baby in the usual sleeping position, which is on the abdomen.
   3. Ask the baby's mother to stay and hold the child.
   4. Request a special nurse to hold the infant.

94. The nurse is doing discharge planning and establishing long-term goals for an infant who had a cleft lip repair. The baby also has a cleft palate. Which long-term goal is most appropriate and necessary for this child?

   1. Prevent joint contractures.
   2. Promote adequate speech.
   3. Promote bowel regularity.
   4. Prevent infection of surgical incision.

95. The nurse is caring for an eight-month-old infant who has had diarrhea for two days. Which is the most useful in assessing the degree of dehydration?

   1. Number of stools

2. Skin turgor

3. Mucous membranes

4. Daily weight

96. An infant who has severe diarrhea and dehydration is hospitalized and is NPO. Intravenous fluids are ordered. What is the immediate goal of care?

   1. Restoration of intravascular volume

   2. Prevention of further diarrhea

   3. Promotion of skin integrity

   4. Maintenance of normal growth and development

97. The nurse is caring for a nine-month-old infant who is allowed only clear fluids. What are the most appropriate liquids for the nurse to offer?

   1. 7-Up and ginger ale

   2. Pedialyte and glucose water

   3. Half-strength formula

   4. Tea and clear broth

98. The nurse is caring for an infant who is being treated for severe diarrhea. Twenty-four hours after admission, the diet is advanced from NPO to clear liquids. After clear liquids are started, the baby has four stools in two hours. What should the nurse do?

   1. Continue oral feedings.

   2. Take the pulse, temperature, and respirations.

   3. Stop feeding the child orally.

   4. Weigh the child.

99. A 12-month-old who was diagnosed at birth as having Hirschsprung's disease has been maintained at home under conservative treatment. The parents have brought the child to the clinic for a well-baby examination. After interviewing the child's parents, the nurse concludes that an appropriate

treatment regime is being followed. Which of the following would indicate this?

   1. Use of tap water enemas and a low-residue diet

   2. Use of soap suds enema and a high-fiber diet

   3. Use of isotonic saline enemas and a high-fiber diet

   4. Use of isotonic saline enemas and a low-residue diet

100. A three-month-old is admitted to the pediatric unit with a diagnosis of Hirschsprung's disease. What is most important when monitoring the infant's status?

   1. Weigh the infant every morning.

   2. Maintain intake and output records.

   3. Measure abdominal girth every four hours.

   4. Check serum electrolyte levels.

101. An infant who has Hirschsprung's disease is scheduled for surgery. Which explanation should the nurse include when discussing the upcoming surgery with the parents?

   1. They will need to learn colostomy care because the child will have a permanent colostomy.

   2. The baby will have tap water enemas until clear before the surgery.

   3. The baby will have a temporary colostomy to allow the bowel time to heal.

   4. They will need to learn how to administer gastrostomy feedings while the colostomy is present.

102. A five-week-old infant is seen in the physician's office for gastroesophageal reflux. What should the nurse suggest to the parents regarding feeding practices?

1. Dilute the formula to facilitate better absorption.
2. Position the child at a 30°–45° angle after feedings.
3. Change from milk-based formula to soy-based formula.
4. Delay burping to prevent vomiting.

103. Which assessment finding would the nurse expect in an infant diagnosed with pyloric stenosis?

1. Abdominal rigidity
2. Ribbon-like stools
3. Visible waves of peristalsis
4. Rectal prolapse

104. An infant has had frequent episodes of green, mucous-containing stools. The nursing assessment reveals that the infant has dry mucous membranes, poor skin turgor, and an absence of tearing. Based on these data, what is the most appropriate nursing diagnosis?

1. Impaired skin integrity related to irritation caused by frequent, loose stools
2. Deficient fluid volume related to frequent, loose stools
3. Impaired comfort related to abdominal cramping and diarrhea
4. Imbalanced nutrition: less than body requirements related to diarrhea

105. The nurse is caring for an infant admitted with diarrhea, poor skin turgor, and dry mucous membranes. Which laboratory data would cause the nurse the most concern?

1. Sodium 140 mmol/l
2. Urine specific gravity 1.035
3. Hematocrit 38%
4. Potassium 4 mmol/l

106. Following surgery for pyloric stenosis, a five-week-old infant is started on glucose water. When will infant formula be started?

1. Following the return of bowel sounds
2. After vital signs are stable
3. When the infant is able to retain clear liquids
4. When there is no evidence of diarrhea

107. The nurse is feeding a newborn infant glucose water. Which finding would make the nurse suspect the infant has esophageal atresia?

1. The infant has projectile vomiting.
2. The infant sucks very slowly.
3. The infant seems fatigued after only a few sucks.
4. The infant chokes after taking a few sucks of water.

108. The parents of an infant who has esophageal atresia ask the nurse how the baby will eat. Which response by the nurse is most accurate?

1. "A tube will be passed from the nose to the stomach."
2. "The doctor will place a tube through the abdomen into the baby's stomach."
3. "Your baby will be given nutrients through a vein."
4. "Your baby can tolerate small feedings given frequently."

109. The nurse is teaching the parents of a child who has celiac disease about the dietary modifications that need to be made. Which foods, if selected by the parents, indicate an understanding of the child's dietary needs?

1. Toast, orange juice, and an egg
2. Rice cake, milk, and a banana
3. Crackers, apple juice, and a hot dog
4. Hamburger, grape juice, and fries

110. A three-year-old child is admitted with a diagnosis of nephrotic syndrome. Which signs and symptoms would the nurse expect the parents to report when the child is admitted?

    1. Jaundiced skin and pale stools
    2. Blood in the urine and high fever
    3. Chest pain and shortness of breath
    4. Puffy eyes and weight gain

111. Which assessment by the nurse would best indicate that a child with nephrotic syndrome is responding appropriately to treatment?

    1. The child has more energy.
    2. The child's pulse rate increases.
    3. The child's appetite improves.
    4. The child weighs less.

112. A three-year-old is admitted with a tentative diagnosis of Wilm's tumor. What nursing action is essential because of the diagnosis?

    1. Avoid palpating the abdomen.
    2. Encourage the child to eat adequately.
    3. Give emotional support to the parents.
    4. Keep the child on strict bed rest.

113. A three-year-old is brought to the physician's office by the parent. The parent states that the child was completely toilet trained but has been "having accidents" recently. The parent also tells the nurse that the child is voiding more often than usual and that the urine has a strong odor. What is the best response by the nurse?

    1. "These could be symptoms of a urinary tract infection. We should obtain a urine specimen for analysis."
    2. "Many preschool children regress when something stressful happens. Has your child been under any stress lately?"
    3. "Accidents like these are not unusual. You have nothing to worry about as long as your child does not have a fever."

    4. "This is very unusual. Your child will probably need to be hospitalized to receive intravenous antibiotics."

114. A four-year-old has been admitted to the nursing unit with a diagnosis of nephrotic syndrome. The symptoms include generalized edema with weight gain, hypoproteinemia, hyperlipidemia, hypotension, and decreased urine output. In developing a nursing care plan for this child, which nursing diagnosis would be highest priority?

    1. Risk for imbalanced nutrition: less than body requirements related to protein loss and poor appetite
    2. Infection related to edema secondary to nephrotic syndrome
    3. Fluid volume excess related to nephrotic syndrome
    4. Disturbed body image related to edema

115. The nurse is caring for an infant born with exstrophy of the bladder. What will be included in the care of this infant?

    1. Give continuous saline irrigations of the exposed bladder.
    2. Cover the exposed bladder with petrolatum gauze.
    3. Insert an indwelling catheter.
    4. Apply a tight-fitting, super-absorbent diaper.

116. A five-year-old had an orchiopexy this morning. Which nursing action is essential?

    1. Tell the parents not to disturb the tension mechanism until the physician removes it in a week or 10 days.
    2. Explain to the parents that the child has a good chance of being sterile.
    3. Teach the parents how to help the child with leg exercises.
    4. Encourage the parents to join a support group related to the child's condition.

117. The parents of a newborn with hypospadias ask the nurse why the doctor told them the baby could not be circumcised. What is the best response?

   1. The infant is not stable enough for the procedure.

   2. The deformity makes circumcision impossible.

   3. The foreskin will need to be used later to repair the defect.

   4. Circumcision is not currently recommended for most infants.

118. A two-year-old has just been diagnosed with a Wilm's tumor. Surgery is recommended. The parents tell the nurse that they feel they are being pushed into surgery and wonder if they should wait and get more opinions. What information is essential for the nurse to include when responding to the parents?

   1. Surgery is one of several options for treating a Wilm's tumor.

   2. Surgery is an essential part of the treatment for Wilm's tumor and must be done immediately.

   3. Surgery can be safely delayed for up to a year after diagnosis.

   4. Wilm's tumor has been successfully treated by chemotherapy and radiation therapy.

119. The parents of a five-year-old ask the nurse in the doctor's office what they should do about their child who is still wetting the bed several nights a week. In addition to reporting this to the physician, what suggestion should be included in the nurse's discussion with the parents?

   1. Do not give the child anything to drink after the evening meal.

   2. Have the child wear diapers to bed.

   3. Suggest that they promise the child a sleepover party if the child stays dry for two weeks.

   4. Punish the child each time he wets the bed.

120. A 13-month-old has just been placed in a hip spica cast to correct a congenital anomaly. Which nursing actions should be included in the plan of care?

   1. Turn the child no more than every four hours to minimize manipulation of the wet cast.

   2. Use only fingertips when moving the child to prevent indentations in the cast.

   3. Assess and document neurovascular function at least every two hours.

   4. Use a hair dryer to speed the cast drying process.

121. A 13-year-old has just arrived on the nursing care unit from the Post Anesthesia Care Unit. This morning, the child underwent a surgical spinal fusion procedure that included the placement of Harrington rods for the treatment of scoliosis. After receiving a report from the PACU nurse, which action should the nurse perform first?

   1. Assess the pain level and administer analgesics as needed.

   2. Offer clear liquids to ensure adequate hydration.

   3. Drain the Hemovac and record the output on the intake and output record.

   4. Notify the child's parents of his/her arrival on the unit.

122. A newborn has been diagnosed as having mild hip dysplasia. The mother asks the nurse why the physician told her to "triple diaper" the baby. What should the nurse include when responding?

1. It is important that there be no contamination of the area.

2. Extra diapers will abduct the hips and help to put the hip in the socket correctly.

3. Triple diapers cause the baby's legs to be sharply flexed and realign the hip.

4. Hip dysplasia can cause abnormal stooling.

123. A six-month-old is placed in bilateral leg casts because she has talipes equinovarus. The mother asks how to bathe the baby. What should the nurse tell the mother?

   1. "Bathe the baby as you usually do."
   2. "Put the baby's buttocks in the bath water, but try to keep the feet out of the water."
   3. "Sponge bathe your baby until the casts are removed."
   4. "Give the baby a bath in the baby bath tub, but limit the time in the water."

124. The nurse is providing home care for an eight-year-old boy who has Legg-Calve Perthes Disease. The boy asks the nurse to let him get out of bed to go to walk to the bathroom. What should the nurse do?

   1. Allow the child to get up and walk to the bathroom.
   2. Explain to him that he must stay in bed so that his hip can heal.
   3. Allow him up to the bathroom if he has no pain.
   4. Encourage his mother to talk with the physician about his desire to be out of bed.

125. The nurse has been asked to set up a program to screen children for scoliosis. What age group should the nurse screen?

   1. Preschoolers
   2. Six-to-eight year olds
   3. Junior high students
   4. College-age students

126. A 12-year-old girl has been diagnosed with scoliosis and is placed in a Milwaukee brace. What instruction should the nurse give about the brace?

   1. "Put the brace on underneath all of your clothes."
   2. "Wear the brace only when you are exercising."
   3. "Wear the brace only when you are in bed or resting."
   4. "Put an undershirt on before putting the brace on."

127. The nurse is caring for a child who has Duchenne's muscular dystrophy. What understanding is correct about the progress of the disease?

   1. The disease is controllable with aggressive treatment.
   2. Most children will die of something else before they die of muscular dystrophy.
   3. Brothers of children with muscular dystrophy should be evaluated for the disease.
   4. Muscular dystrophy causes its victims to become incoherent and often violent.

128. The nurse is caring for a child who is diagnosed as having Lyme disease. The mother asks how the child got this disease. Which explanation about Lyme disease is correct?

   1. It is transmitted by a mosquito.
   2. It is inherited through a recessive gene.
   3. It is caused by a deer tick bite.
   4. It is caused by contact with the oil from plant leaves.

129. The nurse is caring for a child who has Lyme disease and one who has rheumatoid arthritis. What problem are they most likely to have in common?

1. Joint pain
2. High fever
3. Risk for urinary tract infection
4. Risk for cardiac dysrhythmias

130. Which of the following children would most likely be diagnosed with pituitary dwarfism?

1. A 13-month-old who weighs 21 pounds
2. A 4-year-old who is 41 inches tall
3. A 9-year-old who has no permanent teeth
4. A 15-year-old girl who has not begun to menstruate

131. A five-year-old has been diagnosed with congenital hypopituitarism. Which should be included when teaching the parents about this child's condition?

1. You will probably need to give him subcutaneous injections of human growth hormone three to seven times a week at bedtime.
2. Your child is unlikely to achieve normal intelligence and will probably need special schooling.
3. All the other children in the family should be evaluated to see if they have any of the same signs of the condition.
4. Your child is likely to have emotional problems related to growth retardation and should be referred to a psychiatrist soon.

132. The nurse at a summer camp for diabetics is assisting a 15-year-old with adjusting her daily insulin dosage. Which factor will have the greatest impact on insulin needs?

1. The weather forecast calls for high temperature and high humidity.

2. Activities scheduled for the day include a hike in the woods, swim time, and tennis.
3. The girl started her period the previous evening.
4. Daily insulin dose should never be changed, because consistency is important.

133. The nurse is working at a summer camp for diabetic children. A seven-year-old comes to the nurse complaining of dizziness and nausea. It is a warm day and the child has just returned from horseback riding, followed by a walk back from the stables. The nurse notes that the child is sweaty. Which action should the nurse take first?

1. Give the child a cool drink of water.
2. Give the child three units of regular insulin and observe for a response.
3. Give the child three crackers to eat and observe for a response.
4. Have the child rest in the infirmary and re-evaluate in 20 minutes.

134. A four-year-old has recently been diagnosed with Insulin Dependent Diabetes Mellitus (IDDM). The parents tell the nurse that they do not understand much about diabetes. Which is the best way to explain IDDM to them?

1. IDDM is an inborn error of metabolism that makes the child unable to burn fatty acids without insulin requirements.
2. IDDM is a genetic disorder that makes the child unable to metabolize protein without insulin supplements.
3. IDDM is a deficiency in the secretion of insulin by the pancreas, which makes the child unable to metabolize carbohydrates without insulin supplements.
4. IDDM is a problem that occurs when children eat too many sweets early in life and then are unable to metabolize sugar without insulin supplements.

135. A one-month-old is seen in the clinic and is diagnosed as having congenital hypothyroidism (cretinism). Her parents ask the nurse if their child will be normal. What is the best response for the nurse?

1. Your child will need to take medication for life but has a good chance of normal development because of the early detection.

2. Cretinism causes both physical delay and mental retardation in the vast majority of children with the condition.

3. There is no way to tell at this point if there is permanent damage; your child will need continual evaluation.

4. Your child will need to take medication until puberty is completed; if there are no serious problems by then, your child should be perfectly normal.

136. A child is seen in the physician's office for a crusty lesion at the corners of his mouth. The lesion has a yellow crust. The arms and legs also have similar lesions. The physician diagnoses impetigo and prescribes an antibiotic. What teaching is appropriate for the nurse who is working with the child and parents?

1. Help the parents understand the need for an elimination diet.

2. Instruct the parents to put antibiotic ointment under the fingernails as well as on the lesions.

3. Describe what the poison ivy plant looks like.

4. Inform the parents not to let the child share a comb or a hat with anyone.

137. The mother of a child who has ringworm asks what kind of worm the child has. How should the nurse respond?

1. Ringworm is caused by a fungus, not a worm. The lesion often takes the form a circle or ring.

2. The same worm that causes pinworms can cause ringworm. Good handwashing is essential to prevent spreading.

3. The worm is often on plants and leaves, such as those that cause poison ivy.

4. Worms that are on house plants and common garden plants can cause ringworm.

138. The mother of a child who has pediculosis says that she plans to use kerosene to wash the child's hair just like her grandmother did for her. What is the best response for the nurse?

1. "Your grandmother was a wise woman. Kerosene is the major ingredient in the special shampoo we recommend."

2. "Kerosene will work, but the shampoo we recommend is less irritating."

3. "Kerosene can cause serious injury to your child. Try using the shampoos which are not dangerous."

4. "Your grandmother was not a physician. Please do what the doctor recommends."

139. A five-year-old child keeps developing poison ivy. The child's mother insists that the child has not been near any poison ivy plants since the first outbreak several weeks ago. What question should the nurse ask the mother?

1. "Has your child been eating any particular food that might be associated with outbreaks?"

2. "Does your child scratch the blisters and touch the liquid that comes out?"

3. "Does your child ever share combs or hats with other children?"

4. "Do you have a cat or a dog that goes outdoors?"

140. A 10-month-old infant is hospitalized with severe eczema. The child has elbow restraints applied. When should the elbow restraints be removed?

1. They should not be removed until the lesions have healed.

2. When someone is holding the baby

3. Once a shift to check for circulation

4. When the baby is asleep

Answers and Rationales

1. (4) Sitting with slight support would be expected in a child of 5 months. All of the other tasks are appropriate for this age.

2. (3) Anything that can be put in the mouth is inappropriate for a child with cleft lip repair. A rattle and beads can go in the mouth. Button eyes are a hazard for any infant because they may swallow them. A mobile with a music box is appropriate for a three-month-old who lays in a crib, and this item cannot be put in the mouth. Note that a colorful rattle is also age-appropriate but not condition-appropriate.

3. (1) Soft, washable toys of smooth, nonallergenic material should be used. Stuffed toys are contraindicated. Puzzles and games are not age-appropriate. Toy cars could be used for scratching and should be avoided. Toy cars are also not age-appropriate.

4. (4) Peek-a-boo is appropriate for an eight-month-old. Peek-a-boo helps the infant with the concept of object permanence; things that are out of sight do exist. An eight-month-old can sit up; once an infant can sit up, the mobiles should be removed as they can strangle an infant who might try to stand up. An eight-month-old infant cannot stack large blocks yet. A colorful rattle is more appropriate for a younger infant.

5. (1) Stringing large beads is appropriate for 12 months. Note that the beads are large and

therefore not subject to being swallowed. A riding toy and small puzzles would be more appropriate for a toddler. Paste, paper, and scissors are appropriate for a preschooler when used with supervision.

6. (2) An 18-month-old child cannot understand explanations. The nurse needs to assess the patient's knowledge and base teaching on that assessment. The nurse should not assume that no teaching is needed just because the child has had the procedure before. There is no data to indicate that the parents upset the child. They do appear to be smothering the child, but at this time the child would probably be more miserable without the parents. The nurse may want to teach parents about growth and development needs of the toddler.

7. (2) An 18-month-old should be able to feed himself and drink from a cup. He may be messy. A five- or six-year-old can usually button a shirt and tie shoes. Cutting with scissors is appropriate for a preschool child. A two-year-old can go up and down stairs with both feet on the same step, and a three-year-old child can go up and down stairs by alternating feet.

8. (1) Temper tantrums are common and normal in a two-year-old because he is developing autonomy. As long as the child is safe, he should be ignored. Giving in to the child's demands is likely to reinforce the negative behavior and create a long-term pattern of behavior. The nurse should not recommend to the parents that they spank a child. Promising a reward to stop crying is bribing the child and should not be recommended. A two-year-old who is having a temper tantrum is not likely to listen to explanations.

9. (3) The child's teddy bear and security blanket will help to give the child a sense of security. Spending the night would be ideal, but it may not be possible for this mother with two children at home. It is part of the normal separation reaction for a three-year-old to be

upset when the mother leaves. The parents should visit even if the child cries when they leave. Buying a gift will provide less security than bringing the child's favorite comfort items to the hospital.

10. (2) It is normal for a three-year-old to cry when the parents leave. The child will probably not wave good-bye even though he/she is able to. The child is not likely to hide under the covers. The child will likely be too upset to ask to go to the playroom.

11. (2) A sandbox is appropriate for outdoor play. A four-year-old is too young for a two-wheeled bike or for climbing a tree without strict supervision. He is probably past the age of pushing a toy lawn mower, which is more appropriate for a toddler.

12. (3) Five-year-old children like cooperative play, such as playing house. The other activities are solitary activities. Note that the child is several days post surgery. Most five-year-olds are not able to read a book by themselves. Playing a board game with a child is not wrong, but it is a solitary activity. Most five-year-olds would prefer to play with other children. There is almost always a better alternative than turning on the television. This child is several days post surgery and is able to be up and play with others.

13. (3) A six-year-old is apt to be loosing baby teeth. This is an important consideration when anesthesia is to be administered and the child will be intubated. The nurse should assess for loose teeth in any school-age child who is admitted for surgery or other procedures requiring intubation of any kind.

14. (4) By discussing with the child the reasons for the child's fears, the child will feel less afraid and less abnormal. Discussion of fears should be individualized. The child is not old enough to make care decisions. The child should, however, be given some input into the care plan. The child might decide which site the nurse will use for an injection but not whether or not the medication will be given. The parents will make those decisions.

15. (1) A six-year-old learns best by doing. A six-year-old can not conceptualize what he/she cannot see. Touring the operating room and surgical ICU can be very frightening for a six-year-old. Drawing pictures of the procedure would be more appropriate post-operatively, when the nurse may want to help him in understanding what happened to him. Drawing pictures is a good way to express feelings that a six-year-old cannot put into words. It is more appropriate post-operatively. Group discussion is more appropriate for an adolescent. A six-year-old does not have the verbal skills to participate in and learn from a discussion group.

16. (3) Craft work allows her to accomplish something while meeting her needs for rest. Industry is the developmental task for school-age children. The joint pains with rheumatic fever tend to be in the large joints, not the small ones, so craft work utilizing finger activity would probably not be painful. Stringing large wooden beads is appropriate for younger children. Pillow fighting requires too much energy for a child on bed rest and is not appropriate for a hospital environment. Watching television is a solitary activity with no sense of accomplishment.

17. (2) Pounding movements allow for the expression of aggression. The other activities would not allow for an expression of aggression. The scenario describes a child who is expressing aggression in a very physical manner. This child is not likely to respond well to writing a story. Writing a story could be used to help a child express aggression, but pounding clay is more appropriate given the child's aggressive behavior.

18. (3) Hero worship is very common among school-age children. Denial would be manifested by saying that his leg really is not broken. Repression is putting an upsetting or

guilt-laden experience deep in the unconscious mind. This behavior does not suggest repression. Fantasy is living in a make-believe world. This boy shows no evidence of living in a make-believe world.

19. (2) Building with popsicle sticks will foster his sense of industry and can be done while he is in bed in traction. Puppets and coloring would be more appropriate for younger children. Watching television will not promote his development, although it can be used as diversion occasionally.

20. (3) The child's behavior is typical of the despair phase of toddler responses to anxiety. The child should cry. Lying quietly, sucking his thumb, and saying nothing are suggestive of severe anxiety, a bad adjustment to the hospital, and no comfort with the nurses. This anxiety response does not suggest a poor relationship with his parents. In fact, his severe separation anxiety may be because he is so close to his parents.

21. (4) Temper tantrums are a normal response to limit setting in a two-year-old child. Answer 1 might be correct if the child were older. However, temper tantrums in a two-year-old child do not indicate regression; rather, they are normal for this age. Tantrums are not suggestive of a poorly developed sense of trust; they are normal. Ignoring the tantrum is preferable to discipline when a two-year-old has a tantrum.

22. (4) The best response is to simply state that it is time for sleep and to give the child her security blanket or toy. Answer 1, telling the child that she isn't loved because she won't listen, is not therapeutic. Answer 2 implies that if you don't go to bed on time, you are not a good child. This is not a good suggestion to implant in a child. Answer 3 is bribery and is not appropriate.

23. (3) An eight-year-old is concerned about pain and mutilation. An eight-year-old has an understanding that death is the end of life as we know it and would be unlikely to respond

with Answers 1 or 2. Answers 1 and 2 are typical of a preschooler. Answer 4 is typical of an adolescent who wants to leave a legacy.

24. (3) A four-month-old should follow objects with her eyes. A four-month-old is not likely to be able to sit up by herself. This behavior is seen at six months of age. Not being able to hold the rattle as well as she did at first is typical of the time after the loss of the grasp reflex and before pincer movement is established. Most newborn reflexes are gone by about four months of age. Spitting up after a feeding is normal four-month-old behavior.

25. (3) Riding a tricycle is three-year-old behavior. Remember "three years, three wheels." Children start to walk at about one year of age. Throwing a large ball and stating his name are two-year-old behaviors. Remember to use developmental trends when determining the most recently acquired behavior: head to tail and simple to complex. Look for a complex lower-body behavior.

26. (2) The child will have an elevated body temperature. Contrary to what you might expect, metabolism is increased following aspirin overdose. The child will be hot and flushed. Hyperpyrexia means high temperature. The child will be in metabolic acidosis from the acid load of the aspirin. Compensation for metabolic acidosis is rapid, deep breathing. The first choice is incorrect; the child will be hyperventilating and will be flushed, not pale. The third choice is not correct, the temperature will be high, not low. Bleeding may occur following aspirin ingestion, but not initially. The fourth choice is not correct. Melena is hidden blood in the stool. It will take some time for a GI bleed to develop and pass through the stool. Bradycardia will not be present. The child will have tachycardia.

27. (4) Since the child is breathing, there is no need for CPR or ventilatory support. Because the child is difficult to arouse, gastric lavage rather than syrup of ipecac will be given.

28. (2) At six months of age, the nurse would expect to administer the third DTP, the third hepatitis B, and the third Hemophilus influenza B (HIB) immunizations. MMR (measles, mumps, and rubella) is not given until 15 months of age. IPV is given at two months and four months and then again at 18 months and preschool. Varicella vaccine is given between the ages of one year and 12 years.

29. (3) Chicken pox is contagious as long as there are fluid-filled vesicles. Scabs are not contagious. The child will have scabs for a while. The fever may be down, but if there are fluid-filled vesicles, the child is contagious.

30. (1) Eating paint is one of the major risk factors for lead poisoning. Temper tantrums are normal in a two-year-old. Most two-year-olds are not toilet trained. Most two-year-olds are messy eaters.

31. (1) Atrial septal defect is not associated with Tetralogy of Fallot. The four defects are pulmonary stenosis, which causes right ventricular hypertrophy, ventricular septal defect, and overriding aorta.

32. (1) The squatting position will help the child with tetralogy to have better hemodynamics. It increases intraabdominal pressure and increases pulmonary blood flow. Placing the child in a lying or standing position will increase his symptoms and be counter-productive. It is not necessary to call for help because this is not an emergency situation.

33. (2) The child will have to learn to cough and deep-breathe post-operatively. Studies demonstrate that pre-operative teaching makes it easier for the client to perform coughing and deep-breathing exercises in the post-operative period. The nurses will do strict hand washing, not the client. Fluids will likely be restricted post-operatively. It is important to teach the client about positions of comfort, but it is more important to teach the child how to deep-breathe and cough.

34. (3) Chest drainage is positioned below bed level to prevent the reflux of material into the chest cavity.

35. (3) Activity intolerance related to feeding is often a key sign of a serious cardiac problem in an infant. Taking only 45 cc of formula in 45 minutes at three weeks of age probably indicates difficulty sucking. This is definitely not normal. The fact that the infant's color is pink at rest does not tell you what happens during exertion, such as with eating. Asking about skin color during feeding is a good first question to ask. Answers 1 and 2 are incorrect because they interpret the infant's behavior as normal, which it is not. Answer 4 is not correct. It does identify the behavior as abnormal but suggests comparing it to the child's siblings. This is not the appropriate question to ask to get the most information.

36. (1) The catheter is passed into the chambers of the heart, and oxygen levels can be measured. The cardiac catheter does not assess pulmonary vascularization. Coronary arteries can be visualized, however. An abdominal aortic aneurysm is diagnosed with an arteriogram, not a cardiac catheterization. A cardiac catheterization gives information about the heart structures but does not give information about activity tolerance.

37. (4) During a cardiac catheterization, a catheter is inserted into the heart; the infection that the client is most at risk for is, therefore, endocarditis. Urinary tract infection, pneumonia, and otitis media are not related to a client undergoing a cardiac catheterization.

38. (3) Weight is the best indicator of fluid balance. Congestive heart failure causes fluid retention. Sacral edema is positionally dependent. Weight will give a better indication of the child's status. Clubbing of the fingers and toes is an indication of chronic hypoxemia, not the status of his current congestive heart failure. Fluid and food intake is a general indicator of his status

and is not particularly related to his current congestive heart failure.

39. (4) The body tries to compensate for chronic oxygen deficiency by making additional red cells to transport oxygen. The additional red cells increase the hematocrit, which is the percent of blood that is RBCs. Chronic infection is more likely to cause anemia. Recent dehydration will cause an elevated hematocrit because there is less fluid in the blood. However, there is no indication that the child is dehydrated, and we are told that he has a cyanotic heart defect, which makes him chronically hypoxic. Therefore, answer 4 is better than answer 2. Answer 3, increased cardiac output, is also incorrect. Increased cardiac output does not cause an elevated hematocrit.

40. (3) A pulse below 100 in a 10-month-old child who is taking digoxin most likely indicates digoxin toxicity. The nurse should withhold the medication and notify the physician. The normal pulse for this age is about 120 or a little more at rest. The pulse rate does not tell us that the child needs to have his/her potassium level checked. If the child is also taking Lasix or another potassium-depleting diuretic, then the potassium should be checked.

41. (3) The child should be on a sodium-restricted diet with high-potassium foods because he is taking Hydrodiuril, a potassium-depleting diuretic. Apricots and bananas are low in sodium and high in potassium. Cheese and ice cream are high in sodium. Hot dogs are high in sodium. Whole milk is high in sodium. Not only is potassium needed, but excessive sodium should be avoided because those with severe heart defects are prone to fluid retention.

42. (1) The knee-chest or squat position increases intraabdominal pressure and increases blood flow to the lungs. Oxygen is also indicated because the child is hypoxic. Positioning on the side is not appropriate because it will not improve the blood flow to the lungs. There is

no need to ask the parents to leave. In fact, they need to know how to handle these episodes if they are not yet comfortable doing so. Children with cyanotic heart defects have hypoxic episodes fairly regularly. Positioning in the squat position is more important at this time than notifying the physician.

43. (2) The child's mother does not let the child play with others and appears to do everything for the child. She seems to be overprotective. Most children with heart defects are capable of doing most age-appropriate activities. There is no evidence to support that the child is mentally retarded. There is no data to support that the child has regressed.

44. (3) Before the nurse can teach the parents, it will be necessary to reassess their needs and concerns. The question asks for the best *initial* action. Initially, the nurse should assess. Later, the nurse may emphasize the toddler's need for autonomy. The nurse may provide the child with opportunities to develop autonomy, although it would be better to teach the parents. The nurse may also discuss the success of the surgery and how well the child is doing, but this is not the initial action.

45. (3) Excessive drooling is a sign of epiglottitis. A child with epiglottitis is apt to have a high fever. Retching is not typical. Retractions could occur if respiratory distress were great enough, but drooling is the hallmark of epiglottitis.

46. (1) Examining the child's throat with a tongue blade may cause the epiglottis to become so irritated that it will close off completely and obstruct the airway. The child should be placed in a semi- to high-Fowler's position. Humidity is not a problem. A nasopharyngeal culture would not cause problems. The nurse should not get a throat culture, however.

47. (3) H. Influenza is the usual causative agent of epiglottitis. A puppy would be more apt to cause asthma than epiglottitis.

48. (2) Sitting upright and leaning forward, supporting self with hands, is the position

typically assumed by children with epiglottitis. It helps to promote the airway and drainage of secretions. Squatting is more typically seen in children who have cyanotic heart defects.

49. (4) The child with an edematous glottis will keep his mouth open with his tongue protruding to increase free movement in the pharynx. In the presence of potential laryngeal obstruction, laryngeal stridor can be heard especially during inspiration. Rales and diminished breath sounds are more typical of croup. Cyanosis is typical of late-stage, extremely critical respiratory distress.

50. (3) In a child with epiglottitis the first signs of difficulty in breathing can progress to severe inspiratory distress or complete airway obstruction in a matter of minutes or hours. The child usually has a high fever, but airway takes precedence. High humidity may also be appropriate, but the highest priority is maintaining an airway.

51. (1) Regular monitoring of cardiac rate is essential, because a rapidly rising heart rate is an initial indication of hypoxia and impending obstruction of the airway. The blood pressure and temperature may well be monitored, but they are not the most important. An IV will be monitored, if present, but is not the highest priority.

52. (4) Pets, smoke, and changes in temperature can all precipitate asthma. A fruit salad is least likely to precipitate an asthma attack. It is possible that someone could be allergic to something in a fruit salad, but these are not common asthma triggers.

53. (2) These are symptoms of an adverse response to aminophylline. The IV should be stopped and the physician notified immediately. The child may be going into shock.

54. (2) Blowing will extend the expiratory phase of respiration and help the child with asthma exhale more completely. Blowing cotton balls

is exhalation, not inhalation. It does not develop accessory muscles of respiration.

55. (1) The most common and serious complication following tonsillectomy is hemorrhage. The nurse should ask about bleeding tendencies. Information about any familial adverse responses may be nice to know but is not as important as information about the child's tendency to bleed. The child's perception of the surgery is also nice to know but is not the most important information. The frequency and type of tonsil infections is nice to know but not essential.

56. (3) Because the child is sleepy, the child should be semi-prone to prevent aspiration in case the child vomits. When the child is alert, she can be in semi-Fowler's. Trendelenburg position is contraindicated because it would cause more swelling in the operative area.

57. (3) Continual swallowing indicates bleeding. The surgeon should be notified at once. None of the other responses is appropriate. The child may be hemorrhaging.

58. (2) The child needs clear, cold liquids that are not red and are not citrus. Red would make it difficult to determine if vomitus was blood or juice.

59. (1) Bronchial constriction occurs in asthma. This increases the airway resistance to airflow. The respiratory difficulty is accentuated during expiration, when the bronchi are supposed to contract and shorten, as opposed to inspiration, when the bronchi are dilating and elongating. Inspiratory stridor is characteristic of croup. Note that answers 2 and 4 both deal with the inspiratory phase. Asthma affects the expiratory phase.

60. (4) Asthma is an allergic condition and frequently follows eczema, also an allergic condition. Relatives having emphysema or lung cancer is not usually related to childhood asthma. Respiratory distress syndrome as an infant does not predispose the child to asthma.

61. (3) Epinephrine is a rapid-acting drug of short duration. The subcutaneous route is the most effective for rapid relief of respiratory distress. The stat dose is not given intramuscular, sublingual, or by nebulizer.

62. (3) The side effects of epinephrine (tachycardia, rise in blood pressure, tremors, weakness, and nausea) are potentiated by isoproteronol. Therefore, when given concurrently, isoproteronol should not be given within one hour after administration of epinephrine.

63. (4) By providing for maximum ventilatory efficiency, the high-Fowler's position increases the oxygen supply to the lungs and helps to relieve dyspnea. This is most important for the asthmatic child who is experiencing a diminished ventilatory capacity.

64. (1) The major concern regarding toys for a child in a croup tent is that there not be any chance of static electricity or a spark, because the croup tent contains oxygen. Cotton does not create static electricity. Wool and synthetic materials create static electricity. A wind-up toy could create a spark.

65. (2) Chest physiotherapy aids in loosening secretions throughout the respiratory tract. Oxygen therapy does not loosen secretions and may be contraindicated, because many children with cystic fibrosis experience carbon dioxide retention and respiratory depression with too high levels of oxygen. Pancreatic enzymes will be given to this child, but to improve the absorption of nutrients, not to facilitate respiratory effort. A diet high in calories is appropriate for a child with cystic fibrosis. However, it does not facilitate respiratory effort.

66. (2) Pancreatic enzymes should be given with meals. They can be mixed with applesauce. The purpose of the enzymes is to help with the digestion and absorption of nutrients. Therefore, they must be given when the child is having food.

67. (3) The child should receive all of the antibiotic medication. Parents are apt to stop giving it to the child when he/she begins to feel better. This encourages recurrence of the infection that may be resistant to antibiotic therapy. Acetaminophen may be given to the infant, but it is for pain and does not prevent recurrence of the infection. There is some evidence that children who live around smokers have a higher incidence of otitis media. This teaching is relevant but not the most important. Children who go to sleep with milk or juice in their mouths after feeding have a higher incidence of otitis media, but this is not the most important nursing action to prevent recurrence of infection.

68. (2) A croup tent is high humidity, and the child's clothes will get wet. When they do, they should be changed so that the child will not get chilled. It is appropriate to explain this to the mother, but the best response is to change the child. Covering the child will not prevent chilling. The nurse should not remove the child from the croup tent just because his clothing is wet.

69. (4) The child with cystic fibrosis has a problem with chloride metabolism and loses excessive amounts of salt in sweat. The child should be given something with high amounts of sodium, such as broth. Ice cream contains some sodium, but not as much as broth. Kool-Aid and lemonade contain no sodium.

70. (3) A child who is 10 months of age should have been sitting without support for several months. This sign indicates a developmental lag and the need for further assessment. The ability to crawl is usually acquired between 9 and 12 months. Saying 2–4 words is normal for a child of 10 months. The development of the pincer grasp is refined by 11 months of age. It is normal for a 10-month-old child to use a crude pincer grasp.

71. (3) Placing a pillow under the head, using padded side rails, and removing sharp or hard objects from the immediate area all

provide for the safety of a child who is having a seizure. No restraints or force should be used during a seizure. Nothing should be put in the mouth of a person who is having a seizure. Although having a waterproof mattress or pad would prevent the bed from being soiled, it has nothing to do with the child's safety.

72. (1) Upright with stabilization of the jaw is important, because jaw control is often lacking in a child with cerebral palsy. Feeding in a semireclining position does not promote swallowing. A child with cerebral palsy does not usually need tube feeding or a gastrostomy. Hyperextending the neck may interfere with swallowing.

73. (4) Bacterial meningitis is infectious. The child should be placed in a private room with respiratory precautions.

74. (1) The first priority is to begin antibiotics as soon as possible. The more quickly antibiotics are started, the better the child's prognosis. The nurse will keep the room quiet and dim and will explain actions to the parents. However, these actions are not as high of a priority as administering the antibiotics. Oxygen is administered only if the child's respiratory status is impaired.

75. (3) It is important to prevent the defect from becoming dry and cracked and allowing microorganisms to enter. Infants with myelomeningocele remain in a prone position to prevent excessive pressure or tension on the defect. In most cases, infants with myelomeningocele cannot be held and cuddled as other babies are. The parents should stroke and touch the infant even if they cannot hold him or her. The infant is not usually in pain.

76. (2) Parents should be taught intermittent, clean catheterization. Parents can begin using this procedure at the age when unaffected children are toilet trained (about 3 years). Children who have myelomeningocele do not usually have bowel and bladder control, so

taking him to the bathroom would serve no purpose. The child does not need to wear diapers until he goes to school. He should be as normal as possible. A three-year-old child is not old enough to learn self-catheterization techniques. He will learn when he is older and has better motor coordination and understanding of the procedure.

77. (1) Head circumference is the most important tool in early identification of hydrocephalus. Head circumference is measured at birth and at all well-baby visits. Measurements above the norm will be seen in infants with hydrocephalus. Weight and length do not have any connection with hydrocephalus. An infant with severe hydrocephalus may have abnormal reflexes, but head circumference will do the most to help with the early identification of infants who might have hydrocephalus.

78. (2) The infant with hydrocephalus should be positioned sitting up in an infant seat to promote drainage as much as possible and reduce intracranial pressure. Side lying, Sims, prone, and supine are not indicated. These positions would increase intracranial pressure.

79. (4) Aspirin given to children, especially those who may have a viral infection, is associated with the development of Reye's syndrome, a very serious problem affecting the brain and the liver that is often fatal. Therefore, we do not give aspirin to children. Acetaminophen is nearly as effective as aspirin in relieving pain and fever; it is not more effective. Aspirin can cause gastritis in anyone, but that is not the reason why we do not give it to children.

80. (3) Tay-Sachs is an autosomal, recessive condition. That means that both parents must have the gene and that there is a one-in-four chance with every pregnancy that the child will have the condition. The disease is not X-linked, so it is not seen more frequently in boys. Hemophilia is X-linked.

81. (1) There is no cure for Tay-Sachs. The child is missing the enzyme hexosaminidase A, which is necessary for all tissues. The child will become blind and lose any skills that he may have developed and will eventually die. There is no cure and no way to stop the progress of the disease. The disease is not communicable; it is genetic. The parents will need genetic counseling, but that is not the goal of care for the child.

82. (1) Infants with meningomyelocele should be positioned prone with a pillow under the lower legs. Every effort is made to avoid putting pressure on the sac. Breaking the sac would likely cause the infant to develop meningitis. All of the other position choices would put pressure on the sac.

83. (2) The child is sensitive to light and may develop seizures. A dimly lit room reduces the chance that seizures will occur. The child does need rest, but that is not the reason for a dimly lit room. The other answer choices are not correct.

84. (4) The condition described is probably pink eye, and it is very contagious. Once antibiotic treatment is started, the child should stay out of school for 24–48 hours.

85. (2) Eye drops should be placed in the conjunctival sac. Gentle pressure should be applied to the inner canthus to prevent the eye drops from entering the tear ducts and causing a runny nose.

86. (2) Difficulty arousing the child from a nap suggests a change in level of consciousness, a cardinal sign of increased intracranial pressure, and should be reported immediately to the charge nurse. The other findings are all normal for a five-month-old infant.

87. (3) Children with cerebral palsy who have athetoid movements are in constant motion during waking hours but move much less during sleep. The nurse should assist the child with ADLs as needed. The child cannot control these movements. The child should not be sedated constantly.

88. (1) The symptoms suggest conjunctivitis or "pink eye," which is very contagious. The child should not go to school and should be seen by his physician today. Conjunctivitis is treated by the pediatrician or primary care physician and does not require an eye doctor.

89. (2) Infants who have meningomyelocele usually have lower body paralysis and bowel and bladder dysfunction. The surgery closes the defect, but when the spinal nerves are in the sac, there is usually permanent damage. Unless there is associated hydrocephalus, the infant may well have normal mental development.

90. (1) The asepto should be placed in the unaffected side of the baby's mouth and back far enough to encourage swallowing. All of the other answers are correct. The baby's mouth should be rinsed with saline after each feeding to minimize the chance of infection. The baby should be held in an upright position and bubbled or burped frequently because the baby tends to swallow air. The baby with a cleft palate is a mouth breather and will have dry lips. Applying lanolin is appropriate.

91. (3) The symptoms suggest ear infection. A child with an ear infection needs to be seen by a physician and probably treated with an antibiotic. Children with cleft palate are very susceptible to infections and need to be treated promptly to reduce the chance of hearing loss from recurrent ear infections.

92. (4) Priority care following cleft lip repair is to keep the child from pulling at the lip repair site. The IV is probably infiltrated. Further assessment of the IV should be done after the restraint has been replaced. The vital signs are normal. Checking to see if the baby has voided is not a priority measure.

93. (3) Having the mother hold the infant would be most comforting to the infant. A child with cleft lip repair cannot have a pacifier and cannot be on the abdomen. A special nurse is not necessary; the mother will do very well.

94. (2) Promoting speech is a very important long-term goal for a child who has a cleft palate, because speech problems are common. Immobilization following a cleft lip repair is brief. Preventing joint contractures is not a long-term goal. Preventing infection at the surgical site is also a short-term goal.

95. (4) Daily weights are the best indicator of fluid balance. The number of stools gives an indication of fluid loss but is not the best indicator of fluid balance. Skin turgor and assessing mucous membranes are helpful, but daily weights are the best indicator of fluid balance.

96. (1) Restoration of intravascular volume is the immediate goal. This will prevent life-threatening fluid and electrolyte imbalances. The others are goals but are not immediate.

97. (2) Pedialyte and glucose water are appropriate. The infant needs clear liquids, and these are age appropriate. Pedialyte gives electrolytes, and glucose water gives sugar. A nine-month-old infant does not drink carbonated beverages such as 7-Up and ginger ale. Half-strength formula is not a clear liquid. Tea is not appropriate for an infant, and broth is too salty for an infant.

98. (3) The bowel still needs rest. Stop the feedings, and notify the charge nurse or the physician. Taking vital signs and weighing the child do not address the issue, which is that oral feedings stimulate diarrhea-indicating the bowel is still irritable and needs further rest.

99. (4) The child should be receiving isotonic saline enemas. Repeated tap water or a soap suds enemas would cause fluid and electrolyte imbalances. A low-residue diet is indicated because the child has no peristalsis. High-fiber diets are contraindicated.

100. (3) In Hirschsprung's disease, a lack of peristalsis in the lower colon causes accumulation of intestinal contents, distention of the bowel, and possible obstruction. Measuring abdominal girth is most important. The other actions are not wrong, but they are not the most important.

101. (3) The baby will have a temporary colostomy to allow the bowel time to heal and return to normal functioning. The usual surgery for Hirschsprung's disease involves a temporary colostomy, not a permanent colostomy. The child will receive enemas prior to surgery, but they will be saline enemas, not tap water enemas. Tap water enemas cause fluid shifts. A gastrostomy tube is unlikely after surgery. Following recovery from anesthesia, the child should return to oral intake and normal feedings.

102. (2) Small, frequent feedings followed by positioning at a 30°–45° angle have been found to prevent gastric distention and vomiting in the infant with gastroesophageal reflux. Diluting the formula is not appropriate. Infants with gastroesophageal reflux do not have a problem with the absorption of nutrients. Gastroesophageal reflux is not related to milk intolerance, so a change in formula is not indicated. Delaying burping can aggravate gastroesophageal reflux. An infant with gastroesophageal reflux needs frequent burping to prevent reflux.

103. (3) Visible waves of peristalsis moving from left to right across the epigastrum are usually seen in infants with pyloric stenosis. Abdominal rigidity is not typical of pyloric stenosis. Ribbon-like stools might be seen in the child with Hirschsprung's disease. The child with pyloric stenosis will have small, rabbit pellet stools. Rectal prolapse is seen in children with cystic fibrosis.

104. (2) The data presented (dry mucous membranes, poor skin turgor, no tearing) suggest a deficient fluid volume related to frequent stools. Impaired skin integrity is a possibility with frequent stooling, but there are no data to confirm this. Pain related to cramping is a possibility, but there are no data to confirm this. Imbalanced nutrition: less than body requirements is also a possibility, but there are no data to confirm this.

105. (2) A urine-specific gravity of 1.035 indicates dehydration. Normal range for an infant is 1.002–1.030. The normal sodium level is 135–146 mmol/l. The normal hematocrit for an infant is 28–42%. The normal potassium for an infant is 3.5–6 mmol/l.

106. (3) Once the infant retains small, frequent feedings of glucose for 24 hours, the nurse may begin small, frequent feedings of formula until the infant returns to a normal feeding schedule. Answer 1 is not correct, because bowel sounds need to be present before starting clear liquids. A decrease in bowel sounds is not normally a problem in the child who has undergone surgical correction for pyloric stenosis, because the surgery does not enter the stomach itself but rather the pyloric muscle. Answer 2 is not correct, because vital signs do not directly affect the initiation of infant formula. Answer 4 is not correct. The absence of diarrhea is not the criterion for beginning formula.

107. (4) With esophageal atresia, the esophagus ends in a blind pouch. The infant will choke after a few sucks of water because it has no place to go. Projectile vomiting, especially at the age of 2 or 3 weeks, is suggestive of pyloric stenosis. Slow sucking and fatigue with sucking would be more suggestive of cardiac problems.

108. (2) Infants with esophageal atresia will need a gastrostomy tube because the esophagus ends in a blind pouch. There is no connection between the esophagus and the stomach, so a nasogastric tube cannot be passed. Intravenous or TPN feedings are not indicated. Gastrostomy tube feedings are much safer. Because there is no connection between the esophagus and the stomach, the infant cannot have anything by mouth.

109. (2) There is nothing in this choice that contains barley, rye, oats, or wheat, which all contain gluten. Toast, crackers, and hamburger rolls all contain wheat, which has gluten, and is not allowed in a child who has celiac disease and cannot tolerate gluten.

110. (4) Nephrotic syndrome is characterized by proteinuria, hypoalbuminemia, and fluid retention with significant edema. Answer 1 suggests liver or gall bladder disease. Answer 2 is more suggestive of acute glomerulonephritis than nephrotic syndrome. Answer 3 is not likely. A child with renal failure and resulting pulmonary edema could experience these symptoms, but that is not likely at this point in the disease process.

111. (4) Diuretics and steroids will have been prescribed. The goal is to decrease edema. This will be demonstrated by a weight loss. He may feel better and have an improved appetite, but weight loss is a better indicator of the specific goal of therapy for a child with nephrotic syndrome.

112. (1) It is essential not to palpate the abdomen because this may cause the encapsulated tumor to spread. Emotional support to the parents and encouraging the child to eat well are nice but not of the highest priority. Strict bed rest is probably not indicated, although the child will not be allowed to run around.

113. (1) The symptoms described (frequency, urgency, and a strong odor to urine) are those of a urinary tract infection. A urinalysis is indicated. It is true that preschool children may regress when they are under stress. However, that does not explain the frequency and the strong odor of the urine. While a recently toilet-trained child may have an occasional "accident," recurring episodes should be further investigated. Not all persons with a UTI have a fever. If the child does have a UTI as suspected, the treatment is usually oral antimicrobial agents. There is no data to suggest that this child needs to be hospitalized.

114. (3) The symptoms described all suggest fluid overload, which is characteristic of nephrotic syndrome. This must be corrected as quickly as possible to prevent further problems. The

child probably already has altered nutrition rather than simply being at risk for it. However, fluid overload is a higher priority. The child is at risk for infection because of the hypoalbuminemia, but there is no evidence to support that the child already has an infection. The child may develop a disturbed body image related to edema. Again, there is no evidence to suggest that the child has a disturbed body image. Even if the child did, fluid volume excess would take priority.

115. (2) Exstrophy of the bladder is when the bladder lies open on the abdominal wall. The exposed bladder should be covered with petrolatum gauze to help prevent skin damage from constant exposure to urine. Continuous saline irrigations are not appropriate. An indwelling catheter would serve no purpose, because the bladder is on the abdominal wall. Diapers should be applied loosely to prevent irritation of the site.

116. (1) An orchiopexy is the surgical procedure done to bring an undescended testicle into the scrotal sac. The key care following this procedure, which may be done on an outpatient basis, is not to disturb the tension mechanism (a "button" in the scrotum that keeps the testicle from going back up into the abdomen) until the physician removes it in 7–10 days. Children who have the surgery by five years of age are not usually sterile. Waiting longer increases the risk of sterility. The child will not probably need leg exercises following this outpatient surgery. This is not a condition that has or needs a support group. Cryptorchidism (undescended testicle) is quite common and sometimes corrects itself. If it doesn't, the surgery (orchiopexy) is safe and simple.

117. (3) Hypospadias is when the urethral opening is on the ventral side of the penis. Surgical repair is likely at about three years of age. The foreskin is the perfect repair tissue. Hypospadias does not cause the infant to be unstable. Circumcision will be done when the surgery is done at age three. Male circumcision is a choice that the parents make. The American Academy of Pediatrics states that it is not necessary but is optional and may slightly reduce the risk of urinary tract infections in infant boys.

118. (2) A Wilm's tumor is an encapsulated tumor on the kidney. Surgery is an essential part of the treatment. There is no option. In addition, the child may receive radiation and or chemotherapy. Surgery must be done immediately before the tumor spreads or the capsule breaks.

119. (1) Not giving the child anything to drink after the evening meal helps, particularly if the child is a sound sleeper. Cola-type beverages have a diuretic effect. Wearing diapers is not appropriate for a five-year-old. That would be devastating to the child's self esteem. Bribing the child by promising a sleepover party is not appropriate. The child should not be punished for wetting the bed. This usually makes the situation worse. Of course, the nurse will report the mother's concerns to the physician and encourage the mother to discuss it with the physician.

120. (3) Neurovascular function must be assessed every two hours. The child should be turned at least every two hours to prevent skin damage and to facilitate cast drying. Fingertips should be avoided when handling a wet cast because they can leave indentations on a wet cast. The nurse should palm the cast. A hair dryer should not be used to dry the cast. This causes the cast to dry from the outside in and may leave the inside wet and soft.

121. (1) Pain management is a high priority. The child probably is not taking liquids at this time. Even if she is taking clear liquids, pain management is a higher priority. The nurse may drain the Hemovac, but that is not the highest priority. The nurse will notify the child's parents, but pain management is of a higher priority.

122. (2) The treatment for hip dysplasia is abduction. Triple diapers are the easiest way to abduct the hips in mild cases. If that is not successful, then a pillow splint or harness can be used. There is no open wound with hip dysplasia and no worry about contamination of the area. Hip dysplasia does not cause abnormal stooling. Triple diapers do not cause increased flexion; they actually cause less flexion. Less flexion is recommended for children with hip dysplasia.

123. (3) The baby who has bilateral casts should not be placed in water but should receive a sponge bath. Answers 2 and 3 put the baby in water and are not correct. The nurse should not tell the mother to bathe the baby as usual without knowing what the usual is. By six months of age, most babies are being bathed in a baby bath tub. This is not appropriate when there are casts.

124. (2) Legg-Calve Perthes Disease is avascular necrosis of the hip. The primary goal is to keep the child on bed rest to allow the hip to heal. New bone will regenerate. There is great risk of permanent damage if the child bears weight on the damaged hip. The child will be on bed rest and will probably be in traction to keep the bed properly aligned. The child often has pain, which needs to be controlled, but the absence of pain does not mean that he can get out of bed. The mother can talk with the physician, but the nurse should understand that the usual treatment involves keeping the child off the affected hip.

125. (3) Junior high girls are the target group for screening for scoliosis.

126. (4) An undershirt should be worn under the brace to prevent skin injury from the brace. The brace is worn 23 hours a day for three years.

127. (3) Duchenne's muscular dystrophy is an X-linked disease. Therefore, it appears in boys. It would be appropriate to assess brothers of children with muscular dystrophy for the condition. The disease is not controllable and will eventually kill its victims. Muscular dystrophy does not affect the mental status of those who have it; it is a muscular problem.

128. (3) Lyme disease is transmitted by the bite of the deer tick. Malaria is transmitted by a mosquito. The mosquito that carries malaria does not live in the United States. Lyme disease is not inherited. Poison ivy is caused by contact with the oil in plant leaves.

129. (1) Both Lyme disease and rheumatoid arthritis case joint pain, which can be severe. High fever is not characteristic of either condition. A urinary tract infection is not characteristic of either condition. The child with stage II Lyme disease is at risk for cardiac dysrhythmias due to the nerve involvement that may occur. The child with rheumatoid arthritis is not at risk for cardiac dysrhythmias.

130. (3) Delayed dentition is a sign of hypopituitarism or pituitary dwarfism due to a lack of growth hormone. Permanent teeth should begin to erupt around age 5. A 13-month-old that weighs 21 pounds is within the normal range. A 4-year-old who is 41 inches tall is within the normal range. Menarche normally occurs between 10½ and 15½ years of age. This child is within normal limits.

131. (1) Human growth hormone is the treatment for primary hypopituitarism. Three to seven times a week is usual. Bedtime is the best time to give it, because that closely simulates the body's normal production. A child with hypopituitarism should achieve normal intelligence. Endocrine workups of children who have no signs of disease are not necessary. While emotional difficulties relating to this condition are possible and the family should be alerted to that possibility, referral to a psychiatrist at this time seems premature.

132. (2) Increase in exercise will affect the insulin dose the most. Heat and humidity might have some effect. Diabetics are taught to adjust

their insulin dose within ranges. An adolescent needs to learn how to do this.

133. (3) The symptoms suggest hypoglycemia, which should be treated with food. Fluids such as juice or milk that contain carbohydrates should be given to treat hypoglycemia, not plain water. Insulin should not be given because the symptoms suggest hypoglycemia, not hyperglycemia. Having him rest for 20 minutes without treating hypoglycemia will make it worse. Rest following the treatment of hypoglycemia is appropriate.

134. (3) IDDM is a lack of insulin secretion by the pancreas, which makes the child unable to metabolize carbohydrates without additional insulin. IDDM is not a metabolic error, and fatty acids are not primarily affected. IDDM is not a genetic disorder, although there may be a hereditary predisposition to the condition, and proteins are not primarily affected. IDDM is not caused by eating too many sweets early in life.

135. (1) Because the child is one month old, there is a good chance that she will develop normally. Maternal thyroid circulates for the first three months. If the child is started on treatment within the first three months of life, there is a good chance for normal development. Untreated cretinism will cause delays in physical and mental development. This child is being treated early, so answer 2 is not correct. Answer 3 is not correct. She will be continually evaluated but should be normal because treatment is being started early. Answer 4 is not correct. She will need to take medication for the rest of her life.

136. (2) Impetigo is usually caused by staph or strep, causes severe itching, and is often spread from one site to the other by scratching. Putting antibiotic ointment underneath the fingernails helps to prevent the child from spreading from one part of his body to another. An elimination diet is appropriate for a child who has eczema. Impetigo is not caused by poison ivy. Pediculosis (head lice) is spread by sharing combs and hats.

137. (1) Ringworm is caused by a fungus, not a worm. It is often called ringworm because the lesion is often in the shape of circle or ring and looks as if a worm was burrowing under the surface.

138. (3) Kerosene is an old folk remedy for pediculosis. It is very irritating to the scalp and the fumes are very dangerous for the child, to say nothing of the risk of fire. Kerosene should not be used.

139. (4) Cats and dogs may run through poison ivy and get the oil on their fur. A susceptible child who pats or hugs the animal may develop the allergic response. Allergic response to foods is associated with eczema, not poison ivy. Pediculosis or head lice is spread by sharing combs or hats. Poison ivy is not spread by the liquid that oozes out of the blisters.

140. (2) The restraints can be removed when someone is holding the baby. They do need to be removed to check for circulation at least every two hours. The baby could scratch when asleep, so the restraints need to be on during sleep.

Unit IV

Special Populations

UNIT OUTLINE

Chapter 14

The Older Adult Client

Sample Questions

1. A 75-year-old man is brought to the auditory clinic by his son, who tells the nurse that his father is having trouble hearing and seems to be a little depressed. The man says, "There's no point in getting a hearing aid. I don't have much time left and didn't use the time I had very good anyway." The nurse recognizes that this behavior indicates that the client might be

   1. Actively suicidal
   2. Suffering bipolar depression
   3. Struggling with generativity versus stagnation
   4. Struggling with development of integrity versus despair

2. An 88-year-old woman in a long-term care facility is having difficulty remembering where her room is. Which of the following solutions would best help her?

   1. Put a light-blue painting on the door to her room.
   2. Assign her a buddy who will help her when she gets lost.
   3. Put her picture and her name in large letters on the door to her room.
   4. Assign her the room next to the nurses' station so that the staff can assist her.

3. The family of an elderly client asks why their father puts so much salt on his food. The nurse should include which information in the response?

   1. The taste buds become dulled as a person ages.
   2. The body is attempting to compensate for lost fluids during the aging process.
   3. Elderly clients need more sodium to ensure adequate kidney function.
   4. The client is confused and does not remember putting salt on the food.

4. A 65-year-old client is seen in an urgent care center for a sprained ankle. The client also tells the nurse, "I don't know what the problem is. I'm tired all the time. I guess it's just a sign I'm getting old." What is the best response for the nurse to make?

   1. "Sixty-five isn't that old. Do you have enough activities to keep you from getting bored?"
   2. "It's normal for someone your age to feel tired like that. Try taking a two-hour nap during the day."
   3. "It's not normal for someone your age to be tired all the time. Have you had a physical exam recently?"
   4. "You sound depressed. Would you like the name of a psychiatrist?"

5. A 64-year-old woman tells the nurse she has vaginal itching and dryness and that she has pain "down there" at times. What should the nurse do?

   1. Reassure the client that these are normal changes that come with aging.

   2. Explain to the client that this situation is of little importance because sexual activity is not likely at this age.

   3. Suggest to the client that she use a vaginal cream for the itching and dryness.

   4. Encourage the client to see her physician.

6. An elderly woman is admitted to the hospital with a productive cough, progressive forgetfulness, an inability to concentrate, and disinterest in her personal hygiene. What should be of greatest priority as the nurse assesses this client?

   1. Her progressive forgetfulness

   2. Her inability to concentrate

   3. Her disinterest in her personal hygiene

   4. Her productive cough

7. The nurse in a retirement home has noticed that Mr. A. and Ms. C. have been holding hands frequently. One day, the nurse enters Mr. A.'s room and finds Mr. A. and Ms. C. having sexual intercourse. Both residents are alert and oriented. What is the most appropriate action for the nurse to take?

   1. Interrupt the couple and send Ms. C. to her room.

   2. Leave the room and close the door.

   3. Notify the relatives of both residents.

   4. Ask Ms. C. if she is all right.

8. A 45-year-old tells the nurse that she is having difficulty reading the newspaper. She states that she holds it away from her but still cannot see it. What is the best response for the nurse to make?

   1. Reassure her that this situation is normal and encourage her to use a magnifying glass.

   2. Ask her if any of her relatives have had this problem.

   3. Suggest that she see an eye doctor for a prescription for reading glasses.

   4. Explain that she can try on reading glasses at the drugstore.

9. An elderly man tells the nurse that all his family members mumble when they talk. How should the nurse respond to this statement?

   1. Refer the family members to speech therapy.

   2. Suggest that the client have his hearing tested.

   3. Discuss with the family how to speak more clearly.

   4. Ask the client if his parents had difficulty hearing.

10. The nurse is discussing the care of a client who has a hearing deficit. Which suggestion is most appropriate to make to those around him?

   1. Speak in a higher tone of voice.

   2. Raise your voice when speaking.

   3. Be sure to stand so there are no bright lights behind you.

   4. Keep the television or radio on when having a conversation.

Answers and Rationales

1. (4) Integrity versus despair is the developmental task of the elderly. This concept includes looking at one's life with some satisfaction for what has been accomplished. This client indicates he is not satisfied with his life. There are no data to suggest that the client is suicidal or bipolar. Generativity versus stagnation is the developmental task for the middle adult.

2. (3) The behavior suggests short-term memory loss. Identifying her room with her picture, probably a picture of her as a younger woman, and her name in large letters so she can easily read it will help her find her room. Older persons are apt to have difficulty with blue, green, and pastel colors. It is not necessary to assign her a buddy, nor is it necessary to put her next to the nurse's station.

3. (1) As people age, the taste buds diminish and become dulled. Many elderly persons put large amounts of salt on food. The other answers do not make sense. If the client loses fluids, thirst is the response, not a desire for more salt. Elderly clients do not need more sodium for renal function or anything else. Confusion could play a role, but the more likely reason is a loss of taste sensation.

4. (3) It is not normal for a 65-year-old to be tired all the time. Chronic fatigue can be a sign of many things, including anemia, diabetes, and so on. The client should be thoroughly evaluated by a physician. Fatigue could be related to boredom or depression, but the nurse should not make that assumption. The client should be evaluated for physical illness first.

5. (4) Dryness is normal for a post-menopausal woman. Itching and pain are not normal, however. The client needs to be seen by a physician. She might have an infection or another problem.

6. (4) The highest priority has to be the productive cough. It could signify a problem that needs immediate treatment. The other concerns are

longer term and should be addressed after the cough.

7. (2) Both residents are alert and oriented. A relationship has existed. There is no evidence of force being used. It would appear to be a mutually consenting act. Leave the room and close the door. There is no need to notify the relatives of this alert and oriented couple.

8. (3) The data suggest presbyopia-the normal loss of accommodation that occurs with aging. The best response is to suggest that the client see an eye doctor for reading glasses. Reading glasses can be purchased at the drugstore. There are other eye conditions that occur with aging, however, so the client should be seen by an eye doctor.

9. (2) When a person says that everyone is mumbling, the problem is usually with the person's hearing. The most appropriate response is to suggest that his hearing be tested. It is doubtful that the family needs speech therapy or instruction in speaking more clearly. Asking the client about a family history of hearing problems is not particularly relevant. Hearing difficulties might or might not be hereditary.

10. (3) Persons with hearing impairments tend to read lips and faces. Standing with a bright light behind the speaker makes it very difficult to read lips. Persons with hearing impairments usually hear lower tones better, so speaking in a higher tone of voice makes it more difficult to hear. Raising the voice tends to raise the pitch and make it more difficult to hear. Background noise makes hearing more difficult.

Chapter 15

The Mental Health Client

Sample Questions

1. When the nurse detects that a client is using defense mechanisms, the nurse should make which of these interpretations of the client's behavior?

   1. The client is attempting to re-establish emotional equilibrium.
   2. The client is using self-defeating measures.
   3. The client is demonstrating illness.
   4. The client is asking for support from significant others.

2. The treatment goal for a client with severe anxiety will have been achieved when the client demonstrates which of these behaviors?

   1. The client recognizes the source of the anxiety.
   2. The client is able to use the anxiety constructively.
   3. The client can function without any sense of anxiety.
   4. The client identifies the physical effects of the anxiety.

3. The nurse is assessing a 22-month-old child who is thought to be autistic. During an interview with the nurse, the child's mother makes all of the following statements about his behavior until he was one year old. Which statement most strongly suggests that the child may be autistic?

   1. "He was a good baby and rarely cried when I left the room."
   2. "He slept very well after each feeding."
   3. "He spit out every new food the first time I gave it to him."
   4. "He started to walk without learning to crawl first."

4. In attempting to establish a therapeutic relationship with a child who may be autistic, the nurse should expect to encounter which of these problems?

   1. Hallucinating
   2. Impaired hearing
   3. Bizarre behavior
   4. Clinging to others

5. To initiate a relationship with a child who may be autistic, the nurse would probably be most effective by using which of these approaches?

   1. Playing peek-a-boo
   2. Having him point to designated body parts
   3. Sitting with him
   4. Playing an action game like Ring Around the Rosy

6. The nurse is caring for a 75-year-old widow admitted to the psychiatric hospital by her daughter, who became concerned when her mother began to talk in a confused manner about her husband who has been dead for seven years. In the hospital, especially at night, the client wanders in the other clients' rooms looking for her husband. What is the most appropriate action for the nurse to take when this woman wanders in the rooms of the other clients?

   1. Lock the door to her room.
   2. Tell her to stay in her room except for meals.
   3. Take her by the hand and guide her back to her room.
   4. Tell her that she will be restrained if she continues to wander.

7. The nurse is caring for an elderly woman admitted with Alzheimer's disease. When her daughter visits, she asks, "Are you my maid?" How should the nurse describe the client's behavior?

   1. Impaired judgment
   2. Disorientation
   3. Impairment of abstract thinking
   4. Delusions

8. An elderly woman is hospitalized with Alzheimer's disease. When her daughter visits, she does not recognize her. The daughter begins to cry and shares her concerns with the nurse. Which statement by the nurse would demonstrate an empathetic response?

   1. "It must be difficult for you to visit your mother when she is confused about who you are."
   2. "If you are going to cry when you come to visit, maybe you should not visit."
   3. "It is not unusual for people in your mother's condition to forget who other people are."
   4. "If these visits upset you, maybe you should telephone your mother instead of visiting."

9. An elderly woman with Alzheimer's disease refuses to eat and begins to lose weight. Which approach by the nurse will likely be most effective in getting the client to eat?

   1. Explaining to her the necessity of eating three meals daily
   2. Asking the client what she thinks should be done about her lack of eating
   3. Telling the client that if she doesn't eat, she will be given tube feedings
   4. Accompanying her to meals and assisting her in eating

10. A 25-year-old woman has admitted herself to the psychiatric unit for treatment of Valium addiction. She is currently taking 150 mg p.o. of Valium per day, which she gets from various doctors or buys off the streets. The first night she is on the unit, she dresses in a short, see-through night gown and approaches the male nurse. She states she is "coming down" and just needs a little comforting and conversation. What is the best initial response by the nurse?

    1. "Please put on your bathrobe and then we can talk."
    2. "I'm very busy now. Maybe one of the other nurses can help you."
    3. "What seems to be the problem?"
    4. "What you are experiencing is very common. It should get better soon."

11. A young woman has admitted herself to the psychiatric unit for treatment of Valium addiction. A schedule of drug withdrawal is ordered by the doctor. Which of the following may the nurse expect to see as the Valium dose is decreased?

    1. Decreased blood pressure
    2. Tremors and hyperactivity
    3. Increase in appetite
    4. Grandiosity

12. Three days after admission for treatment of Valium addiction, a young woman briefly left the hospital to talk to a visitor. Her psychiatrist has threatened to discharge her for noncompliance with the treatment program. The client seems very depressed and refuses to get out of bed. The evening nurse finds the client crying, "I've screwed everything up. It's hopeless. It's no use." In responding to the client, which of the following would be most appropriate?

    1. "You've screwed everything up?"
    2. "Why do you feel it's no use?"
    3. "Sometimes we have to hit bottom before things get better."
    4. "You sound like you're feeling very sad. Are you thinking about harming yourself?"

13. A woman is admitted to the detoxification unit. She admits to drinking increasingly larger amounts of alcohol for the past five years. What question is most important for the nurse to ask initially?

    1. "How much alcohol do you drink daily?"
    2. "When was your last drink?"
    3. "When did you last eat?"
    4. "What type of alcoholic beverages do you drink?"

14. The morning after admission for withdrawal from alcohol, a client is restless, tremulous, and somewhat agitated. The nurse should take which of these actions at this time?

    1. Offer her medicinal whiskey.
    2. Observe her behavior closely.
    3. Darken the client's room.
    4. Prepare to place her in restraints.

15. Two nights after admission for alcohol withdrawal, the client runs out of her room. She is confused and disoriented and says, "Let me out of here. Bugs are crawling all over that room." The nurse should take which of these actions?

    1. Escort her back to her room and show her that there is nothing to fear.
    2. Assist her back into bed and then search her room for alcohol.
    3. Take her to a quiet area and ask her if she usually has nightmares.
    4. Have a staff member stay with her and notify the physician.

16. An adult woman is admitted to the detox unit for alcohol withdrawal. Her husband tells the nurse that he is fed up. Either she gets treatment, or he is leaving her. Two days later the woman develops delirium tremens. At this time, which of these nursing diagnoses should be given priority in caring for this client?

    1. Potential for physical injury related to impulsiveness
    2. Noncompliance with medical regimen related to denial of illness
    3. Anticipatory grieving related to her husband's threat of abandoning her
    4. Translocation syndrome related to transfer to a strange environment

17. Following withdrawal from alcohol, the client agrees to participate in group therapy sessions for a period before being discharged. Initially, group therapy may have which of these effects on the client?

    1. She will develop insight into her reasons for needing alcohol.
    2. She will experience periods of extreme anxiety.
    3. She will be able to set realistic goals for herself.
    4. She will be able to identify the personality traits she needs to change.

18. Following withdrawal from alcohol, a client is to receive disulfiram (Antabuse). The medication is prescribed for which of these purposes?

    1. To minimize the effects of alcohol
    2. To improve detoxification of alcohol by the liver
    3. To increase utilization of vitamins
    4. To help the client refrain from drinking alcohol

19. A client asks the nurse about participation in Alcoholics Anonymous. In addition to arranging for a visit by someone from Alcoholics Anonymous, the nurse should explain that the primary purpose of the organization is to:

    1. Explore the individual member's need for dependence on alcohol.
    2. Help members abstain from alcohol.
    3. Teach members how to manage social situations without the need for alcohol.
    4. Increase public awareness of the results of alcoholism.

20. Chlorpromazine hydrochloride (Thorazine) is prescribed for a young adult with schizophrenia. For three days, the Thorazine is to be administered intramuscularly. Before administering Thorazine intramuscularly to the client, the nurse should make which of these assessments?

    1. Checking his blood pressure
    2. Testing his urine for glucose
    3. Testing his patellar reflexes
    4. Checking laboratory results for his serum potassium level

21. The client who is taking Thorazine should be observed for which of these symptoms?

    1. Pseudoparkinsonism
    2. Dehydration
    3. Manic excitement
    4. Urinary incontinence

22. A 23-year-old premedical student is admitted to a psychiatric hospital in a withdrawn, catatonic state. For two days prior to admission, she remained in one position without moving or speaking. On the unit, she continues to exhibit waxy flexibility as she sits all day. What is the first priority for the nurse during the initial phase of hospitalization?

    1. Watch for edema and cyanosis of the extremities.
    2. Encourage the client to discuss her concerns, which may have led to the catatonic state.
    3. Provide a warm, nurturing relationship with a therapeutic use of touch.
    4. Identify causes for her illness.

23. A woman has been having auditory hallucinations. When the nurse approaches her, she whispers, "Did you hear that terrible man? He is scary!" Which would be the best response for the nurse to take initially?

    1. "Tell me everything the man is saying."
    2. "I don't hear anything. What scary things is he saying?"
    3. "Who is he? Do you know him?"
    4. "I didn't hear a man's voice, but you look scared."

24. A man who is being treated for paranoia walks toward the nurse's desk and observes the nurse making a telephone call. A few minutes later, he accuses the nurse of having called the police. How should the nurse interpret his behavior?

1. Projection
2. Reaction formation
3. Transference
4. Ideas of reference

25. A woman is admitted to the hospital because of recent overactive behavior. She enters the dining room for lunch after everyone is seated and eating. She runs around telling everyone that she has just been invited to speak at an important political meeting. She then sits down and starts to eat. After taking a few bites, she gets up and walks quickly out of the dining room. What initial action should the nurse take to meet the client's nutritional needs?

1. Serve her meals in her room.
2. Give her finger foods to eat.
3. Sit with her while she eats.
4. Discuss with her the importance of eating.

26. Lithium carbonate is ordered for a client with overactive behavior. The nurse should observe her for which of these side effects?

1. Diarrhea
2. Rhinitis
3. Glycosuria
4. Rash

27. A man who is severely depressed following the death of his wife sits in the dayroom for hours at a time, not speaking to anyone and showing no interest in unit activities. He does not answer when spoken to. Which action should the nurse take to help him at this time?

1. Encourage him to talk about his children.
2. Start playing a game in which he can participate.
3. Turn on the television for him to watch.

4. Speak to him briefly from time to time without expecting an answer.

28. A woman is being treated for severe depression. During the acute phase of her illness, which of these measures should have priority in her care?

1. Keeping her in seclusion
2. Repeating unit routines to her in detail
3. Urging her social interaction with other clients
4. Providing her with physical care

29. A woman who is severely depressed begins to improve. Which of these behaviors may be indicative of an impending suicide attempt?

1. Responding sarcastically when asked about her family
2. Avoiding conversation with some clients on the unit
3. Identifying with problems expressed by other clients
4. Appearing detached when walking about the unit

30. A young woman was referred to the psychiatrist by her family physician because she is fearful of getting into elevators. During the course of therapy, it was discovered that her initial fear was of men and that it had changed to elevators. Which of the following mechanisms is demonstrated by this change?

1. Repression
2. Identification
3. Projection
4. Displacement

31. A young woman who is fearful of getting into elevators is admitted. Two days after admission, she is scheduled for group therapy sessions that meet on the sixth floor. Her room is on the second floor. The other clients and the nurse go to the sixth floor on the elevator. The client starts trembling and refuses to get on the elevator. Which action is most therapeutic for the nurse to take?

1. Firmly insist that she get on the elevator with the other clients.

2. Explain to her that the elevator is safe and take her on a separate elevator from the rest of the group.

3. Excuse her from group therapy until she will get on the elevator.

4. Assign someone to walk up the stairs with her.

32. A 40-year-old man is admitted to the psychiatric unit for treatment of anxiety neurosis. For several weeks, he has had increasingly frequent periods of palpitations, sweating, chest pain, and choking. His nursing diagnosis is "severe anxiety, stressor unidentified." Which of these measures is appropriate during the client's attacks?

1. Supporting and protecting him

2. Engaging him in group activities

3. Having him review the circumstances that precipitated the symptoms

4. Ignoring him until the symptoms subside

33. Which nursing action would help to reduce stress and to aid an obsessive-compulsive client in using a less maladaptive means of handling stress?

1. Provide varied activities on the unit, because a change in routine can break a ritualistic pattern.

2. Give him unit assignments that do not require perfection.

3. Tell him of changes in routine at the last minute to avoid the buildup of anxiety.

4. Provide an activity in which positive accomplishment can occur so he can gain recognition.

34. After the nurse has had several brief conversations with a newly admitted client, the client suddenly says, "I'm afraid to ride in an elevator, I know it's silly, but I can't help it." Which of these responses by the nurse would be the best example of acknowledgment?

1. "It's hard to manage without using elevators."

2. "Being afraid to ride in elevators seems unreasonable to you."

3. "Perhaps you should consider why you are afraid to ride in an elevator."

4. "The speed of elevators frightens you."

35. A client with severe anxiety manifested by many somatic complaints starts psychotherapy. She becomes increasingly anxious, and her physical symptoms intensify. The nurse should make which of these interpretations of her observations?

1. The client needs to be involved in modifying the goals of therapy.

2. The client may be developing a physical illness unrelated to her emotional problems.

3. The client is responding to therapy as expected at this time.

4. The client is probably beginning to have insight into her behavior.

36. A young man who is admitted with antisocial behavior seeks the attention of a young, attractive nurse, and he finds many excuses to involve the nurse in conversation. The nurse should have which of these understandings of this situation?

1. The nurse should help him in any way possible.

2. The nurse is responsible for maintaining a therapeutic relationship with him.

3. The nurse should prepare to act as an advocate for him.

4. The nurse is uniquely able to gain his confidence.

37. A client says to the nurse, "I have something to tell you because I know you can keep a secret." To respond to his statement, the nurse should make which of these remarks?

1. "It's nice that you trust me to keep a secret."

2. "I would like to hear your secret."

3. "I cannot promise that I can keep your secret."

4. "A secret is not a secret when it is repeated."

38. A 75-year-old woman has been widowed for 12 years. She was forced to vacate her apartment several months ago and has been wandering about the city, begging, and sleeping on park benches. One day she enters the bus terminal and creates a disturbance. The police are called, and she is brought to a psychiatric unit. To plan care for this woman, which of these actions should be taken first?

1. Determine her interests.

2. Obtain information about her family.

3. Identify her emotional needs.

4. Evaluate her physical condition.

39. A homeless woman is admitted to the hospital. When she is admitted, she is asked to keep her possessions in a locker that is in her room. She insists on removing several articles to carry around with her. Following nursing interventions, she continues to carry most of her possessions around with her. The nurse should make which of these interpretations of this behavior?

1. The client needs to keep busy.

2. The client needs to maintain her identity.

3. The client needs to be a focus of attention.

4. The client needs a means of becoming involved with others.

40. A young woman who has a washing ritual has been late for breakfast each of the three days since admission. What is the most appropriate nursing intervention?

1. Give her a choice of getting to breakfast on time or not eating breakfast.

2. Restrict her privileges if she is late again.

3. Get her up early so she can complete her washing ritual before breakfast.

4. Insist that she stop washing her hands and go to breakfast.

41. A 15-year-old girl is brought to the hospital by her parents. She is 5 feet, 7 inches tall and weighs 80 pounds. This evening she is very difficult to arouse and had to be carried into the emergency room. She is diagnosed with anorexia nervosa. Which of the following is most likely to be present in the client?

1. Enlarged breasts

2. Scanty pubic hair

3. Elevated temperature

4. Tachycardia

42. An adolescent with a diagnosis of severe anorexia nervosa is now on the adolescent psychiatric unit after being in intensive care. In developing the nursing care plan, which will be of highest priority?

1. Weighing her before and after each meal

2. Observing her for two hours after each meal

3. Teaching her the elements of good nutrition

4. Recording her food intake

43. A 52-year-old man is admitted to the psychiatric unit. He states he does not sleep well, has not been eating, and has no energy. He tells the admitting nurse, "I don't think you can make me feel better. There's no use in talking to me. Leave me alone." What is the most appropriate interpretation of his behavior? The client:

1. Needs solitude. The nurse should leave him alone.
2. Is depressed. The nurse should stay with him.
3. Needs encouragement. The nurse should assure him that he will get well soon.
4. Is in a bad mood. The nurse should tell him to cheer up.

44. An adult man is being treated for depression and has been taking amitriptyline (Elavil) for three days. His wife says to the nurse, "I don't think the medicine is doing anything for him. He is still depressed." What is the best response for the nurse to make?

1. "I will observe him carefully and make a full report to the physician."
2. "Depression takes a while to clear. We are seeing small behavior changes."
3. "The medicine takes two to three weeks to be effective. It is too soon to see behavior changes."
4. "His doctor is pleased with his progress. Have patience."

45. An adult male is being treated for depression. He has been in the hospital for three weeks. Which observation by the nurse is indicative of improvement in his condition?

1. He appears for breakfast unshaven.
2. He says, "I now have the answer to my problems."
3. He refuses to eat, saying, "I don't like hospital food."
4. He initiates a conversation with another client.

46. An adult is being treated for depression. One day he appears at the nursing station and gives one of the nurses his favorite book. He smiles happily and says, "I want you to have this." The nurse's response is based on which understanding?

1. Nurses should not accept gifts from clients.
2. His actions indicate an improvement in communication skills.
3. The nurse should support actions that bring the client obvious pleasure.
4. Giving away objects of personal importance is a suicidal warning sign.

47. A client with cancer states he has no reason to live anymore. What is the most therapeutic response for the nurse to give at this time?

1. "You feel as though you have no reason to live?"
2. "Your wife needs you and wants you to live."
3. "Your children care about you."
4. "I care about what happens to you."

48. A young woman is admitted for the first time with a diagnosis of catatonic schizophrenia and is receiving Thorazine daily. She is to go home for a weekend pass. What is the most important instruction to give her relative to her medications?

1. "Use a sunscreen lotion, and do not drink alcoholic beverages."
2. "Do not drink wine or beer or eat hard cheeses."
3. "Stay away from persons with colds and infections and report any rashes immediately."
4. "Drink plenty of orange juice, and take your pills with milk."

49. A male client who has not spoken for years is diagnosed as having paranoid schizophrenia. One day, when a female client was standing facing the elevator, the male client approached

her from behind and reached for her as if to strangle her. What is the most appropriate action for the nurse to take at this time?

1. Grab the male client by the arm to stop him.
2. Ask other clients to assist the nurse.
3. Say, "Sir, that is not appropriate behavior."
4. Get the male client's attention and call for help.

50. Thorazine is prescribed for a client. Which of the following, if observed in the client, would suggest Thorazine toxicity?

1. Tremors
2. Sore tongue
3. Rash
4. Hoarseness

Answers and Rationales

1. (1) Defense mechanisms are measures that the client uses to re-establish emotional equilibrium. Some are self-defeating, and some are good.

2. (2) Anxiety can be used constructively as a learning and motivating tool. The goal is not to eliminate anxiety but to have the client respond appropriately to it and not be overwhelmed by it.

3. (1) The child with autistic behavior reveals a disturbance in the development of social relationships. There is often an absence of responsive behavior toward the approach of the parents, and typically the child seems as content alone as in the presence of the parents.

4. (3) The child often demonstrates peculiar motor behavior in the form of spinning, rocking, head banging, and repetitive arm movements. Hallucinations are not evident in the autistic child. Failing to respond to parents' voices is not evidence of impaired hearing. Autistic children tend to respond well to music. The child with autism does not relate to others so will not be seen clinging to others.

5. (3) Because of the autistic child's avoidance of interpersonal contact and the disturbance in language development that typically occurs, a therapeutic approach to the child offers the nurse's presence without making demands for a response or imposing personal closeness.

6. (3) Gently providing guidance allows her to maintain her esteem and communicates supportive caring. Locking the door to her room is not safe for the client and interferes with her independence. Telling the client to stay in her room is ineffective because she has a memory impairment. Restraints increase feelings of helplessness, frustration, and inadequacy.

7. (2) The client is unable to recognize her daughter. The symptom of disorientation in organic mental disorders such as Alzheimer's is characterized by the inability to recall day or time, place, who they are, or the person or position of the person to which they are relating. Impaired judgment and impaired abstract thinking may be seen in organic mental disorders, but it is not the behavior described. They are both examples of impaired intellectual functioning, characterized by the inability to recall and use general knowledge in decision making and problem solving. Perceptual impairments such as delusions may occur in organic mental disorders, manifested by a fixed idea for which there is no factual basis. This is not the behavior described.

8. (1) This is empathetic, because it lets the daughter know that the nurse has an understanding of what the daughter must be feeling. Answers 2 and 4 are incorrect, because the nurse is giving advice and neglects the daughter's feelings. Answer 3 is not correct because it generalizes and minimizes the daughter's feelings.

9. (4) This approach conveys caring, support, and helpfulness. It also ensures that the patient knows where and when to eat. Impaired intellectual functioning that is evident in organic mental disorders interferes with the

person's ability to reason or solve problems. Answer 3 will increase frustration and anger.

10. (1) The client's behavior suggests an attempt at manipulation. Manipulative behavior is best handled by setting limits. Asking her to put on a robe sets limits. Answers 2 and 3 are incorrect because they avoid the problem. Answer 4 does not address the problem behavior, which is manipulation.

11. (2) Tremors and hyperactivity are common symptoms of Valium detoxification. Although blood pressure should be monitored, it generally does not decrease. Increased appetite and grandiosity are not symptoms of detoxification.

12. (4) The nurse is identifying the overall feeling tone of the client's communication and is directly asking for feedback about her suicide potential. Most suicide clients will give truthful information when directly asked. Answer 1 is a reflective statement and can allow her to continue talking, but it is appropriate after her suicide potential is assessed. Answer 2 asks for an analysis and may be distracting to the theme. Answer 3 invalidates the client's thoughts and feelings.

13. (2) The nurse must determine when the client had her last drink to help anticipate when withdrawal symptoms will occur.

14. (2) Physiological dependence on alcohol is responsible for the syndrome that occurs when alcohol is withdrawn. The syndrome includes the symptoms of tachycardia, elevated blood pressure, nausea, restlessness, tremors, hallucinations, convulsions, and ultimately may progress to delirium tremens. The client who is being detoxified must be monitored carefully for the development of these symptoms so that adequate measures can be taken to prevent injury, to meet metabolic and nutritional needs, and to minimize anxiety. Medicinal whiskey is not used during detoxification. Although the client in withdrawal may become confused and agitated, the use of physical restraints should be avoided if possible because they tend to

increase agitation. The room should not be darkened, this tends to promote shadows that may be misintrepreted (this client is prone to illusions).

15. (4) Visual and tactile hallucinations are indicative of the development of delirium tremens. The presence of a staff member offering reassurance and orientation may reduce the client's growing sense of panic and prevent self-injury. The physician should be informed of the client's condition so that the use of a tranquilizer may be considered. Showing her that there is nothing to fear is not appropriate when the confusion is due to withdrawal. There is no need to search her room for alcohol. The behavior suggests withdrawal, not intoxication or nightmares.

16. (1) When a client is in delirium tremens, the potential for physical injury may be life-threatening. Protective measures are a priority. All of the other diagnoses could be appropriate at some point in the care, but not at this time.

17. (2) It is expected that any client beginning group therapy will experience a period of uncertainty, during which considerable anxiety will be felt. Only when the client has progressed through this phase, and through the phases of aggression and regression, will she arrive at the adaptation phase-during which she may develop insight into her behavior. It is important to understand the phases through which participants move in group therapy.

18. (4) The purpose of Antabuse is to help the client abstain from alcohol. The client who takes Antabuse regularly will experience symptoms of nausea, vomiting, and palpitations when even a small amount of alcohol is consumed. The drug is usually used for only a limited time in conjunction with other treatment methods.

19. (2) Self-help and peer support are offered by AA in an ongoing education program that assists the members to achieve abstinence from alcohol. The other purposes may be secondary,

but the primary purpose is to help members abstain from alcohol.

20. (1) The hypotension caused by Thorazine is more severe when the drug is administered IM. The other choices do not relate to side effects of Thorazine.

21. (1) Pseudoparkinsonism is one of the extrapyramidal side effects that occur with phenothiazine drugs. If this is severe, an antiparkinsonian drug is prescribed. The other choices are not side effects of Thorazine. The client is more apt to experience urinary retention than incontinence.

22. (1) Circulation may be severely impaired in a client with a waxy flexibility who tends to remain motionless for hours unless moved. She does not speak and will not be able to discuss her concerns or identify predisposing factors during the initial stages. Touch is not used at this stage.

23. (4) This is a reality-based response as well as one that acknowledges the client's nonverbal reaction. The nurse should not focus on the "voice," because that reinforces the hallucination and does not place doubt. Answer 2 voices doubt but focuses on the voice, not the client's feelings.

24. (4) Ideas of reference are a common symptom in paranoid disorders. The person interprets an event occurring in the environment as having particular significance or reference to himself.

25. (2) The client is too active to eat and at the moment is unable to control this overactivity. Nursing actions to meet nutritional needs include giving her finger foods that she can eat while moving about.

26. (1) Diarrhea is a common side effect of lithium carbonate and may indicate toxicity. Rhinitis (runny nose), glycosuria (sugar in the urine), and rash are not side effects of lithium.

27. (4) This client is severely depressed and needs an environment that places few demands on him. His self-esteem will be raised by knowing that someone cares enough about him to speak to him. In time, he may respond. Note that the scenario states twice that he does not speak; therefore, encouraging him to talk about his children is not appropriate.

28. (4) During the acute phase of depression, the client is not meeting her physical needs. The nurse must meet these needs.

29. (4) As the depressed client begins to improve, the risk of suicide is increased because the person now has a greater amount of energy. Behaviors that may indicate that the client is planning a suicide attempt include a sudden lightening of mood, an air of relaxation, or the appearance of detachment.

30. (4) The original fear of men was displaced onto elevators, a safer object.

31. (4) Her anxiety is high when faced with the elevator. Forcing her to get on the elevator may precipitate an anxiety attack or panic reaction. Note that this is early in the course of her hospitalization. The nurse must not force her to get on the elevator.

32. (1) He needs support during this time. He will be unable to pay attention to details or to think clearly during an anxiety attack. Note that his symptoms include chest pain and choking.

33. (4) Positive accomplishment will help to boost self-concept and self-confidence. A client with ritualistic behavior will do best when routine activities are set up and anxiety-producing changes are avoided. Perfection-type activities bring satisfaction (cleaning and straightening a linen closet). He needs to know changes in routine in advance in order to cope with the anxiety produced by the changes.

34. (2) Acknowledgment is really restating what the client says. This answer is a restatement of "I'm afraid to ride in an elevator, I know it's silly, but I can't help it."

35. (3) In the initial stage of psychotherapy, as clients begin to confront the conflicts that are the source of their symptoms, it is common for them to experience an intensification of anxiety

and defensive behavior. The nurse should anticipate this phenomenon.

36. (2) It is common for the client with an antisocial personality disorder to single out a staff member whom he will attempt to manipulate for the gratification of his wishes. The nurse must be aware of the client's motivations and of the responses that he may be attempting to elicit from the nurse. The nurse may mistakenly interpret the client's desire to communicate as an expression of real interpersonal closeness, or the nurse may engage in fantasies about saving the client from his destructive behavior. The realistic assessment of the situation is based on the understanding that the nurse can establish guidelines of the plan of care.

37. (3) The nurse cannot promise not to tell a client's secret. The client may tell of a suicide plan or something else that must be shared with the physician or other staff members.

38. (4) Since, in some cases, the symptoms of organic mental disorder are attributable to systemic illness, nutritional disorders, and effects of drugs, it is imperative that the client be given a thorough physical examination so that physiologic problems that may be causing her behavior or may simply coexist can be addressed.

39. (2) The nurse should understand that the client's possessions represent an extension of herself and an affirmation of her personal identity in an alien environment. It is most therapeutic to allow the client to use this coping behavior as long as she is not dangerous.

40. (3) In the early part of hospitalization, the nurse should allow the client to perform the ritual and still eat. Given a choice, the obsessive-compulsive client would choose the ritual. Restriction privileges this early in treatment is not reasonable. Insisting that she stop washing her hands could precipitate a panic attack.

41. (2) Secondary sex characteristics tend to disappear. Her breasts will get smaller. She will have bradycardia, not tachycardia. Her temperature will not be elevated.

42. (2) Observing her to be sure she does not induce vomiting is the highest priority.

43. (2) He is exhibiting the classic symptoms of depression, and the nurse should stay with him. He should be evaluated for suicide potential.

44. (3) Elavilisa tricyclic antidepressants take 2–3 weeks for therapeutic effects to be seen.

45. (4) This indicates that he is less withdrawn. Answer 1 indicates poor self esteem. Answer 2 may be a suicidal warning sign.

46. (4) Giving away items may be a sign he is going to commit suicide.

47. (1) This response opens communication and encourages him to express his feelings.

48. (1) Thorazine causes photosensitivity. Because it is a central nervous system drug, alcohol should not be taken.

49. (4) The nurse should get the male client's attention so that he will release the other client. Help is needed.

50. (1) Tremors suggest Thorazine toxicity.

Chapter 16

The Perioperative Client

Sample Questions

1. When informed consent is obtained for surgery, who must explain the surgical procedure to the client?

   1. Physician
   2. Nurse on the surgical unit
   3. Anesthesiologist
   4. Operating room nurse

2. A 19-year-old unmarried college student is admitted unconscious following a car accident. He is hemorrhaging from severe internal injuries. Which statement is true concerning obtaining informed consent for treating him?

   1. Emergency care can be given because his injuries are life threatening.
   2. He can sign his own consent form because he is older than 18.
   3. Parental consent must be obtained before treatment is started.
   4. The hospital must obtain a court order before treating him.

3. An adult is to have abdominal surgery this morning. Immediately, preoperatively the nurse must assure that he

   1. Is comfortable
   2. Has an empty bowel
   3. Practices coughing
   4. Voids

4. A woman who is to have surgery tomorrow denies any fears or worries about the upcoming surgery. She talks incessantly about trivial matters and is constantly rearranging the items on her bedside stand, however. What is the most appropriate action for the nurse to take?

   1. Listen to her trivial talk.
   2. During preoperative teaching, encourage her to ask questions and express concerns.
   3. Assume that she is well prepared for surgery and discuss it very little.
   4. Probe deeply to find out what is bothering her.

5. What is the primary reason that surface hair is removed from the skin prior to surgery?

    1. To enhance vision of the surgical field
    2. To reduce the chance of infection as the skin is opened
    3. To prevent postoperative discomfort from adhesive tape
    4. To prevent itching in the postoperative period

6. Preoperative orders for an adult client include pentobarbital. This drug is administered primarily to

    1. Control secretions
    2. Control pain
    3. Promote sedation
    4. Provide anesthesia

7. An adult was given meperidine HCl (Demerol) 75 mg and Atropine Sulfate 0.4 mg as a preoperative medication. On her arrival in the operating room, she says to the nurse, "My mouth is very dry." What is the best response for the nurse to make?

    1. "I will tell the doctor about that."
    2. "That is a normal response to your medication."
    3. "Have you ever had an allergic reaction to any other drugs?"
    4. "Everything is going to be all right."

8. What is the primary problem that can occur as a result of vomiting in the immediate postoperative period?

    1. Electrolyte imbalance
    2. Dehiscence
    3. Aspiration
    4. Wound contamination

9. An adult has returned to the surgical floor following an abdominal cholecystectomy and an uneventful stay in the post-anesthesia room.

Which nursing action should be the highest priority?

    1. Encourage her to take deep breaths.
    2. Ask her to flex and extend her feet.
    3. Assist her in performing range-of-motion exercises.
    4. Irrigate her T-tube with normal saline.

10. A young man had an emergency appendectomy for a ruptured appendix. He is in the post-anesthesia care unit. He has not yet awakened. An IV is running. A penrose drain is in place. How should the nurse position this client?

    1. Semi-Fowler's position
    2. Supine with head turned to the side
    3. Prone with head and neck extended
    4. Right Sims

11. A young man had an emergency appendectomy for a ruptured appendix and is in the post-anesthesia care unit. A penrose drain is in place. After he recovers from anesthesia, how should he be positioned?

    1. Right Sims
    2. Dorsal
    3. Trendelenburg
    4. Semi-Fowler's

12. The nurse is planning care for a woman who had an abdominal hysterectomy and bilateral salpingectomy and oophorectomy. The nurse knows that because of the location of her surgery, the client is at risk for the development of

    1. Thrombophlebitis
    2. Pneumonia
    3. Stress ulcers
    4. Wound infection

13. An adult client is admitted to the post-anesthesia care unit following an

abdominoperineal resection. Which action should the nurse take initially?

1. Assess respiratory function.
2. Monitor IV fluids.
3. Check abdominal and perineal dressings.
4. Apply antithromboembolic stockings.

14. The nurse is caring for a woman who just delivered a healthy baby. She received a saddle block anesthesia during delivery. She is admitted to the postpartum unit. Which nursing action is most appropriate?

1. Encourage her to ambulate as soon as sensation and motion have returned.
2. Keep her flat and quiet for eight hours.
3. Keep her NPO for four hours.
4. Position her in the semi-Fowler's position as soon as she is alert.

15. A man who is recovering from a prostatectomy complains of pain in his left calf. The nurse observes slight ankle swelling and elicits Homan's sign. What is the best action for the nurse to take at this time?

1. Tell him to stay in bed and notify the charge nurse.
2. Massage his leg to relieve the pain.
3. Place a blanket roll under his left knee.
4. Encourage active ambulation.

Answers and Rationales

1. (1) Explaining the surgical procedure is the physician's responsibility. The nurse teaches about deep breathing, coughing, turning, pain management, and so on.

2. (1) Emergency care can be given without informed consent when there is a life-threatening emergency. He is older than 18 and could sign a consent form if he were conscious. The hospital will attempt to get consent from his parents for continuing medical care if he

remains unconscious after the emergency care is rendered.

3. (4) The key word is *immediately*. An enema can be given the evening before surgery to assure an empty bowel. Comfort is not the highest priority. Neither is coughing immediately preoperatively. The client should go to surgery with an empty bladder.

4. (2) The nurse should open communication with this client who is exhibiting anxious behavior. The nurse never assumes and should not probe deeply. Listening is appropriate, but trivial means unimportant.

5. (2) While there is some controversy about the need to shave a client prior to surgery, the primary reason that it is done is to reduce the chance of infection.

6. (3) Pentobarbital is a barbiturate and promotes sedation. Atropine is given to control secretions. Demerol will control pain. Scopolamine in large doses promotes anesthesia.

7. (2) Atropine is an anticholinergic drug given for the purpose of reducing secretions to prevent the possibility of aspiration.

8. (3) The key word is *immediate*. Aspiration is the primary problem associated with vomiting before the client is alert. Electrolyte imbalance could occur as the result of prolonged vomiting. Dehiscence might occur after violent vomiting.

9. (1) Persons who have a cholecystectomy are especially prone to the development of respiratory complications, because the incision is located under the ribcage.

10. (2) Before clients have awakened from anesthesia, they should be positioned either on their back with their head turned to the side or semi-side lying.

11. (4) The semi-Fowler's position promotes drainage. The client has a penrose drain.

12. (1) Pelvic surgery is a significant risk factor in the development of thrombophlebitis.

13. (1) Assessing airway function is of prime importance immediately following surgery and anesthesia. The other actions will all be done but only after the nurse is assured that the client has an adequate airway.

14. (2) A saddle block is a spinal anesthesia. Because of the loss of cerebrospinal fluid (CSF) during this procedure, it is necessary to keep the client flat for eight hours to prevent the development of a spinal headache. Choice 1 is appropriate for a client who has had an epidural anesthesia. Fluids should be encouraged to promote the formation of CSF.

15. (1) Homan's sign (pain in the calf when the ankle is dorsiflexed) and ankle swelling are suggestive of thrombophlebitis. The client should be placed on bedrest, and the physician should be notified. Massaging and ambulating are contraindicated because these activities might cause a thrombus to become an embolus. Placing a blanket roll under a knee causes venous stasis and clot formation.

Chapter 17

The Client with Cancer

Sample Questions

1. The nurse is caring for a client who is being treated for cancer. Which question by the client indicates that the client is not ready for teaching?

   1. "Am I going to lose my hair?"
   2. "Should I get a second opinion?"
   3. "Will this make me really sick?"
   4. "Will I have to stop exercising at the gym?"

2. The nurse caring for a client who is receiving chemotherapy is concerned about the client's nutritional status. What should the nurse encourage the client to do?

   1. Increase the amount of spices in the food.
   2. Avoid red meats.
   3. Medicate with Compazine before meals.
   4. Eat foods that are hot in temperature.

3. In planning care for a client with a platelet count of 8,000 and a WBC of 8,000 the nurse can expect to

   1. Remove flowers from the room
   2. Encourage fresh fruit and vegetables
   3. Use a strict hand-washing technique
   4. Take the client's temperature frequently

4. The nurse is teaching a client with a WBC of 1,400. Which statement made by the client indicates an understanding of the teaching?

   1. "I will eat fresh fruits and vegetables to avoid constipation."
   2. "I will stay away from my cat."
   3. "I will avoid crowded places."
   4. "I will wash all my fruits and vegetables before I eat them."

5. In evaluating the client with cancer what best indicates that the nutritional status is adequate?

   1. Calorie intake
   2. Stable weight
   3. Amount of nausea and vomiting
   4. Serum protein levels

6. An adult client with newly diagnosed cancer says, "I'm really afraid of dying. Who's going to take care of my children?" What is the best initial response for the nurse to make?

   1. "What makes you think you are going to die?"
   2. "How old are your children?"
   3. "This must be a difficult time for you."
   4. "Most people with your kind of cancer live a long time."

7. A client with terminal cancer yells at the nurse and says "I don't need your help, I can bathe myself." Which stage of grief is the client most likely experiencing?

    1. Projection
    2. Denial
    3. Anger
    4. Depression

8. The nurse can expect a client with a platelet count of 8,000 and a WBC count of 8,000 to be placed

    1. In a private room
    2. On protective isolation
    3. On bleeding precautions
    4. On neutropenic precautions

9. Which statement made by the client indicates understanding of the needs related to external radiation therapy?

    1. "I'll stay away from small children since I am radioactive."
    2. "I won't wash these marks off until after my therapy."
    3. "I'll put lotion on my skin to keep it moist."
    4. "I'll flush the toilet twice each time I use the bathroom."

10. When teaching and preparing a client for a bone marrow biopsy, the nurse should

    1. Check for an iodine allergy
    2. Position the client in the fetal position with his or her back curved
    3. Have the client sign the consent form
    4. Have the client remain NPO

11. An adult says to the nurse, "The doctor said I have a carcinoma and my friend has a sarcoma. What is the difference?" What should the nurse include in the response?

    1. Carcinoma is usually more serious than a sarcoma.

2. Carcinoma indicates that the tissue involved is epithelial, such as the GI tract or breast; sarcoma indicates that the tissue involved is connective tissue, such as the bone.

3. Carcinoma is a malignancy that usually appears early in life, while individuals who develop a sarcoma of any type are usually older.

4. Carcinomas are not as likely to metastasize to distant sites as sarcomas are.

12. The nurse is teaching a group of persons in the community about risk factors for cancer. Which is not a risk factor and should not be included in the teaching?

    1. A change in bowel habits
    2. Difficulty in swallowing
    3. Unexplained weight gain
    4. Nagging hoarseness

13. A woman who has had surgery for colon cancer asks the nurse why the doctor has her come back for a blood test called CEA. What is the best response for the nurse to make?

    1. "You should ask your physician about specific tests."
    2. "High levels of CEA are found in cancers of the colon; continued low levels after surgery indicate there is probably not a recurrence."
    3. "CEA is used to monitor your blood to be sure you are not getting side effects from the treatment."
    4. "CEA levels should increase as your general health increases."

14. An adult is undergoing diagnostic tests for possible cancer. A liver scan is scheduled. The client asks whether she will need to stay away from people because she is radioactive following the test. What should be included in the nurse's response?

1. She will be radioactive after the scan and should avoid small children and pregnant women.

2. The radioisotope doses used in the scan are very small, and she will not be a hazard to others.

3. Radioopaque substances are used, not radioisotopes, so there is no radioactivity.

4. Because the liver is being scanned, the breakdown of the substances will be delayed, so caution is needed.

15. The client has been receiving chemotherapy for cancer and has stomatitis. What nursing care is indicated because the client has stomatitis?

   1. Have the client rinse his or her mouth well with Listerine or other mouthwash before and after eating.

   2. Use meticulous care when cleaning the stoma and applying the drainage bag.

   3. Maintain NPO status until the condition improves.

   4. Encourage the client to use viscous lidocaine mouthwash as needed.

16. An adult woman is scheduled to start chemotherapy next week. In anticipation of alopecia, which recommendation is appropriate?

   1. Encourage the client to cut her hair and buy a wig.

   2. Recommend the client wash her hair carefully daily to prevent hair loss.

   3. Suggest that the client have a color photograph taken before starting chemotherapy so that hair color can be matched if necessary.

   4. Explain to the client that she should plan to have a hair transplant following chemotherapy.

17. The client is receiving cancer chemotherapy. Metoclopramide (Reglan) is also ordered. She asks the nurse why she is receiving Reglan. What nursing response is most accurate?

   1. Reglan is a stool softener and will help with the constipation the chemotherapy might cause.

   2. Reglan will help prevent alopecia.

   3. Reglan helps prevent diarrhea.

   4. Reglan will help control nausea and vomiting.

18. Allopurinol (Zyloprim) is ordered for the client who is receiving cancer chemotherapy. What instruction should the nurse give the client because allopurinol is ordered?

   1. Drink several additional glasses of water each day.

   2. Avoid foods containing folic acid.

   3. When you get up from lying down, sit on the edge of the bed for a few minutes before standing up.

   4. Avoid caffeine-containing products.

19. Which instruction is appropriate for the nurse to give the client who is undergoing external radiation therapy?

   1. Avoid gas-forming foods such as beans and cabbage.

   2. Be sure to get outdoors in the sun for a few minutes each day.

   3. Do not apply powders, deodorants, or ointments to your skin.

   4. Tight-fitting clothes will give you the most support.

20. The nurse is caring for a person who has radiation pellets inserted in the mouth to treat oral cancer. One of the pellets falls out. What should the nurse do initially?

    1. Put on rubber gloves and pick up the pellet and place it in the utility room.

    2. Use long-handled forceps to pick up the pellet and place it in a lead-lined container.

    3. Call the Nuclear Medicine Department.

    4. Replace the pellet in the mouth.

Answers and Rationales

1. (2) This statement indicates denial of his illness. The question states that he has cancer. All of the other comments indicate an interest in what is going to happen to him.

2. (1) Because taste buds are affected, increasing the spices will improve flavor.

3. (2) Fresh fruits and vegetables will help the client prevent constipation, which could cause bleeding. All of the other choices are appropriate for a low WBC, but this WBC is normal. The problem for this client is a low platelet count.

4. (3) Crowded places predispose to client infection. Choice 1 is related to low platelet count. The client should not eat fresh fruits and vegetables even if they are washed.

5. (2) Stable weight indicates adequate nutritional status.

6. (3) This empathetic response will open communication. Choice 1 is really a "why" question, which would put the client on the defensive. Choices 2 and 4 do not focus on the client's feelings.

7. (3) Yelling at the nurse would be typical of anger. Projection is putting his feelings on the nurse: "You are angry at me." Denial would be denying that he was terminally ill or that he had cancer. A client who is depressed would be apathetic and would probably not have the energy to yell at the nurse.

8. (3) The platelet count is very low. Normal is 150,000–500,000. Platelets clot the blood. The client must be on bleeding precautions. A WBC of 8,000 is within the normal range, so neutropenic precautions, protective isolation, and a private room are not indicated.

9. (2) It is important that the client not wash off the marks until after therapy is finished. The marks outline the tumor and show where the radiation should be concentrated. The client who is receiving external radiation is not radioactive and should not put anything on the skin. While flushing the toilet after each use is good hygiene, it is not related to external radiation. There is no radioactivity in the waste of a person who is receiving external radiation.

10. (3) A bone marrow biopsy is an invasive procedure that requires a legal consent form to be signed. No iodine dye is used. The usual site is the iliac crest; the client will not be placed in the fetal position. That is the position for a lumbar puncture. There is no need for the client to be NPO. Only a local anesthetic is used.

11. (2) Carcinoma indicates that the tissue involved is epithelial, such as the GI tract or breast; sarcoma indicates that the tissue involved is connective tissue, such as the bone. No general statement about the difference in severity or age of onset can be made because the terms indicate the type of tissue involved. Both types of cancers can metastasize.

12. (3) An unexplained weight loss is a possible sign of cancer. Unexplained weight gain is not usually associated with undetected cancer. A change in bowel habits, difficulty in swallowing, and nagging hoarseness are all possible warning signs of cancer.

13. (2) High levels of CEA are found in cancers of the colon; continued low levels after surgery indicate that there is probably not a recurrence. When cancers of the GI tract are present or when they have been removed and recur, the

Carcinoembryonic Antigen (CEA) levels rise. CEA levels are monitored following surgery to pick up a possible spread or recurrence early. The nurse should know this information and should not have to refer to the physician for general information about this test. CEA tests do not monitor the side effects of cancer treatment; a *complete blood count* (CBC) would pick up bone marrow depression. CEA levels do not increase with improvement in general health.

14. (2) Radioisotopes are used when most scans (except CT scans) are performed. The doses are so small, however, that the client is not considered radioactive—and no special precautions need to be taken.

15. (4) Stomatitis is a sore mouth and is commonly seen in persons who are receiving cancer chemotherapy. Lidocaine is a local anesthetic and will help relieve the pain of stomatitis. Listerine mouthwash contains alcohol and is contraindicated for a person who has mouth sores. Stomatitis refers to mouth sores, not a colostomy stoma. There is no need to maintain NPO status.

16. (1) The client should be encouraged to cut her hair and buy a wig if desired before starting chemotherapy. Alternatively, she could purchase scarves and use them to cover her head. When the hair falls out, it is easier to manage the loss of short hair than long hair. Washing hair will not prevent hair loss from chemotherapy. Having a color photograph taken before chemotherapy to match hair color is not the best answer. It would be better to match hair color in a wig before starting chemotherapy than waiting until after the hair is gone. Hair usually grows back following chemotherapy. It might not be the same color or have the same characteristics, however. A hair transplant is not indicated.

17. (4) Reglan is an antiemetic and will help control nausea and vomiting caused by the chemotherapy. It is not a stool softener and does not prevent alopecia or diarrhea.

18. (1) Allopurinol is given to help the client excrete uric acid, which might accumulate when cancer chemotherapeutic agents are given. The client should drink several additional glasses of water each day to help the kidneys flush the uric acid out of the system. There is no need to avoid foods containing folic acid because the client is taking allopurinol. This measure might be indicated depending on the chemotherapeutic agent the client is taking. Allopurinol does not cause orthostatic hypotension. Antiemetics might cause orthostatic hypotension. There is no need to avoid caffeine-containing products because the client is taking allopurinol.

19. (3) The client should put nothing on the skin. Deodorants and powders usually contain heavy metals, such as aluminum or zinc, and block radiation rays. Lotions and ointments should not be applied to the skin because they might further irritate the skin. There is no major reason to avoid gas-forming foods. That instruction is more appropriate for a person who has had a colostomy. If the client becomes nauseated, she should avoid any irritating food. Sun will irritate the client's sensitive skin. The person should wear loose-fitting clothes to avoid skin irritation, not tight-fitting clothes.

20. (2) The nurse should use long-handled forceps to pick up the pellet and place it in a lead-lined container. Afterward, the nurse should call the Nuclear Medicine Department. The nurse should never touch the pellet directly. Rubber gloves give no protection from radiation.

Unit V

Health Promotion and Drug Therapy

UNIT OUTLINE

Chapter 18

Nutrition & Special Diets

Sample Questions

1. The nurse knows that the client understands a low-sodium diet when the client selects which of the following menus?

    1. Lobster salad, corn bread, and milk
    2. Hot roast beef sandwich, celery sticks, and coffee
    3. Sliced chicken, fresh tomatoes, and beets
    4. Liver and onions, creamed carrots, and a biscuit

2. An adult has chronic renal failure and asks why sodium must be limited. What is the best answer for the nurse to make?

    1. "Sodium causes high blood pressure, which is not good for your kidneys."
    2. "Kidneys normally help the body eliminate sodium. Your kidneys are not doing that now."
    3. "Sodium tends to increase the workload of the kidneys. Your kidneys need rest."
    4. "Sodium causes hypotension, which is dangerous when your kidneys don't work."

3. A low-sodium, low-fat diet has been prescribed for a client who recently had a myocardial infarction. Which of the following menu selections would be most appropriate for this client?

    1. Hot dog and roll, tossed salad with blue cheese dressing, and chocolate chip cookies
    2. Roast beef with gravy, baked potato, and sliced carrots
    3. Cream of mushroom soup, tuna sandwich, and sliced tomatoes
    4. Baked chicken, green beans, and mashed potatoes

4. Digoxin and furosemide (Lasix) have been prescribed for a client who is in congestive heart failure. Which snack would be best for the client?

    1. Crackers
    2. Honeydew melon
    3. Apple
    4. Carrots

5. Which foods should be omitted from the diet of a client who has gout?

   1. Eggs and cheese
   2. Lobster and liver
   3. Bread and peanut butter
   4. Apricots and melons

6. A client who is on a special diet for the treatment of gout asks the nurse why a special diet is prescribed. What is the best answer for the nurse to give?

   1. "When purines are used by the body, they break down into uric acid that deposits in your joints and causes pain."
   2. "Proteins make your lungs work harder and cause you pain."
   3. "Your heart cannot handle extra fluids."
   4. "Fats cause oxalates to deposit in your toes and legs, decreasing circulation."

7. A 10-year-old has a lactose intolerance. The child's mother asks the nurse for assistance in meeting calcium needs. What is the best nursing response?

   1. "Serve broccoli and other dark green vegetables frequently."
   2. "Give her ice cream."
   3. "Have Susan drink skim milk."
   4. "Serve carrots and other yellow vegetables frequently."

8. The wife of a man who has coronary artery disease asks the nurse how she can prepare foods that will be good for her husband. What should the nurse include when talking with this woman?

   1. Encourage her to use cream sauces to enhance the flavor of foods.
   2. Tell her to shop exclusively at health food stores.
   3. Suggest she substitute salmon or other fish for meat several times a week.
   4. Encourage her to use onion salt and celery salt to foods.

9. A client who has hypertension makes all of the following statements. Which statement indicates a need for more teaching?

   1. "I eat fresh fruit every day."
   2. "I just love dill pickles with my sandwich at lunch."
   3. "I prefer broiled meats to fried food."
   4. "I enjoy one cup of decaffeinated coffee at lunch."

10. An adult who has hypertension is taking furosemide (Lasix). The client has been placed on a low-sodium, high-potassium diet. What is the reason for the potassium alteration?

    1. To prevent sodium loss from the renal tubules
    2. To replace potassium lost from the kidneys
    3. To prevent osteoporosis secondary to diuresis
    4. To maintain an acid-base balance

11. Ferrous sulfate has been prescribed for a woman who is pregnant. The nurse should advise her to take the medication at which time?

    1. Upon arising
    2. With meals
    3. Immediately following meals
    4. At bedtime

12. A pregnant woman asks why iron has been prescribed for her. How should the nurse reply?

    1. "Iron helps to prevent sickle cell anemia in your baby."
    2. "Iron will help your baby to develop more intelligence."
    3. "Your body needs a lot of iron to make red blood cells for you and your baby."

4. "Your morning sickness will be less if you have plenty of iron."

13. A pregnant woman asks the nurse for help in planning her diet to include iron sources. Which suggestion would be best?

    1. Be sure to eat at least one egg white a day.
    2. Drink orange juice with your morning egg.
    3. Drink milk with every meal.
    4. A peanut butter sandwich is a good snack.

14. A young mother is concerned about providing an adequate diet for her children and asks the nurse how to be sure they get enough B vitamins. Which response is best?

    1. Provide a glass of milk with every meal.
    2. Offer whole grains and cereals.
    3. Give citrus fruits as snacks.
    4. Offer carrots and melons.

15. An adult says to the nurse, "The doctor told me that I should have plenty of the healing vitamin to help my operation heal." What foods would best meet this prescription?

    1. Apple juice
    2. Strawberries
    3. Hamburger
    4. Peanut butter

16. An adult is on a low-sodium, low-fat diet for hypertension. What question is most important for the nurse to ask when starting to teach the client?

    1. "How do you prepare your foods?"
    2. "When do you eat your meals?"
    3. "Who eats with you?"
    4. "When do you sleep?"

17. Which of these meals would the nurse recommend to provide the highest amount of protein and calories?

    1. Vegetable soup, cottage cheese on crackers, applesauce, and a hot chocolate
    2. Cheeseburger, French-fried potatoes, carrot sticks, cantaloupe balls, and milk
    3. Fresh fruit plate with sherbert, buttered muffin, slice of watermelon, and a fruit-flavored milk drink
    4. Chicken noodle soup, cream cheese and jelly sandwich, buttered whole kernel corn, orange sherbert, and a cola drink

18. Mothers should be instructed that diets for infants and toddlers who drink a lot of milk and few other foods will most likely result in the development of a deficiency in which of these nutrients?

    1. Iron
    2. Carbohydrate
    3. Vitamin D
    4. Vitamin K

19. Following surgery, a clear liquid diet is ordered. Which of these foods would be contraindicated for this person?

    1. Tea with lemon
    2. Ginger ale
    3. Milk
    4. Gelatin desert

20. A 4-year-old child has phenylketonuria and must follow a special diet. Which food is allowed on this diet?

    1. Bread and butter
    2. Strawberries
    3. Peanut butter sandwich
    4. Hamburger

21. A low-residue diet is ordered for a man who has ulcerative colitis. The nurse knows that he understands his diet when he selects which foods?

   1. Spinach salad and roast beef

   2. Mashed potato and chicken

   3. Green beans and pork chop

   4. Lettuce salad and spaghetti

22. The nurse is to teach a client about a low-purine diet. What should the nurse do initially?

   1. Provide a list of foods to be avoided.

   2. Ask the client what he has eaten for the last three days.

   3. Obtain baseline weight and height measurements.

   4. Explain why he must follow this diet.

23. A woman who is in the seventh month of pregnancy has symptoms of preeclampsia. When discussing diet, the nurse instructs the client to eat a high-protein diet and to avoid foods that have a high sodium content. Which of these foods, if selected by the client, would be correct?

   1. Creamed chipped beef on dry toast

   2. Cheese sandwich on whole-wheat toast

   3. Frankfurter on a roll

   4. Tomato stuffed with diced chicken

24. An adolescent has been recently diagnosed as having type I insulin-dependent diabetes. She asks the nurse if she will ever be able to go out with her friends for pizza or ice cream. Which of these responses by the nurse would give accurate information?

   1. "You can go with the group, but you cannot eat pizza or ice cream."

   2. "You can have pizza but not ice cream."

   3. "If you eat when out with your friends, you will have to skip the next meal."

   4. "It is important for you to be with your friends. We will help you learn how to choose foods."

25. A pregnant woman tells the nurse she is constipated. What suggestion is best for the nurse to give the woman?

   1. Reduce your fluid intake.

   2. Reduce your intake of fruits.

   3. Increase your intake of raw vegetables.

   4. Increase your intake of rice.

Answers and Rationales

1. (3) Chicken is lower in sodium than seafood and beef. Fresh tomatoes are low in sodium. Canned tomato products are not. Beets are not high in sodium. Seafood is high in sodium. Foods containing baking soda, such as corn bread and biscuits, are high in sodium. Milk and milk products are high in sodium. Creamed foods are high in sodium. Celery sticks and carrots are naturally high in sodium.

2. (2) This best explains the reason for reducing sodium in the diet of someone who has chronic renal failure. There is some truth to answer 1. Sodium is probably related to hypertension in some individuals, and hypertension is not good for the kidneys. However, answer 2 is better. Answer 3 is not correct. Answer 4 is not correct. Sodium causes hypertension, not hypotension.

3. (4) Chicken is lower in sodium and fat than beef and other meats. Green beans and mashed potatoes are low in sodium. Hot dogs are high in sodium and fat. Blue cheese dressing is high in sodium and fat. Chocolate chip cookies are high in sodium and fat. Roast beef and gravy are both high in sodium and fat. Carrots are naturally high in sodium. Creamed products are high in sodium and fat. Soups have about 1,000 mg of sodium per serving. Tuna is high in sodium. Bread contains about 200 mg of sodium per slice.

4. (2) Furosemide is a potassium-depleting diuretic. Melons are high in potassium. Crackers have very little potassium. An apple is not high in potassium. Carrots are high in sodium.

5. (2) Lobster and liver are high in purines. The other foods are not particularly high in purines.

6. (1) The prescribed diet for gout is a low-purine diet. Purines break down into uric acid. Persons who have gout do not excrete the uric acid normally, and it deposits in joints and causes severe pain. Answer 2 makes no sense. Extra fluid volume is not the problem in gout. Gout is faulty purine metabolism, not faulty oxalate metabolism.

7. (1) Broccoli and other dark green vegetables are high in calcium. The person who has lactose intolerance usually cannot eat ice cream or skim milk, both of which contain lactose (milk sugar). Carrots and yellow vegetables are high in Vitamin A but are not high in calcium.

8. (3) Salmon and fish contain omega 3 fatty acids, which are "heart healthy" and help to increase HDL and lower LDL. Meat is high in omega 6 fatty acids, which raise the bad cholesterol (LDL). Cream sauces are high in fat and should be avoided if a person has coronary artery disease. There is no need to shop exclusively at health food stores. Onion salt and celery salt contain salt and are usually limited for a person who has coronary artery disease.

9. (2) The person who has hypertension should have a diet low in sodium and fat and avoid caffeine. Dill pickles are extremely high in sodium. Each slice of bread has about 200 mg of sodium. Sandwiches should be avoided on a low-sodium diet. Fresh fruit is low in sodium. Meats, when eaten, should be broiled, not fried. Decaffeinated coffee is recommended for persons who have hypertension.

10. (2) Furosemide (Lasix) is a potassium-depleting diuretic. Persons taking furosemide should increase their intake of potassium to replace the potassium lost in the urine. A high-potassium diet does not prevent sodium loss from the renal tubules. Sodium loss from the renal tubules is the mechanism by which furosemide works. Potassium in the diet does not prevent osteoporosis secondary to diuresis. Dietary potassium is not increased to maintain acid-base balance.

11. (2) Taking ferrous sulfate (iron) with meals helps to reduce nausea associated with the medicine. Absorption is best on an empty stomach. However, many people experience nausea when taking iron.

12. (3) The mother has to supply the iron needed for her increase in blood volume during pregnancy, for the baby's blood, and a six-month supply of iron for the newborn. Iron does not prevent sickle cell anemia. Iron does not increase intelligence. Iron does not reduce morning sickness. In fact, iron can cause nausea if it is taken on an empty stomach.

13. (2) Egg yolk contains iron. Iron is best absorbed when taken with a Vitamin C source, such as orange juice. Egg white contains no iron. Milk contains no iron. A peanut butter sandwich is not a good source of iron.

14. (2) The best sources of B vitamins are whole grains and cereals. Milk contains good amounts of calcium. Citrus fruits are good sources of vitamin C and potassium. Carrots and melons are good sources of vitamin A.

15. (2) Strawberries are high in Vitamin C. The other choices are not high in Vitamin C. Vitamin C is called "the healing vitamin."

16. (1) A low-fat, low-sodium diet involves low salt and baking or broiling, not frying. The other questions are not particularly relevant to a low-sodium, low-fat diet.

17. (2) Protein is in the cheeseburger and the milk. The calorie load is high. The other choices have less protein and fewer calories.

18. (1) Milk contains no iron.

19. (3) Milk is not a clear liquid. All of the other choices are clear liquids.

20. (2) The PKU diet eliminates phenylalanine. Phenylalanine is a protein. The person should avoid all meats and protein foods. Bread contains small amounts of protein and should be avoided on a PKU diet.

21. (2) Mashed potatoes and chicken are low in residue. Residue sources have skins, seeds, and leaves. Spinach, green beans, and lettuce are all high in residue.

22. (2) Nutrition teaching should start with a diet history.

23. (4) Chicken contains protein and is relatively low in sodium. Fresh tomatoes are low in sodium. Creamed chipped beef on toast, a cheese sandwich, and a hot dog all contain protein but are also very high in sodium.

24. (4) This answer recognizes the adolescent's need to be with her friends and explains that she will learn how to choose foods. The other answers do not give accurate information.

25. (3) Constipation is best prevented by increasing fiber intake. Fresh vegetables and fruits are good sources of fiber. Fluid intake should be increased, not reduced. Rice tends to cause constipation.

Chapter 19

Pharmacology

Sample Questions

1. The nurse is administering an IM injection to a client. When the nurse aspirates, there is a blood return. What is the most appropriate action for the nurse to take?

   1. Continue to administer the medication.
   2. Withdraw the needle and administer in another site.
   3. Withdraw the needle, discard the medication, and start over.
   4. Change the needle before administering the medication in another site.

2. The nurse is to administer a subcutaneous injection. Which technique is correct?

   1. Pull the skin taut. Insert a 21-gauge needle at a 90-degree angle.
   2. Pinch the skin. Insert a 25-gauge needle at a 45-degree angle.
   3. Stretch the skin taut. Insert a 27-gauge needle at a 10-degree angle.
   4. Pinch the skin. Insert a 21-gauge needle at a 60-degree angle.

3. The nurse is to administer an IM injection to a six-month-old. What is the most appropriate site to utilize?

   1. Vastus lateralis
   2. Dorsal gluteal
   3. Ventral gluteal
   4. Iliac crest

4. Ringers Lactate is running at 125 ml/hr. The administration set has 15 drops/ml. What should the drip rate be?

   1. 8 drops/min.
   2. 31 drops/min.
   3. 50 drops/min.
   4. 67 drops/min.

5. A two-year-old child who weighs 33 pounds is to receive a total daily dose of 25 mg/kg of a medication. It is to be administered in three evenly divided doses. The label reads 150 mg/ml. How many ml will be injected per dose?

   1. 0.5 ml
   2. 0.8 ml
   3. 3.75 ml
   4. 155 ml

6. An adult is receiving gentamicin IV q 8 h. Which laboratory tests does the nurse expect that the client will have done regularly?

   1. CBC and hemoglobin
   2. BUN and creatinine
   3. SGOT and SGPT
   4. Urine and blood cultures

7. Which observation, if reported by a client, is most suggestive of an adverse reaction to gentamicin?

   1. A WBC of 8000
   2. Ringing in the ears
   3. Itching
   4. Nasal stuffiness

8. Penicillin V Potassium (Pen-Vee-K) 500 mg PO qid is ordered for an adult client. He reports that he took penicillin for the first time two months ago. What should the nurse do?

   1. Be sure that skin testing for a penicillin allergy has been done.
   2. Observe for signs of an allergic response.
   3. Withhold the penicillin.
   4. Notify the physician.

9. The nurse in the physician's office is instructing an adult about taking penicillin V potassium (Pen-Vee-K) qid. When should the nurse tell him to take the medicine?

   1. With meals and at bedtime
   2. Once a day at 10 A.M.
   3. On an empty stomach at six-hour intervals
   4. With orange juice at four-hour intervals

10. A 10-month-old has been diagnosed as having acute otitis media. The pediatrician prescribed amoxicillin suspension. What instructions should the nurse give the child's mother?

    1. When your child's temperature has been normal for two days, discontinue the medicine.
    2. Discard any unused medication.
    3. If your child has symptoms of an ear infection again, start giving her the leftover medication.
    4. Give your child all of the medication in the bottle.

11. Keflex 250 mg PO q 6 h is ordered for an adult. The nurse notes that her history indicates that she has an allergy to penicillin. What is the most appropriate initial action for the nurse?

    1. Notify the physician.
    2. Observe the client carefully after giving the medication.
    3. Administer the Keflex IV instead of PO.
    4. Ask the client to describe the reaction that she had to penicillin.

12. Which of the following persons would be least likely to receive tetracycline?

    1. An adolescent with acne
    2. A woman with chlamydia who is seven months pregnant
    3. A 10-year-old with Rocky Mountain Spotted Fever
    4. A 32-year-old man with walking pneumonia

13. An adult is receiving Gantrisin 1 GM PO qid for a urinary tract infection. Which statement that she makes indicates a need for more teaching?

    1. "If I get a rash, I will apply calamine lotion."
    2. "I will take my pills with a full glass of water."
    3. "I will take all the pills even if I feel better."
    4. "I will stay out of the sun while I am taking the pills."

14. An adult client is seen in the clinic, and methenamine mandelate (Mandelamine) is prescribed. Which information is most appropriate for the nurse to include in the teaching?

    1. You should drink several glasses of cranberry juice each day.
    2. If it upsets your stomach, try taking it with an antacid.
    3. Avoid going out in the sun while taking Mandelamine.
    4. Take the tablets with orange juice or milk.

15. An adult client has pulmonary tuberculosis. He is receiving INH 300 mg PO and Ethambutol 1 GM PO daily and streptomycin 1 GM I.M. three times a week. When he comes in for a checkup, he tells the nurse that he hates getting shots and his ears ring most of the time. What is the best interpretation for the nurse to make regarding the client's complaints?

    1. He may be receiving too much Ethambutol.

    2. He should be evaluated for adverse reaction to streptomycin.

    3. Tuberculosis may have spread to the brain.

    4. He is experiencing a reaction commonly seen when INH and Streptomycin are given at the same time.

16. An adult client has pulmonary tuberculosis. He is receiving INH 300 mg PO and Ethambutol 1 GM PO daily and streptomycin 1 GM I.M. three times a week. When he comes in for a checkup, he tells the nurse that he hates getting shots and his ears ring most of the time. What advice does the nurse expect will be given to this client?

    1. Take pyridoxine (Vitamin B6) daily.

    2. Expect orange-colored urine and feces.

    3. Stop the medications when his cough is gone.

    4. Take streptomycin by mouth instead of by injection.

17. An adult client is being treated for genital herpes with acyclovir (Zovirax) tablets. Which statement she makes indicates that she understands her therapy?

    1. "It is safe now to have sexual relations."

    2. "I will stay home from work until the blisters are gone."

    3. "This medicine will cure the herpes infection."

    4. "If the blisters come back, I will start taking the pills immediately."

18. The clinic nurse is teaching an adult male who has AIDS. He is receiving zidovudine. Which statement he makes indicates that he understands the medication regimen?

    1. "If I get a sore throat and it is hard to swallow my capsules, I can empty the capsule into applesauce."

    2. "I am hopeful that this drug will get rid of this awful disease."

    3. "I understand I might need a transfusion."

    4. "I should take acetaminophen (Tylenol), not aspirin, if I get a fever."

19. An adult client has been diagnosed as having rheumatoid arthritis and is started on Piroxicam (Feldene) 20 mg daily. Two days later, the client calls the nurse and says that her joints still hurt. What is the best response for the nurse to make?

    1. "It may take up to two weeks before results are seen with Feldene."

    2. "Take aspirin with the Feldene. It has an additive effect."

    3. "Come in to see the physician. You should have pain relief by now."

    4. "You may need more medication. Take one additional pill each day."

20. A 13-month-old child is admitted to the emergency room with salicylate poisoning. Her mother found her beside the empty bottle of adult aspirin. She says there were "about 10" aspirin left in the bottle. What manifestations would the nurse most expect to see in the child?

    1. Bradypnea and pallor

    2. Hyperventilation and hyperpyrexia

    3. Subnormal temperature and bleeding

    4. Melena and bradycardia

21. A toddler who has swallowed several adult aspirin is admitted to the emergency room. When admitted, the child is breathing but is difficult to arouse. What is the immediate priority of care?

   1. Administration of syrup of ipecac
   2. Cardiopulmonary resuscitation
   3. Ventilatory support
   4. Gastric lavage

22. An adult client is on call for the operating room. The pre-op medication order is for meperidine HCl (Demerol) 100 mg IM and atropine 0.4 mg IM. The operating room calls at 11 A.M. and requests that the client be medicated. The nurse notes that the client last received meperidine for pain at 10 A.M. What is the most appropriate action for the nurse to take?

   1. Give the pre-op medication as ordered.
   2. Give half the dose of meperidine and all of the atropine.
   3. Check with the anesthesiologist before administering the medication.
   4. Withhold both the meperidine and the atropine.

23. An adult client had an abdominal hysterectomy this morning. Meperidine HCl (Demerol) 75 mg IM q 3–4 hrs prn for pain is ordered. At 9 P.M., she complains of lower abdominal pain. She was last medicated at 5:45 P.M. What is the most appropriate initial action for the nurse to take?

   1. Offer her a bed pan and a back rub.
   2. Reposition her.
   3. Administer meperidine HCl 75 mg IM.
   4. Encourage her to perform relaxation and breathing exercises.

24. An adult client has rheumatoid arthritis. Aspirin 975 mg q 4 hrs prn is ordered for pain. At 2 P.M. the client requests pain medication. Aspirin was last given at 9:30 A.M. What is the most appropriate initial action for the nurse to take?

   1. Give the aspirin as ordered.
   2. Question the order because it is a higher-than-normal dosage.
   3. Attempt to divert the client's attention from the pain.
   4. Assess the nature of the pain.

25. A 68-year-old man has been diagnosed as having Parkinson's Disease. He is started on Cogentin 0.5 mg PO daily. Which nursing action is most essential at this time?

   1. Monitor his blood pressure and pulse.
   2. Encourage cold beverages and hard candies.
   3. Observe for rashes.
   4. Monitor his stools for fluid loss.

26. A young adult, 20 years old, who is hospitalized for the first time with schizophrenia, is receiving chlorpromazine (Thorazine) 75 mg PO tid. The client is to go home for a weekend pass. Which statement that the client makes indicates a need for nursing intervention?

   1. "I won't drink any alcohol this weekend."
   2. "It will be good to taste home-cooked food again."
   3. "We plan to go dancing."
   4. "I'm looking forward to sunbathing at the beach."

27. An adult client is receiving Lithium 600 mg PO tid for the treatment of bipolar disorder. The client should be taught that it is important to have adequate amounts of which substance?

   1. Potassium
   2. Sodium
   3. Calcium
   4. Magnesium

28. An elderly adult is scheduled for repair of a fractured femur this morning. The nurse goes in to administer pre-op medication of Demerol 75 mg and Atropine 0.4 mg I.M. The client asks the nurse if he should take his eye drops before surgery. What is the best initial response for the nurse to make?

1. "You can take them when you get back from surgery."
2. "I'll give them to you now."
3. "Let me check with your physician."
4. "What kind of eye drops are you taking?"

29. A 68-year-old client was admitted with congestive heart failure, has been digitalized, and is now taking a maintenance dose of Digoxin 0.25 mg PO daily. The client is to be discharged soon. Which assessment is of most immediate concern to the nurse?

1. The client's apical pulse is 66.
2. The client says that he is nauseous and has no appetite.
3. The client says that he will take his pill every morning.
4. The client has lost eight pounds since his admission one week ago.

30. An adult has angina and is to be discharged on transdermal nitroglycerin. Which statement by the client indicates that the client needs additional teaching?

1. "I am glad that I can continue walking."
2. "I will change the site each day."
3. "I will be able to continue to drink alcoholic beverages."
4. "I will need to get up slowly."

31. A 48-year-old man is in the emergency room. He has crushing substernal pain, is diaphoretic, apprehensive, and ashen gray in color. The cardiac monitor shows runs of premature ventricular contractions. Which drug is most likely to be given to this client?

1. Lidocaine
2. Verapamil
3. Digitalis
4. Nitroglycerine

32. A 60-year-old client has been hospitalized for deep vein thrombosis. The client is to be discharged on warfarin 5 mg PO daily. Which statement that the client makes indicates the best understanding of the medication routine?

1. "I will take aspirin for my arthritis."
2. "I love to eat spinach salads."
3. "I will get a blood test next week."
4. "I made an appointment to have my teeth pulled."

33. A 67-year-old client is to be discharged from the hospital. The client is taking digoxin and furosemide daily. Which instruction is most essential for the nurse to give this client?

1. Take your medicine early in the day.
2. Be sure to drink orange juice and eat bananas or melons every day.
3. Avoid foods that are high in sodium.
4. Drink plenty of milk.

34. An adult client who has been taking furosemide (Lasix) 40 mg PO every day for several weeks is complaining of muscle weakness and lethargy. Which test will be of greatest value in assessing the client's condition?

1. Serum electrolytes
2. Urinalysis
3. Serum creatinine
4. Five-hour glucose tolerance test

35. An adult receives NPH insulin at 7 A.M. When is a hypoglycemic reaction most apt to develop?

    1. Mid morning
    2. Mid afternoon
    3. During the evening
    4. During the night

36. A 17-year-old has been recently diagnosed as having diabetes mellitus Type I. Insulin is prescribed. The client asks why insulin can't be taken by mouth. What is the best answer for the nurse to give?

    1. "Insulin is irritating to the stomach."
    2. "Oral insulin is too rapidly absorbed."
    3. "Gastric juices destroy insulin."
    4. "You can take it by mouth when the acute phase is over."

37. An adult received regular insulin at 7 A.M. At 10 A.M., she is irritable and sweaty, but her skin is cool. What is the most appropriate action for the nurse to take?

    1. Have her lie down for a rest.
    2. Give her a cola drink.
    3. Give ordered insulin.
    4. Encourage exercise.

38. A woman who is taking cortisone for an acute exacerbation of rheumatoid arthritis is upset about the fat face she has developed. She says to the nurse, "I'm going to quit taking that cortisone." The nurse's response should be based on which understanding?

    1. Cortisone does not cause a fat face.
    2. The symptoms will lessen as her body adjusts to the medication.
    3. The drug should be immediately discontinued when adverse effects occur.
    4. Cortisone should never be abruptly discontinued.

39. An adult woman has been diagnosed as having hypothryoidism. She is taking Cytomel (liothyronine sodium) 50 mcg daily. Which of the following side effects should the nurse be especially alert for?

    1. Angina
    2. Fatigue
    3. Rash
    4. Gastritis

40. A 19-year-old has just started taking birth control pills. She calls the clinic nurse to say that her breasts are tender and she is nauseous. The nurse's response is based on which understanding?

    1. These are serious side effects.
    2. These effects usually decrease after three to six cycles.
    3. Taking the pill in the morning reduces its side effects.
    4. Taking the pills every other day reduces its side effects.

41. A young woman delivered a 7 lb., 8 oz. baby boy spontaneously. Ergotrate 0.4 mg q 6 hr for five days is ordered. A half hour after the nurse administers the first dose she complains of abdominal cramping. The nurse's best response is based on which understanding?

    1. Cramping indicates a serious adverse reaction.
    2. Cramping can be reduced by abdominal breathing.
    3. The medication is having the desired effect.
    4. The dosage needs to be reduced.

42. Aluminum hydroxide gel (Amphojel) is ordered for an adult who has acute renal failure. What is the primary reason for administering this drug to this client?

    1. To prevent the development of Curling's ulcers
    2. To bind phosphates

3. To maintain normal pH

4. To prevent diarrhea

43. An adult is hospitalized for an acute attack of gout. Which medication should the nurse expect to administer?

   1. Morphine

   2. Colchicine

   3. Allopurinol

   4. Acetaminophen

44. An adult is scheduled for a left cataract extraction. Homatropine and Cyclogel eye drops are ordered. What is the expected action of these drops?

   1. Mydriasis

   2. Miotic effects

   3. Relaxation of eye muscles

   4. Prevention of infection

45. When administering eye drops, the nurse should administer the drops into which place?

   1. The pupil

   2. The conjunctival sac

   3. The inner canthus

   4. The cornea

46. Ear drops have been ordered for a 10-month-old. How should the nurse teach the mother to pull the baby's ear to straighten the ear canal?

   1. Down and back

   2. Down and forward

   3. Up and forward

   4. Up and back

47. A client who has Hodgkin's Disease receives a weekly IV dose of nitrogen mustard. Which nursing order is most appropriate?

   1. Encourage mouth care with an astringent mouth wash and dental floss after every meal.

2. Encourage organ meats and dried beans and peas.

   3. Monitor vital signs daily.

   4. Encourage fluid intake to 3,000 cc.

48. A woman who is receiving cancer chemotherapy exhibits all of the following. Which is most indicative of bone marrow depression?

   1. Alopecia

   2. Petechiae

   3. Stomatitis

   4. Constipation

49. A six-year-old is seen in the emergency room after stepping on a rusty nail. He has received no immunizations. What should the nurse expect to give him immediately to prevent a tetanus infection?

   1. Tetanus toxoid

   2. DPT

   3. Immune serum globulin

   4. Penicillin

50. A woman is two months pregnant when her five-year-old child develops rubella. What is most likely to be given to her?

   1. Immune serum globulin

   2. MMR

   3. RhoGam

   4. Rubella antitoxin

Answers and Rationales

1. (3) The nurse should not inject medication that has blood in it. Blood may interact with the medication and cause an adverse response.

2. (2) The skin should be pinched, and a 25-gauge needle should be inserted at a 45-degree angle. Answer 1 describes an IM injection. Answer 3 describes an intradermal injection.

3. (1) Infants and small children do not have enough muscle in the gluteal area to use that site. The iliac crest is a site used for subcutaneous injections, not IM.

4. (2) Divide 125 ml/hr by 60 min./hr and multiply by 15 drops/ml.

5. (2) Break the problem down into steps. First, determine the child's weight in kilograms. Divide the number of pounds by 2.2 obtaining 15 kg. Then, multiply 15 kg by 25 mg/kg and obtain 375 mg. Next, divide 375 mg by three daily doses, coming up with 125 mg/dose. The last step is to perform a desired over have calculation to determine the dose. Divide the desired dose (125 mg) by the have-on-hand amount (150 mg), obtaining .83 ml.

6. (2) BUN and creatinine are tests of renal function. Gentamicin is nephrotoxic. All persons receiving gentamicin should have these tests done regularly to assess for toxicity. Elevated levels indicate toxicity. CBC and hemoglobin tests are done to indicate anemia or bone marrow suppression. SGOT and SGPT are liver function tests. Cultures are done before and after antibiotic treatments, not during treatment.

7. (2) Gentamicin is ototoxic (ears). Ringing in the ears suggests possible damage to the eighth cranial nerve, the auditory nerve. A WBC of 8,000 is normal.

8. (2) The client does not have a history of allergic response to penicillin, so there is no need to skin test or withhold the medication. However, the nurse knows that allergic responses rarely occur with the first administration of a medication. Most allergic responses occur following the second or later dose. In the United States, routine skin testing for penicillin allergy is not done. Skin testing is done when there is a question about whether the person has really had an allergic response.

9. (3) Penicillin V potassium (Pen-Vee-K) should be taken on an empty stomach at six-hour intervals.

10. (4) The nurse should tell the mother to give the child all of the medication in the bottle. The bottle contains the prescribed amount. Stopping the medication when the child begins to feel better is likely to cause antibiotic resistant strains of the microorganism to develop. There should be no unused medication. The amoxicillin suspension is only good for two weeks.

11. (4) The nurse knows that there is often a cross allergy between penicillin and the cephalosporins, like Keflex. The initial response by the nurse should be to determine what type of reaction the client had. The nurse should then notify the physician and describe the reaction. Reactions such as nausea or diarrhea are not allergic responses. A reaction such as hives or anaphylaxis would prevent giving Keflex.

12. (2) Tetracycline causes gray tooth syndrome in children under eight years of age. Tooth buds are developing during the third trimester of pregnancy and can be damaged if the mother takes tetracycline then. Tetracycline is effective for chlamydia but should not be given because the woman is pregnant. Tetracycline is often given to adolescents with acne. Tetracycline is effective against Rocky Mountain Spotted Fever. Note that the child is older than eight. Walking pneumonia is probably a mycoplasma infection; tetracycline is effective against mycoplasma.

13. (1) The client should be taught that a rash might be an adverse reaction to Gantrisin, and it should be reported to the physician, not self medicated. Gantrisin is a sulfa medication and should be taken with a full glass of water. Photosensitivity is common; the client should stay out of the sun. All antimicrobials should be taken for the full course of treatment even if the person feels better.

14. (1) Mandelamine is used to treat urinary tract infections. It works most effectively in an acid environment. The urine should be acidified by drinking cranberry juice. Antacids should not be taken with mandelamine; neither should

orange juice and milk, which leave an alkaline urine. Photosensitivity is not a concern with mandelamine.

15. (2) A major toxic response to streptomycin is damage to the eighth cranial nerve, the auditory nerve. Ringing in the ears suggests streptomycin toxicity. Ethambutol might cause color blindness.

16. (1) Persons who are taking INH should also be taking pyridoxine (Vitamin B$_6$) daily to prevent peripheral neuritis. Rifampin causes red-orange colored urine and feces. This client is not on Rifampin. A person with active tuberculosis will be on medication for a year or more. Streptomycin is not available in an oral form because it is not systemically absorbed when given orally.

17. (4) Persons with recurrent genital herpes should start taking their prescription acyclovir tablets at the first sign of an infection. This shortens the outbreak and makes it less severe. The client should avoid sexual relations whenever lesions are present. There is no need to stay home from work with genital herpes. The medicine shortens the outbreaks and makes them less severe but does not cure herpes infections.

18. (3) Zidovudine causes such a decrease in red blood cell count that transfusions are often necessary. The capsules should not be opened. Zidovudine does not cure AIDS. The client should not take over-the-counter medications such as acetaminophen when taking zidovudine.

19. (1) It takes up to two weeks for Feldene to reach therapeutic levels. The other options are not appropriate nursing interventions.

20. (2) Aspirin overdose causes an increase in metabolic rate and metabolic acidosis. The child will have an increased temperature (hyperpyrexia) from the increased metabolic rate. The pulse will be up. Compensation for metabolic acidosis is hyperventilation to blow off the acid. The child will be warm, flushed, tachycardic, and hyperventilating. The child is

at risk for bleeding. Melena (blood in the stools) is unlikely at this time. Enough time has not elapsed for a GI bleed and hidden blood in the stool.

21. (4) The child is breathing, so CPR and ventilatory support are not needed. Once the child is breathing, the first priority is to remove the poison. The child is difficult to arouse, so gastric lavage is used, not syrup of ipecac, which induce vomiting.

22. (3) The client was medicated one hour ago. It is too soon to give meperidine again. The nurse should call the physician for instructions.

23. (3) The client has pain in the operative area and the time interval is appropriate, so medicate her. A back rub, repositioning, and relaxation and breathing exercises alone are not likely to relieve pain on the day of surgery.

24. (4) The client asked for pain medication, but there is no indication of where the client hurts. The nurse cannot assume that the pain is arthritis pain without asking. The aspirin dose is not high for someone with rheumatoid arthritis. The nurse should not divert attention from pain without first assessing.

25. (1) Cogentin can affect the blood pressure and pulse. The nurse must monitor vital signs. The client probably will also have a dry mouth as a result of taking Cogentin, and cold beverages and hard candies are also indicated. However, they are not the priority intervention. Rashes are not common side effect of Cogentin. He is likely to be constipated.

26. (4) Sunbathing should be avoided. Photosensitivity is a common side effect of Thorazine. The client should not drink alcohol. It is MAOIs that have food contraindications. There is no contraindication to dancing.

27. (2) Lithium is excreted from the body as a sodium salt. The client should be taught to have adequate amounts of sodium and water so that lithium can be excreted in the urine and not cause toxicity.

28. (4) The nurse knows that atropine is contraindicated in persons who have glaucoma. The client is elderly and takes eye drops. The nurse should determine the type of eye drops and the reasons for them before administering the preoperative medication.

29. (2) Anorexia and nausea are signs of digoxin toxicity. A pulse of less than 60 indicates possible toxicity. The client should take his pill every morning. Digoxin is not a diuretic effect, but the increase in pumping effectiveness of the heart will help to pump the accumulated fluid from congestive heart failure to the kidneys for excretion. A weight loss is normal when the client who has heart failure starts taking dioxin.

30. (3) The client who is taking nitroglycerin should not drink alcohol. He should be able to walk. The site should be changed daily. He will need to get up slowly, because orthostatic hypotension is a common reaction to the vasodilating effects of nitroglycerin.

31. (1) The client is having premature ventricular contractions. Lidocaine is the drug of choice for frequent PVCs. Verapamil is a calcium channel blocker and is not the drug of choice for PVCs during an MI. Digitalis is used for heart failure and atrial dysrhythmias. Nitroglycerine is used to treat angina. This client more likely has a myocardial infarction.

32. (3) Persons who are taking warfarin must have prothrombin times done on a regular basis. This indicates understanding. Aspirin is an anticoagulant and should not be taken by the person who is taking coumadin unless specifically ordered as part of the anticoagulant regimen. Spinach is high in Vitamin K, a coagulant and the antidote for coumadin. Spinach should not be eaten in large amounts. The person who is taking anticoagulants should not have any teeth removed because of the possibility of hemorrhage.

33. (2) Furosemide (Lasix) is a potassium-depleting diuretic. The client who is also taking digoxin is at greater risk for digoxin toxicity when the serum potassium is low. The person must replace the potassium lost by eating foods high in potassium and possibly by taking a potassium supplement. The client should also be told to take the diuretic early in the day to prevent diuresing during the night and interfering with sleep. However, potassium replacement is of greater importance and takes priority. The client will also probably be told to avoid high-sodium foods, but that is not the highest priority. There is no need to tell the client to drink milk.

34. (1) The symptoms suggest hypokalemia. The client is at risk for hypokalemia because he is taking furosemide, a potassium-depleting diuretic. A urinalysis is used for many things, including picking up urinary tract infections. There is no indication of that in this client. Serum creatinine is the blood test for renal failure. There is no indication for that test. A five-hour glucose tolerance test is the definitive test for diagnosing diabetes. There is no indication for that in this question.

35. (2) Hypoglycemic reactions are most likely to occur at peak action times, when the insulin is taking the glucose out of the blood stream into the cells. Peak action time of NPH insulin is 6–8 hours after the dose. That would be 1–3 P.M. Mid afternoon is the best answer. The peak action for regular insulin would be mid morning.

36. (3) Gastric juices break down insulin, which is a protein.

37. (2) The symptoms suggest hypoglycemia. The peak action of regular insulin is 2–4 hours after administration, and the client took regular insulin three hours ago. The treatment for hypoglycemia is to administer sugar in some form—fruit juice, milk, cola drinks. Insulin would make her worse.

38. (4) When high doses of cortisone are taken, the body decreases its own production. If the client abruptly stopped the cortisone, she would develop Addisonian crisis. Cortisone does cause a moon face. The symptoms will not

disappear until she stops the medication. Cortisone should never be abruptly discontinued.

39. (1) Angina is a frequent side effect when thyroid medication is started. Thyroid increases the metabolic rate and the heart rate. Persons with hypothyroidism are also likely to have atherosclerosis. When the heart rate increases, angina may result. Clients starting on thyroid medication should be instructed to call the physician if they develop chest pain or dysrhythmias.

40. (2) Breast tenderness and nausea are common side effects of the progesterone in birth control pills. These effects usually decrease after three to six cycles. Taking the pill at night reduces the nausea. If the client is sleeping, she is not aware of it. The pill must be taken to be effective. Skipping doses renders the regimen ineffective.

41. (3) Ergotrate is an oxytocic and is given to cause uterine contractions or cramping and prevent postpartum bleeding.

42. (2) Aluminum hydroxide gel binds phosphates when given to a client in renal failure. It can also help prevent the development of Curling's (stress) ulcers and is used as an antacid. Constipation is a side effect. It can be used as an antacid.

43. (2) Colchicine is given for acute gout. Allopurinol is given to prevent recurring attacks of gout. Morphine and acetaminophen are not indicated.

44. (1) Homatropine and Cyclogel are mydriatic drugs; that is, they dilate the pupil. Cyclogel also paralyzes the ciliary muscles so that the pupil cannot constrict.

45. (2) Eye drops should be placed into the conjunctival sac.

46. (1) For infants and small children, the ear should be pulled down and back to straighten the ear canal. For older children and adults, the ear should be pulled up and back.

47. (4) The client should drink plenty of fluids and empty her bladder frequently to prevent hemorrhagic cystitis. Mouth care with an astringent mouth wash and dental floss are contraindicated because of mouth sores and the risk of bleeding with cancer chemotherapeutic agents. Organ meats and dried peas and beans are high in folic acid. The drug antagonizes folic acid. Daily vital signs are not often enough.

48. (2) Bone depression causes a decrease of white cells, red cells, and platelets. Petechiae (small, pinpoint bruises) are indications of bleeding and a decrease in platelets.

49. (3) A person who has stepped on a rusty nail is at risk for tetanus infection. He has received no immunizations. He needs immune serum globulin to give him an immediate, passive immunity. Later, he will receive tetanus toxoid to help him develop antibodies for future needs. Penicillin will not prevent tetanus.

50. (1) Immune serum globulin will give her a passive immunity and help keep her from developing rubella, which can have devastating effects on the unborn child. MMR is a live virus and is not given to pregnant women. RhoGam prevents anti Rh antibody development. There is no such thing as rubella antitoxin.

Unit VI

Practice Tests

UNIT OUTLINE

Practice Tests

Comprehensive Practice Tests

This section contains five 100-question practice tests that are similiar in structure and concept to those you will find on the NCLEX-PN® examination. At the end of each test are the correct answers and rationales for the correct answers, as well as rationales explaining the incorrect answers. Also included are the identifiers for the clinical problems solving process, or nursing process (NP), the categories of client needs (CN), and the subject area (SA) for each question.

The following codes are used for the answers and rationales as identifiers to categorize the test items:

NP	=	CLINICAL PROBLEM SOLVING PROCESS (NURSING PROCESS)	Ps	=	Psychosocial Integrity
			Ps/5	=	Coping and Adaption
Dc	=	Data collection	Ps/6	=	Psychosocial Adaption
Pl	=	Planning	Ph	=	Physiological Integrity
Im	=	Implementation	Ph/7	=	Basic Care and Comfort
Ev	=	Evaluation	Ph/8	=	Pharmacological and Parental Therapies
CN	=	CLIENT NEED			
Sa	=	Safe Effective Care Environment	Ph/9	=	Reduction of Risk Potential
Sa/1	=	Management of Care	Ph/10	=	Physiological Adaption
Sa/2	=	Safety and Infection Control	SA	=	SUBJECT AREA
He	=	Health Promotion and Maintenance	1	=	Medical/Surgical
He/3	=	Growth and Development through the Lifespan	2	=	Psych/Mental Health
			3	=	Female Reproductive
He/4	=	Prevention and Early Detection of Disease	4	=	Pediatrics
			5	=	Pharmacology
			6	=	Nutrition

The following sample answer should help you understand how to interpret these codes. The correct answer is listed first and is in bold type.

ANSWER	RATIONALE	NP	CN	SA
#1. 4.	**Sterile gloves must be worn during the dressing change.**	Im	Sa/2	1
1.	This is not good practice. Sterile technique must be carried out during a dressing change.			
2.	Talking over a sterile field can cause bacteria to enter the wound.			

3. This would be allowed if an irrigating solution were ordered by the physician. Do not irrigate any wound unless ordered by a physician.

The elements of this previous example read as follows:

Number 1 is the question of the item number in the test; Number 4 is the correct answer.

The first rationale explains the correct rationale and appears in bold print.

The remaining rationales explain the incorrect answers.

The phase of the clinical problem solving process (nursing process) is implementation.

The category of client need is Safe Effective Care Environment and Safety and Infection Control.

The subject area is Medical/Surgical.

Practice Test One

1. The client is being admitted for surgery. During the admission assessment the client states she usually has 8–10 alcoholic drinks a day. How should the nurse reply?

   1. What type of alcohol do you drink?
   2. How long have you been drinking alcohol?
   3. When was your last drink?
   4. Why do you drink so much?

2. The nurse is caring for a woman who had a mastectomy following a diagnosis of breast cancer. When the nurse enters the room, the curtains are drawn and the client is lying with her body turned toward the wall away from the nurse. When the nurse approaches her, the client says, "Just leave me alone. I'm no use to anyone. I'm not even a real woman." How should the nurse respond?

   1. Leave the room.
   2. Open the curtains.
   3. Say, "You sound upset."
   4. Say, "Women are more than breasts."

3. The nurse is providing home care to a 78-year-old woman who has early dementia. The client tells the nurse, "My daughter is mean to me." What should the nurse do initially?

   1. Report suspected elder abuse to the supervisor.
   2. Report elder abuse to the authorities.
   3. Ask the daughter about the mother's comment.
   4. Ask the client to describe what the daughter does to be mean to her.

4. The nurse is inserting an indwelling catheter in a female. The nurse knows the urethral meatus is located where?

   1. Between the clitoris and the vagina
   2. Between the vagina and the rectum
   3. Above the clitoris
   4. Below the rectum

5. The nurse is caring for an adult male who is diagnosed with probable appendicitis. Which assessment finding is most consistent with the diagnosis?

   1. Pain in the right upper quadrant
   2. Decreased white blood count
   3. Nausea and vomiting
   4. High fever

6. How should the nurse position the client who has just had a liver biopsy?

   1. On the left side
   2. On the right side
   3. Semi-Fowler's
   4. Low Fowler's

7. An adult is to have a paracentesis performed today. What should the nurse do before the procedure?

   1. Encourage the client to drink large amounts of fluids.
   2. Ask the client to empty her bladder just before the test.
   3. Keep the client NPO until after the procedure.
   4. Premedicate the client as ordered.

8. The physician has ordered an oil retention enema and a cleansing enema for a client. How should the nurse plan to carry out these orders?

   1. Administer the cleansing enema first and several hours later give the oil retention enema.

   2. Administer the oil retention enema first and give the cleansing enema an hour later.

   3. Mix the oil and the cleansing enema and give together.

   4. Give the cleansing enema today and the oil retention enema tomorrow.

9. The nurse observes a certified nursing assistant (CNA) placing a hot water bottle directly on the skin of a 90-year-old client. What action should the nurse take initially?

   1. Report the act to the patient care supervisor.

   2. Interrupt the procedure.

   3. Talk to the CNA when the procedure is finished.

   4. Notify the physician.

10. The nurse is planning care for all of the following clients. Which client should be cared for first?

   1. A 60-year-old, who is three days post-op and needs a dressing change and ambulation.

   2. A 75-year-old, who had a suprapubic prostatectomy yesterday and says, "Take that tube out of me, I have to pee."

   3. A 90-year-old, who had a total hip replacement two days ago and is to get out of bed today.

   4. A 50-year-old, who had an abdominal cholecystectomy yesterday and is asking for pain medication.

11. An adult is admitted with advanced cancer of the GI tract. What question must be included in the admission assessment?

   1. "What foods do you like best?"

   2. "Do you have advance directives?"

   3. "Do you want CPR if you go into cardiac arrest?"

   4. "Do you understand the serious nature of your illness?"

12. The nurse is providing home care for an immobile client who has a stage IV decubitus ulcer that is not healing. Assuming all of the following are available, which person would be most appropriate to consult re: care of the wound?

   1. Physician

   2. Physical therapist

   3. IV therapist

   4. Enterostomal therapist

13. A woman reports to the physician's office complaining of urinary frequency and pain and burning on urination. The nurse expects which procedures will be ordered for this client?

   1. Urine for culture and sensitivity

   2. CBC, BUN

   3. Routine urinalysis

   4. BUN, creatinine

14. A 38-year-old who has mitral stenosis is hospitalized for a valve replacement. Which condition is the client most likely to report having had earlier in life?

   1. Meningitis

   2. Syphilis

   3. Rheumatic fever

   4. Rubella

15. Following cardiac surgery, a client's urine output for the last hour is 20 cc. The nurse

understands this indicates which of the following?

1. Possible hyperkalemia
2. Insufficient cardiac output
3. Inadequate fluid replacement
4. Diuresis is occurring

16. A 20-year-old woman is admitted to the hospital following an accident. Her uncle, a physician from out of state, visits her and asks to see her chart. How should the nurse respond?

1. Comply with the request and give the chart to the physician.
2. Explain that written permission from his niece is needed first.
3. Suggest that he discuss the case with the attending physician.
4. Give him the chart but do not let him remove it from the nurse's station.

17. An adult is admitted for surgery today. Immediately after administering the pre-operative medication of meperidine and atropine, the nurse notes that the operative permit has not been signed. Which action should the nurse take?

1. Have the client sign the operative permit immediately before the medication takes effect.
2. Have the client's next of kin sign the permission form.
3. Ask the client if he/she is willing to undergo surgery and sign the form for the client and indicate your name as witness to the client's verbal consent.
4. Report it to the physician so the surgery can be delayed until the client can legally sign a consent form.

18. The nurse is administering hygienic care to an elderly client in her home. What should the nurse wash first?

1. Perineal area
2. Face
3. Upper torso
4. Hands

19. The family of a 90-year-old resident in a long-term care facility asks the nurse why the client only gets a shower three times a week. What information is most important for the nurse to include when answering the question?

1. The staff members have limited time and must schedule all the residents.
2. The client's skin is dry; too many showers will dry the skin further.
3. The client has limited energy and must conserve it.
4. The client is not very active and doesn't get very dirty.

20. The nurse is giving home care to an elderly client with angina pectoris and Type II diabetes mellitus. Which observation is of most concern and should be reported immediately?

1. The client reports chest discomfort yesterday while taking a walk.
2. The nurse observes several brown spots on the client's arms and legs.
3. The client reports an ingrown toenail that is getting more painful.
4. The client reports shortness of breath when climbing stairs.

21. All the following clients assigned to LPN/LVN ring their call bells. Which client needs the most immediate attention?

    1. A 72-year-old diabetic who is blind says she has to go to the bathroom.
    2. A 75-year-old client who has rheumatoid arthritis asks for pain medication.
    3. A client who has a blood transfusion running says her chest hurts.
    4. A post-operative client who says he is in pain and wants a pain shot.

22. The nurse notes all of the following. Which should be attended to first?

    1. A blind client is calling out stating she cannot find the call bell.
    2. There is a water spill on the floor near the bed of an elderly client who ambulates regularly.
    3. A post-operative client is asking for pain medication.
    4. A diabetic client is asking for a glass of water.

23. The nurse is to insert an indwelling catheter in a male. Which action is appropriate?

    1. Cleanse the meatus before preparing the catheter for insertion.
    2. Wash hands before starting the procedure.
    3. Hold the penis at a 45-degree angle during insertion of the catheter.
    4. Inflate the balloon immediately before inserting the catheter.

24. A 75-year-old woman who is hospitalized with congestive heart failure falls out of bed. She has a bruise on her leg but X-rays reveal no fractures. How should the nurse record the incident in the client's chart?

    1. "Client fell out of bed at 10 A.M. Physician notified. Incident report completed."

    2. "Client found on floor beside bed at 10 A.M. Alert and oriented times 3. States she slipped as she was standing up. Bruise (3 inches by 2 inches) on left hip. Denies pain. Dr. _____ examined client. X-rays taken."
    3. "Client fell while getting out of bed. Seems okay. Charge nurse examined client. Doctor notified and incident report filed."
    4. "Found client on floor beside bed. Responds to questions. Red area on left hip. Notified charge nurse and physician."

25. The nurse is caring for a 78-year-old woman in a long-term care facility. The client is sitting in a geriatric chair with the attached tray in place. The client is agitated and appears to be sliding down in the chair. What is the best action for the nurse to take?

    1. Ask the supervisor for advice.
    2. Put a jacket restraint on the client.
    3. Tie a sheet around the client's waist.
    4. Use foam wedges beside the client.

26. The nurse is observing a Certified Nursing Assistant (CNA) caring for a client who has AIDS. Which action, if observed, is not correct?

    1. The CNA wears gloves when cleaning the client after an episode of fecal incontinence.
    2. The CNA uses chlorine bleach to wipe up blood after the client cut himself shaving.
    3. The CNA is observed giving the client a back rub without gloves on.
    4. The CNA wears a mask whenever entering the client's room.

27. An adult who has COPD is receiving oxygen at home via nasal cannula. In addition to instructing the client and his family about not smoking when oxygen is in use, what should the nurse plan to include in the teaching?

1. If the prescribed liter flow does not relieve his difficulty breathing, increase the liter flow by up to 2 liters/minute every four hours.

2. Try not to shuffle across the carpeted floor.

3. Clean the nasal cannula with alcohol several times a day.

4. Increase the oxygen flow rate if you develop shortness of breath.

28. An adult had major abdominal surgery this morning under general anesthesia. When the client arrives in the recovery room she is very lethargic and restless. Her BP is 150/98; pulse, 110 and irregular; respirations, 30 and shallow. Post-operative orders include meperidine (Demerol) 75 mg I.M. for operative site pain; reinforce dressings p.r.n.; O₂ at 6 liters/min p.r.n.; irrigate nasogastric tube q 2 hours and p.r.n.; IV 2500 cc D5W in 24 hours. What should the nurse do next?

1. Carefully inspect the dressings for any drainage.

2. Irrigate the nasogastric tube.

3. Administer meperidine (Demerol) as ordered.

4. Administer oxygen.

29. An adult client who had major abdominal surgery is returned to her room on the surgical nursing unit. The post-anesthesia nurse reports that the client is awake and has stable vital signs. She has an NG tube in place that is attached to intermittent suction. How should the nurse position the client?

1. Supine

2. Semi-Fowler's

3. Dorsal recumbent

4. Prone

30. The nurse is to open a sterile package. How should the nurse plan to open the first flap?

1. Toward the nurse

2. Away from the nurse

3. To the right side

4. To the left side

31. A 66-year-old woman is being evaluated for pernicious anemia. Which assessment findings would be most apt to be present in a client with pernicious anemia?

1. Easy bruising

2. Pain in the legs

3. Fine red rash on the extremities

4. Pruritus

32. A Schilling test has been ordered for a client. What is the nurse's primary responsibility in relation to this test?

1. Collect the blood samples.

2. Collect a 24-hour urine sample.

3. Assist the client to X-ray.

4. Administer an enema.

33. A throat culture is positive for streptococcus. An antibiotic is prescribed. Which question is it essential for the nurse to ask the client before administering the medication?

1. Has the client ever had an adverse reaction to sulfa drugs?

2. Is the client currently taking vitamins?

3. Does the client drink alcoholic beverages?

4. Is the client allergic to penicillin?

34. The nurse is caring for an adult who had a kidney transplant. He is taking maintenance doses of cyclosporine and prednisone. Which of the following is the greatest cause for concern to the nurse?

    1. Moon face

    2. Acne

    3. Sore throat

    4. Mood swings

35. During a home visit the nurse observes a man who is recovering from a left total hip replacement. Which observation indicates the client understands his care?

    1. He is sitting in a soft, overstuffed easy chair.

    2. He bends over to pat his cat.

    3. He crosses his legs when sitting.

    4. He holds the cane in his right hand when walking.

36. A 17-year-old client is admitted following a seizure. That evening the nurse goes into the room and notes that the client has obviously been crying. The client says to the nurse, "Now that I have epilepsy, I am a freak." What is the best initial response for the nurse to make?

    1. "It must be very difficult for you to realize you have epilepsy."

    2. "Don't say that. You might be having a few seizures now but I'm sure the doctor will be able to control them."

    3. "Don't think like that. You're still a bright, good-looking, young person."

    4. "Many famous athletes and actors have epilepsy, and they can still do anything they used to do."

37. The physician orders phenytoin (Dilantin) and phenobarbital for a client admitted with a cerebrovascular accident. The nurse knows

these drugs are administered for what purpose?

    1. To prevent seizures

    2. To promote sleep

    3. To stop clots from forming

    4. To stop bleeding

38. An adult who has cholecystitis reports clay-colored stools and moderate jaundice. The nurse knows that which is the best explanation for the presence of clay-colored stools and jaundice?

    1. There is an obstruction in the pancreatic duct.

    2. There are gallstones in the gallbladder.

    3. Bile is no longer produced by the gallbladder.

    4. There is an obstruction in the common bile duct.

39. Following a cholecystectomy, drainage from the T tube for the first 24 hours post-operative was 350 cc. What is the appropriate nursing action?

    1. Notify the physician.

    2. Raise the level of the drainage bag to decrease the rate of flow.

    3. Increase the IV flow rate to compensate for the loss.

    4. Continue to observe and measure drainage.

40. The nurse is caring for a client who had a total thyroidectomy. What should the nurse plan to observe the client for after his return to the nursing care unit?

    1. Hoarseness

    2. Signs of hypercalcemia

    3. Loss of reflexes

    4. Mental confusion

41. The nurse is caring for a woman who has diabetic neuropathy. The nurse knows the client needs more instruction when the client makes which statement?

    1. "I'll use a hot water bottle if my feet hurt."
    2. "I should dry my feet and toes carefully."
    3. "I go to the podiatrist to have my toenails cut."
    4. "The Tegretol seems to help my leg pain."

42. The nurse is auscultating an elderly bedridden client's breath sounds and hears crackles. What is the best interpretation of this finding?

    1. This is normal for the client's age.
    2. This is suggestive of an immediately life-threatening condition.
    3. This is an indication the client needs to take deep breaths.
    4. This is an indication the client may need nasal oxygen.

43. The nurse is providing home care to an elderly woman who had a cerebral vascular accident several weeks ago. All of the following need to be done. Which should the nurse plan to do first?

    1. Auscultate lung fields.
    2. Hygienic care.
    3. Assist with ambulation.
    4. ROM exercises.

44. An older adult is seen in clinic. During the assessment process all of the following are expressed or noted. Which is of most immediate concern to the nurse?

    1. The client's daughter says the client has become increasingly forgetful.
    2. The client has a productive cough.
    3. The client ambulates slowly.
    4. The client says "My arms aren't long enough for me to read the paper."

45. All of the following need to be done. Which should the nurse do first?

    1. A client who had surgery earlier today asks for pain medication.
    2. A person who is two days post-operative needs a dressing change.
    3. A client who had a cerebrovascular accident needs a bed bath.
    4. A person scheduled for surgery tomorrow needs an enema.

46. The nurse is about to medicate a client who is to have surgery today. The client says, "I do not understand what the doctor is going to do," and asks the nurse to explain specific details of the surgery. The client has already signed an operative permit. What is the best action for the nurse to take at this time?

    1. Attempt to answer the client's questions.
    2. Notify the physician of the client's concerns prior to medicating the client.
    3. Reassure the client that the physician is well respected and very competent.
    4. Suggest that the client ask the physician her questions when in the operating room.

47. The nurse has completed teaching the client about his low-sodium, low-fat diet. Which menu, if selected by the client, would indicate to the nurse that the client understands his diet?

    1. Mashed potatoes, spinach, and meat loaf.
    2. Swordfish with Hollandaise sauce, carrots, and rice pilaf.
    3. Baked chicken, wild rice, and broccoli.
    4. Roast beef with gravy, baked potato with sour cream, and creamed peas.

48. The afternoon following a thyroidectomy, the client experiences all of the following. Which one indicates to the nurse the client is experiencing a serious complication?

    1. A sore throat
    2. Pain at the surgical site
    3. Temperature of 100.2°F
    4. Sudden hoarseness

49. The nurse is caring for a client who had a colostomy. Which comment by the client indicates that she is showing an interest in learning about her colostomy?

    1. "Why did this problem have to happen to me?"
    2. "What is the bag of water for?"
    3. "When will I get rid of this thing?"
    4. "The doctor didn't really do a colostomy."

50. The client is scheduled for a paracentesis. What should the nurse expect to do prior to the procedure?

    1. Insert an indwelling catheter.
    2. Have the client void.
    3. Keep the client NPO.
    4. Administer an enema.

51. The nurse is caring for a client who is to be on bed rest for two weeks. What should the nurse do to prevent atelectasis?

    1. Encourage the client to deep-breathe and cough every two hours.
    2. Encourage the client to flex and extend her feet every two hours.
    3. Apply antiembolism stockings as ordered.
    4. Perform range-of-motion exercises several times a day.

52. The nurse is administering tuberculin skin tests. How should the nurse insert the needle when administering the skin test?

    1. At a ten-degree angle
    2. At a thirty-degree angle
    3. At a sixty-degree angle
    4. At a ninety-degree angle

53. The nurse is teaching a community group about healthy lifestyles to prevent cancer and heart disease. Which comment by a member of the group indicates a need for more teaching?

    1. "Smoking is not good for you."
    2. "Reducing fat intake helps reduce the risk of heart disease."
    3. "Walking every day puts a strain on your heart."
    4. "Eating lots of fruits and vegetables helps keep me healthy."

54. The parents of a child who is in for a one-year well-baby check ask what immunizations the child needs. The nurse checks the child's record and determines that the child has had immunizations as recommended during the first year. What should the nurse reply?

    1. MMR and DTP
    2. Hepatitis B and polio
    3. Hemophilous and chickenpox
    4. Pneumonia and tetanus

55. The nurse is providing home care. Which assessment finding would suggest to the nurse that the elderly client should be evaluated for abuse?

    1. The client says, "My daughter takes some of my Social Security money. She says it's to pay for my food and medicine."
    2. The client has several bruises on her arms and legs.
    3. The client says her family is mean because they hire someone to stay with her when they go out.

4. The client has several bruises and circular marks that look like cigarette burns on her back.

56. The nurse is assessing the client's abdomen. Which should the nurse do first?

    1. Auscultate
    2. Percuss
    3. Inspect
    4. Palpate

57. The nurse is teaching a young woman how to perform self breast examination. Which comment, if made by the client, indicates the teaching has been effective?

    1. "I should examine my breasts every year."
    2. "I need to see the doctor every six months for a breast exam."
    3. "I don't need to worry about breast cancer for a few years."
    4. "I should examine all parts of my breasts both lying down and standing up."

58. The parents of an infant ask the nurse in the physician's office what diseases the DPT shot protects against. What should the nurse include when replying?

    1. Diarrhea, polio, and typhoid
    2. Diphtheria, whooping cough, and tetanus
    3. Diarrhea, pertussis, and typhus
    4. Diphtheria, paralysis, and tetany

59. The nurse is providing home care to a post-operative client who has a wound infection. What is essential to include when teaching the family about infection transmission?

    1. The client should stay isolated from the rest of the family.
    2. No one who is pregnant should care for the client.

3. The family should wash hands before and after caring for the client.
4. The client should not be allowed to have any visitors.

60. An adult is scheduled for surgery today and has signed an operative permit. As the nurse is about to administer the client's pre-operative medication, the client says that she has changed her mind and no longer wishes to have the surgery. How should the nurse respond?

    1. "Once you have signed the permit form you cannot change your mind."
    2. "I will give you the medication and call your doctor about your change of mind."
    3. "I will call your doctor so you can discuss it with her."
    4. "This is a safe procedure; you do not need to be afraid."

61. The nurse is providing home care to a confused client. The client's family is using a restraint to keep the client from pulling out her indwelling catheter. What should the nurse plan to include when teaching the family?

    1. Remove the restraints for one hour three times a day.
    2. Check the restrained extremities every two hours for circulation.
    3. Remove the restraints whenever someone is with the client.
    4. Do not remove the restraints unless the nurse is present.

62. A client who has Parkinson's disease is having difficulty ambulating. The nurse knows the client and his family understand safety issues when the client is seen wearing which type of shoe?

   1. Rubber-soled shoe.
   2. Smooth-soled shoes
   3. Elevated shoes
   4. Open-toed shoes.

63. The nurse administered an intramuscular injection to an adult. How should the nurse dispose of the needle and syringe?

   1. Immediately place syringe and needle in the disposal container.
   2. Recap the needle and place syringe and needle in the disposal container.
   3. Separate the syringe and the needle and place in the appropriate disposal containers.
   4. Recap the needle and cut the syringe before placing in disposal container.

64. The nurse is caring for a client who is receiving oxygen therapy. A visitor yells at the nurse saying there is a fire burning in the wastebasket on the other side of the room. What should the nurse do initially?

   1. Go for help.
   2. Ask the visitor to go for help while the nurse calms the client.
   3. Turn off the oxygen and remove the client from the room.
   4. Grab the nearest fire extinguisher and try to put out the fire.

65. A young woman comes to the physician's office seeking contraceptive advice. The client reports all of the following. Which contraindicates the use of oral contraceptives?

   1. A gonorrhea infection last year
   2. Thrombophlebitis in the legs six months ago
   3. A family history of diabetes
   4. A bladder infection last month

66. When planning care for a woman who is admitted in labor, it is most important for the nurse to obtain which of the following information about the client?

   1. Age of the client and due date
   2. Frequency and duration of contractions
   3. Whether the membranes have ruptured
   4. Who will be assisting the woman during labor

67. A woman who is 32 weeks gestation comes to her physician's office. Which finding is of most concern to the office nurse?

   1. Trace of glucose in the urine
   2. Weight gain of 4 pounds in one month
   3. Swelling around the client's eyes
   4. Ankle and foot edema

68. The nurse is planning care for a group of senior citizens. The nurse should plan activities that promote achievement of which developmental task?

   1. Identity
   2. Intimacy
   3. Generativity
   4. Ego integrity

69. A young couple asks the nurse what method of contraception they should use. What information is most important for the nurse to have before giving an answer?

   1. The exact age of the couple
   2. The sexual history of both partners
   3. The method they find most acceptable
   4. How soon they want to start a family

70. The nurse is making a home visit to the mother of an eight-pound baby boy born five days ago. Which observation indicates the mother understands the care of the newborn?

    1. The mother is concerned about the fact the baby has a soft stool after every breast feeding.
    2. The mother cleans the cord stump with alcohol when changing the diaper.
    3. The mother cleans the circumcised penis with alcohol when changing the diaper.
    4. The mother nurses the baby hourly.

71. The nurse in a college health clinic is teaching the male students self testicular examination. Which statement made by one of the young men indicates a need for more teaching?

    1. "I should do a self testicular examination every month."
    2. "When I am taking a shower is a good time to do the self exam."
    3. "If I feel any lumps I should report it to the physician."
    4. "Testicular cancer is usually found in older men."

72. The nurse has been interacting for several weeks with a client on the psychiatric unit. The nurse is to be transferred to another unit. Which comment by the client indicates separation anxiety?

    1. "We had a good time at the party last night. You should have been here."
    2. "Some of us are going to the museum next week. Too bad you can't go."
    3. "I was thinking about my friend last night; the one who died in the car crash."
    4. "I was telling my wife what a good nurse you are."

73. The nurse is caring for a client who is very demanding. She frequently rings the bell and asks to have her pillow fluffed or the water glass filled. Which response by the nurse will likely be most effective?

    1. Answer the bell quickly each time she rings.
    2. Tell her you do not have time to be in her room constantly.
    3. Say, "Why are you so upset?"
    4. Say, "You seem concerned about something."

74. An elderly client is severely dehydrated. Which is the best way to assess the effectiveness of fluid restoration therapy?

    1. Assess the client's skin turgor every shift.
    2. Record weights daily.
    3. Ask the client if she is thirsty.
    4. Record all intake.

75. The nurse is caring for a client who is recovering from a cerebrovascular accident and is partially paralyzed on the right side. How should the nurse position the chair when getting the client out of bed?

    1. On the right side of the bed facing the foot of the bed
    2. On the right side of the bed facing the head of the bed
    3. On the left side of the bed facing the foot of the bed
    4. On the left side of the bed facing the head of the bed

76. An adult woman who broke her right ankle is seen in the physician's office one week after the cast was applied. Which observation indicates to the office nurse that the client is using crutches correctly?

    1. The client moves the left crutch forward, then the right foot, then the right crutch, and finally the left foot.
    2. The client moves the left crutch and the right foot together, and then moves the right crutch and the left together.
    3. The client moves the left foot and the crutches forward while bearing weight on the right foot.
    4. The client bears weight on the left foot and moves the right foot and the crutches forward.

77. The nurse observes a certified nursing assistant (CNA) moving a client up in bed. Which action by the nursing assistant indicates a need for more instruction in how to move a client?

    1. Using a pull sheet
    2. Asking another nursing assistant to help
    3. Lowering the head of the bed
    4. Pulling the client by the shoulders

78. The client tells the nurse she is having trouble falling asleep. What initial nursing action is least appropriate?

    1. Asking the physician for a sleeping medication
    2. Offering the client a back rub
    3. Asking the client if she is concerned about something
    4. Repositioning the client

79. The nurse is caring for a client who is ordered to be on bed rest for a prolonged period of time. What should be included in the nursing care plan to prevent venous stasis?

    1. Deep-breathe and cough every two hours
    2. Range-of-motion exercises every shift
    3. Antiembolism stockings on legs
    4. Turn every two hours

80. The nurse is caring for a client who is receiving intravenous fluid therapy. Which observation needs to be reported to the charge nurse?

    1. The client says the IV fluid feels cool when it goes in.
    2. The infusion site is covered with clear tape.
    3. The client is ambulating while the IV infusion is running.
    4. The area around the infusion site is cool and blanched.

81. The nurse is to administer the daily dose of digoxin to an adult client. What is it essential for the nurse to do before administering the medication?

    1. Check the client's temperature
    2. Check the client's blood pressure
    3. Check the client's respirations
    4. Check the client's apical pulse

82. An adult client who has a fractured tibia is ordered one baby aspirin a day. He says to the nurse, "I don't think the aspirin is doing any good. I still have pain." What should the nurse include when replying to this client?

    1. "The aspirin is given to prevent clots from forming."
    2. "The aspirin is given to keep your temperature normal."
    3. "The aspirin is given to control your pain and should be helping."
    4. "The aspirin is given to decrease inflammation at the fracture site."

83. A client who is about to be discharged from the acute care facility is receiving warfarin (Coumadin). The nurse should plan to teach the client which of the following?

1. Take the medication on a full stomach.

2. Do not take any over-the-counter medications without checking with your physician.

3. Take aspirin if you need an analgesic.

4. Avoid prolonged exposure to the sun while taking warfarin.

84. A spansule is ordered twice a day for a client in the outpatient clinic. What should the nurse teach the client about taking a spansule?

1. Take the spansule before breakfast and dinner.

2. If the spansule is difficult to swallow, open it up, and put the contents in food.

3. Spansules should be taken at 12-hour intervals.

4. Spansules can safely be cut for partial doses.

85. The client says to the nurse, "I don't see why I should live any longer." How should the nurse respond initially?

1. Ask the client why she doesn't want to live any longer.

2. Ask the client if she is considering suicide.

3. Tell the client that life is precious and worth living.

4. Help the client see the good things that she has in her life.

86. A client who has had a right below-the-knee amputation refers to himself as "a freak " and "old peg-leg." What initial response by the nurse is most therapeutic?

1. "You are not a freak."

2. "Lots of people have amputations and live a normal life."

3. "You feel like a freak."

4. "You shouldn't say that, you are very attractive."

87. The nurse is caring for a client who is suffering from severe anxiety. What must the client do first when learning to deal with his anxiety?

1. Recognize that he is feeling anxious.

2. Identify the situations that precipitated his anxiety.

3. Understand the reason for his anxiety.

4. Select a strategy to use to help him cope with his anxiety.

88. The nurse is caring for a client who had a right below-the-knee amputation three days ago. The client complains of pain in the right foot and asks for pain medication. What nursing action is appropriate initially?

1. Elevate the stump.

2. Administer a placebo.

3. Administer ordered medications.

4. Encourage the client to discuss his feelings.

89. An adult woman has obsessive-compulsive disorder. She continually washes her hands and misses meals because she has not completed her washing rituals. What should be in the nursing care plan for this woman?

1. Interrupt the ritual and insist the woman go to meals.

2. Bring meals to the client if she is unable to get to the dining room.

3. Remind her an hour before meals so she can perform her washing ritual.

4. Give her a choice of performing her washing ritual or going to meals.

90. An eight-month-old infant is admitted with head injuries and suspected child abuse. Which comment, if made by the mother, would be most suggestive of child abuse?

    1. "He always cries just to irritate me."

    2. "I get worried when he cries, and I don't know what he wants."

    3. "When he cries I usually just feed him and hope that is what he wants."

    4. "I wish he could talk to me and tell me what he wants."

91. An 82-year-old woman who has Alzheimer's disease is admitted to the acute care unit. She frequently gets out of bed and wanders in the hall, unable to find her way back to her room. She even gets in the beds of other clients. What nursing action is most appropriate for this client?

    1. Restrain her so she will not wander in the halls.

    2. Ask her roommate to call the nurse whenever she leaves the room.

    3. Punish her when she gets in a bed other than her own.

    4. Put her favorite picture on the door to her room.

92. A 35-year-old woman with three children is seen in the emergency room for a broken arm and facial lacerations. This is the third emergency room visit in the last three months for injuries. Each time she tells the staff that she fell. This time she confides to the LPN/LVN that "my husband accidentally pushed me." What should the LPN/LVN do with this information?

    1. Ask the client why she stays with a man who has caused her to get hurt.

    2. Notify the charge nurse so the client can receive a referral.

    3. Ask the client if she wants a referral to a divorce lawyer.

    4. Tell the client that she has rights and does not have to put up with abuse.

93. An adult is receiving external radiation as part of her treatment for cancer. She asks what precautions are necessary for her to take because of the radiation therapy. The nurse replies that the client should not be around which of the following persons?

    1. Pregnant women

    2. People who are sick

    3. People who have pacemakers

    4. Elderly persons

94. An adult client is showing signs of developing hypovolemic shock. Which finding is most likely to be present?

    1. Elevated systolic and lowered diastolic blood pressure

    2. Decreased heart rate

    3. Decreased urine output

    4. Decreased respiratory rate

95. The nurse finds a person unresponsive on the floor. What is the initial nursing action?

    1. Start chest compressions.

    2. Assess respirations and pulse.

    3. Place on a hard surface.

    4. Start mouth-to-mouth breathing.

96. A home care client is scheduled for dialysis. He asks the nurse if he should take his antihypertensive medication before going for dialysis. How should the nurse respond?

    1. He should take all regularly scheduled medications.

    2. Antihypertensives should not be taken before dialysis because the blood pressure drops during dialysis.

    3. He should check with the physician because it varies from person to person.

4. He should take it with him and take it if his blood pressure rises during the treatment.

97. During suctioning of the client's tracheostomy tube the catheter appears to attach to the tracheal wall and creates a pulling sensation. What is the best action for the nurse to take?

   1. Release the suction by opening the vent.
   2. Continue suctioning to remove the obstruction.
   3. Increase the pressure.
   4. Suction deeper.

98. The client has a chest tube attached to a portable chest drainage system. Four hours after the chest tube is inserted the nurse notes there is no bubbling in the water seal compartment. What is the most likely explanation for this?

   1. The lung has re-expanded.
   2. There is an obstruction in the tubing coming from the pleural cavity.
   3. There is an air leak in the drainage system.
   4. The suction is not turned on.

99. An adult client was admitted for congestive heart failure today. An IV is running. The nurse enters the room and notes the client is having increased difficulty breathing. Before calling the physician, what action should the nurse take?

   1. Increase the IV drip rate.
   2. Place the client in a supine position.
   3. Ask the client if this has happened before.
   4. Raise the head of the bed.

100. An adult client is receiving oxygen at 6 liters/min. The client asks the nurse why the oxygen is running through bubbling water. What should be included in the nurse's reply?

   1. The water cools the oxygen and makes it more comfortable.
   2. Oxygen is very drying to tissues; the water humidifies it.
   3. The water prevents fires when oxygen is in use.
   4. The water helps to prevent infections from developing in the tubing.

Answer	Rationale	NP	CN	SA

#1. **3.** **Admitting to 8–10 alcoholic drinks a day is suggestive of alcoholism. It is important to know when the client last had a drink of alcohol in order to anticipate the onset of withdrawal symptoms.** — Dc — Ps/6 — 1

1. The type of alcohol the client drinks is not the key issue. The key issue is when to anticipate withdrawal symptoms.
2. The key issue is when to anticipate withdrawal symptoms, not how long the client has been drinking.
4. The key issue is when to anticipate withdrawal symptoms, not why the client drinks so much. "Why" questions are usually not therapeutic because they make the client defensive.

#2. **3.** **Acknowledging the client's feelings is an appropriate response to this common grief reaction following the loss of a body part.** — Im — Ps/5 — 2

1. Leaving the room would reinforce the client's perception that she is useless.
2. Opening the curtains does not address the client's concerns; it merely forces the nurse's perception of appropriateness on the client.
4. While this statement is true, it is not an appropriate response to the client. The nurse should recognize the client's feelings, not put them down.

#3. **4.** **The client's statement is very vague and needs to be clarified. Initially the nurse should ask the client what the daughter does that is mean to her. Examples of behavior are important in evaluating whether the client is the victim of abuse or whether the client's dementia is affecting her perceptions.** — Dc — Ps/6 — 2

1. The nurse does not have enough data at this point to report the client's claim.
2. The nurse does not have enough data at this point to report the client's claim.
3. Initially the nurse should clarify the accusation with the client. After doing that, it would be appropriate to discuss the issue with the daughter.

#4. **1.** **The urethral opening is located between the clitoris and the vagina.** — Dc — Ph/7 — 1

2. The urethral opening is located between the clitoris and the vagina.
3. The urethral opening is located between the clitoris and the vagina.
4. The urethral opening is located between the clitoris and the vagina.

#5. 3.   Nausea and vomiting are typically seen in persons who have appendicitis.   Dc   Ph/10   1

  1.   The pain of appendicitis is in the right lower quadrant, not the right upper quadrant.

  2.   The white blood count is elevated in the person with appendicitis.

  4.   The temperature of a person with appendicitis is likely to be a low-grade fever, not a high fever.

#6. 2.   The person who has had a liver biopsy should be positioned on the right side so that there is pressure on the liver to stop any potential bleeding. The liver is located on the right side.   Im   Ph/9   1

  1.   The person who has had a liver biopsy should be positioned on the right side so that there is pressure on the liver to stop any potential bleeding. The liver is located on the right side.

  3.   The person who has had a liver biopsy should be positioned on the right side so that there is pressure on the liver to stop any potential bleeding. The liver is located on the right side.

  4.   The person who has had a liver biopsy should be positioned on the right side so that there is pressure on the liver to stop any potential bleeding. The liver is located on the right side.

#7. 2.   The client should empty her bladder before a paracentesis so the bladder will not be in the abdominal cavity during the procedure. This reduces the risk of accidental puncture of the bladder.   Im   Ph/9   1

  1.   The bladder should be empty during a paracentesis to avoid accidental puncture.

  3.   A paracentesis is usually done at the bedside with only a local anesthetic prior to insertion of the needle. There is no need to keep the client NPO.

  4.   A paracentesis is usually done at the bedside with only a local anesthetic prior to insertion of the needle. There is no need to premedicate the client.

#8. 2.   The oil retention enema is given first to soften the feces. An hour later a cleansing enema is given to help remove the feces.   Pl   Ph/7   1

  1.   The oil retention enema is given first to soften the feces. An hour later a cleansing enema is given to help remove the feces.

  3.   The oil retention enema is given first to soften the feces. An hour later a cleansing enema is given to help remove the feces.

  4.   The oil retention enema is given first to soften the feces. An hour later a cleansing enema is given to help remove the feces.

#9. 2. Applying heat directly to skin with no barrier is dangerous. The   Im   Sa/1   1
client, especially an elderly client, is at risk for skin burn. The
nurse's first responsibility is for the safety of the client. The act
must be stopped before the client is injured.

1. The nurse should first stop the dangerous act, then discuss it with the
CNA. If the problem cannot be resolved, the nurse should talk with
the patient care supervisor.

3. The nurse cannot wait until after the heat has been applied. Applying
heat directly to skin with no barrier is dangerous. The client,
especially an elderly client, is at risk for skin burn. The nurse's first
responsibility is for the safety of the client. The act must be stopped
before the client is injured.

4. The nurse should first stop the dangerous act. There is no need to
notify the physician unless the CNA carries out the improper
procedure and the client's skin is damaged.

#10. 2. An urgent feeling of having to urinate in a client who has a   Pl   Sa/1   1
suprapubic tube or an indwelling catheter suggests the tube may
be blocked. The nurse should further assess the client immediately
and irrigate the catheter if ordered or notify the physician if no
irrigation order is present.

1. This client's needs can wait for a few minutes.

3. This client's needs can wait a few minutes.

4. This client's needs can wait a few minutes. Caring for a blocked
catheter is of higher priority than administering pain medication.

#11. 2. All persons should be asked upon admission if they have advance   Dc   Sa/1   1
directives.

1. All persons should be asked upon admission if they have advance
directives. Asking about favorite foods might be appropriate in some
situations but is not something that must be included in an initial
assessment.

3. All persons should be asked upon admission if they have advance
directives. CPR is only one item that may be included in advance
directives. Initiation of a feeding tube might be an issue with this
client, for instance.

4. All persons should be asked upon admission if they have advance
directives. At some point in the course of caring for this client, it
might be appropriate to ask if they understand the serious nature of
the illness, but it is not something that must be done during the
admission assessment.

#12. 4. **An enterostomal therapist is a Registered Nurse who is an expert**   Im   Sa/1   1
in wound care, including stomas such as colostomies and
decubitus ulcers.

    1. Most physicians are not expert on the care of decubitus ulcers. The
enterostomal therapist is the expert in wound care.

    2. A physical therapist is not an expert in wound care. The enterostomal
therapist is the expert in wound care.

    3. An IV therapist is not an expert in wound care. The enterostomal
therapist is the expert in wound care.

#13. 1. **The symptoms suggest a urinary tract infection. A clean catch**   Pl   Ph/9   1
urine for culture and sensitivity will most likely be done to
confirm the diagnosis.

    2. CBC and BUN are not the tests most likely to be ordered for this
client. An elevated BUN is a sign of renal failure. However, the client's
signs and symptoms suggest urinary tract infection. An elevated
WBC indicates infection. However, the diagnostic test for UTI is urine
for C&S.

    3. The symptoms suggest a urinary tract infection. A clean catch urine
for culture and sensitivity will most likely be done to confirm the
diagnosis.

    4. The symptoms suggest a urinary tract infection. A clean catch urine
for culture and sensitivity will most likely be done to confirm the
diagnosis. BUN and serum creatinine are done to diagnose renal
failure. The client's findings suggest urinary tract infection.

#14. 3. **The most common cause of mitral valve stenosis is rheumatic fever.**   Dc   Ph/9   1

    1. Meningitis is not a cause of mitral valve stenosis. Sequelae from
meningitis would most likely be neurological problems.

    2. Tertiary syphilis can cause cardiovascular problems such as aortic
aneurysm. However, this would be unlikely at age 38. The most
common cause of mitral valve stenosis is rheumatic fever.

    4. Rubella in the mother can cause cardiac defects in the unborn child.
While any viral infection has the potential to cause heart problems,
mitral stenosis is not a common sequela of rubella.

#15. 2. **Urine output below 30 ml/hr indicates the onset of shock.**   Dc   Ph/10 1
        Remember that urine is made from blood. If there is insufficient
        blood flow to the kidneys there will be a decrease in urine output.

   1. Hyperkalemia is not characterized by decreased urine output. Renal
       failure could cause hyperkalemia.

   3. Inadequate fluid replacement could cause a decrease in urine output;
       however, there is not enough data to suggest that. More likely, the
       heart is not beating effectively.

   4. The urine output is less than normal. Diuresis would be characterized
       by an increase in urine output.

#16. 2. **The client's right to confidentiality requires that only persons with**   Im   Sa/1   1
        a need to know have access to her chart. If she wants her physician
        uncle to read the chart, she needs to sign written permission.

   1. The client's right to confidentiality requires that only persons with a
       need to know have access to her chart. The physician uncle who is
       from out of state is clearly not actively involved in the case. If she
       wants her physician uncle to read the chart, she needs to sign written
       permission.

   3. The client's right to confidentiality requires that only persons with a
       need to know have access to her chart. The physician uncle who is
       from out of state is clearly not actively involved in the case. If she
       wants her physician uncle to read the chart, she needs to sign written
       permission. The client needs to give permission for her physician to
       discuss the case with her physician uncle.

   4. The client's right to confidentiality requires that only persons with a
       need to know have access to her chart. The physician uncle who is
       from out of state is clearly not actively involved in the case. If she
       wants her physician uncle to read the chart, she needs to sign written
       permission.

#17. 4. **A consent form must be signed before surgery can be legally**   Im   Sa/1   1
        performed. A client who has been medicated may not sign the
        consent form. The surgery will be delayed or postponed until the
        client is free of the influence of mind-altering medications and can
        legally sign a consent form.

   1. Even though the client has just received the medication, the client can
       not legally sign documents until free of the influence of mind-altering
       drugs.

   2. If the client is otherwise able to sign the consent form (the client is of
       age and alert and oriented before being medicated), the next of kin
       are not authorized to sign for her.

   3. If the client is not legally able to give written consent, the client is not
       legally able to give verbal consent for surgery.

#18. 2.   The nurse should start the bath by washing the eyes and face first.   Im   Ph/7   1

   1.   The perineal area is the last to be washed. The nurse should start the
         bath by washing the eyes and face first.

   3.   The upper torso is washed after the face and hands and arms have
         been washed. The nurse should start the bath by washing the eyes
         and face first.

   4.   The hands are washed after the face. The nurse should start the bath
         by washing the eyes and face first.

#19. 2.   Elderly clients usually have dry skin. Bathing every day is not   Im   Ph/7   1
         recommended for persons with very dry skin. Showers two or
         three times a week are usually recommended.

   1.   Elderly clients usually have dry skin. Bathing every day is not
         recommended for persons with very dry skin. Showers two or three
         times a week are usually recommended. The nurse should not tell
         family members that the staff does not have time to care for their
         loved one.

   3.   Elderly clients usually have dry skin. Bathing every day is not
         recommended for persons with very dry skin. Showers two or three
         times a week are usually recommended. The client may have limited
         energy but from the data given, the primary reason for showering
         only three times a week is the client's dry skin due to aging.

   4.   Elderly clients usually have dry skin. Bathing every day is not
         recommended for persons with very dry skin. Showers two or three
         times a week are usually recommended. It may also be true that the
         client does not get very dirty, but the primary reason for showering
         only three times a week is the client's dry skin due to aging.

#20. 3.   An ingrown toenail in a person who has diabetes can be very   Dc   Ph/9   1
         serious. Diabetics have poor circulation and are prone to infection,
         especially in the feet and legs. An ingrown toenail should be
         reported immediately to the nurse supervisor so an appropriate
         referral can be made.

   1.   Chest discomfort while exercising is a common occurrence in persons
         who have angina.

   2.   Brown spots on the arms and legs are common in elderly persons;
         these are sometimes called age spots.

   4.   Shortness of breath when climbing stairs occurs frequently in
         persons who are elderly and who have angina. The nurse should note
         this so comparisons can be made to see if the shortness of breath is
         getting worse. However, the greatest concern at the moment is the
         painful ingrown toenail.

#21. 3. **Chest pain in a person receiving a transfusion may indicate a transfusion reaction that could be immediately life-threatening. The transfusion should be stopped immediately and the charge nurse notified.**   Im   Sa/1   1

   1. Assisting a blind person to ambulate to the bathroom is important; however, a possible transfusion reaction could be immediately life-threatening and takes priority.

   2. Administering pain medication is important; however, a possible transfusion reaction could be immediately life-threatening and takes priority.

   4. Administering pain medication is important; however, a possible transfusion reaction could be immediately life-threatening and takes priority.

#22. 2. **A water spill on the floor next to the bed of an elderly client who ambulates creates an immediate hazard and should be wiped up immediately. Wiping up the spill is not a time-consuming process and immediately assures the safety of the client. The other clients can safely wait until the immediate hazard has been dealt with.**   Im   Sa/2   1

   1. The blind client obviously can speak to get attention. The need for the call bell is not an immediate safety need. A water spill on the floor next to the bed of an elderly client who ambulates creates an immediate hazard and should be wiped up immediately.

   3. A post-operative client who needs pain medication is not an immediate safety concern. A water spill on the floor next to the bed of an elderly client who ambulates creates an immediate hazard and should be wiped up immediately.

   4. A diabetic client who asks for a glass of water is not an immediate safety need and can wait for a few minutes. A water spill on the floor next to the bed of an elderly client who ambulates creates an immediate hazard and should be wiped up immediately.

#23. 2. **Hands should be washed before starting any procedure.**   Im   Ph/7   1

   1. The nurse should lubricate the catheter and test the balloon before touching the client. Once the nurse touches the client's penis to cleanse the area, that hand is contaminated.

   3. The penis should be held at a 90-degree angle to insert the catheter.

   4. The nurse may test the balloon before draping and cleansing the client. However, the balloon is not inflated during insertion of the catheter. It would be dangerous, if not impossible, to try to insert a catheter with an inflated balloon.

		NP	CN	SA

#24. 2. This answer is most complete. The client's mental status is described; the bruise is described; and the actions taken are described.

NP: Im CN: Sa/1 SA: 1

  1. The notes are too vague. The nurse should not make reference to an incident report in the written notes. However, an incident report should be completed. The purpose of the incident report is for the hospital to follow untoward events. The client's chart is a legal record.

  3. The notes are too vague. The nurse should not make reference to an incident report in the written notes. However, an incident report should be completed. The purpose of the incident report is for the hospital to follow untoward events. The client's chart is a legal record.

  4. The notes are too vague. Answer Number 2 gives more information.

#25. 4. The nurse should use only one form of restraint. The tray is considered a restraint. Foam wedges and pillows are not considered restraints.

NP: Im CN: Sa/2 SA: 1

  1. The nurse should be able to solve this problem without asking a supervisor.

  2. The nurse should use only one form of restraint. The tray is considered a restraint. A jacket restraint is a second form of restraint.

  3. The nurse should use only one form of restraint. The tray is considered a restraint. Tying a sheet around her waist is a second form of restraint.

#26. 4. There is no reason to wear a mask whenever entering the room of a person who has AIDS. A mask might be worn when suctioning if the client had a lot of secretions.

NP: Ev CN: Sa/2 SA: 1

  1. This action is correct. Gloves should be worn when there is contact with any body fluids.

  2. This action is correct. Chlorine bleach 1:10 dilution should be used to clean up blood spills.

  3. This action is correct. There is no need to wear gloves when touching the client's intact skin such as when giving a backrub.

#27. 2. Shuffling across a carpet may create static electricity and the possibility of fire with oxygen running.

NP: Pl CN: Sa/2 SA: 1

  1. Persons with COPD should not have oxygen at levels above 2–3 liters because their drive to breathe is a low oxygen level.

  3. The nasal cannula can be cleaned with soap and water but should not be cleaned with alcohol, which is flammable.

  4. Persons with COPD should not have oxygen at levels above 2–3 liters because their drive to breathe is a low oxygen level.

#28. 4. **Most cases of restlessness in combination with lethargy are due to hypoxia. Hypoxia will cause an irregular pulse and rapid shallow respirations. The client may be in pain. However, the priority is to treat anoxia first and then reassess the client before giving analgesia.**
 Im   Ph/9   1

    1.   The nurse will inspect the wounds for drainage on a regular basis. The data do not suggest an immediate need to inspect the wound. The data are more consistent with hypoxia.

    2.   There is no data to suggest the nasogastric tube needs irrigating.

    3.   The data are more consistent with hypoxia than pain. Airway takes precedent over pain.

#29. 2. **Semi-Fowler's position will facilitate respirations, take pressure off the abdominal incision, and aid drainage if a drain is in place. Semi-Fowler's position is indicated when a client has a nasogastric tube in place to prevent backflow of gastric juices.**
 Im   Ph/9   1

    1.   A person who has a nasogastric tube should not be placed in the supine position because of the risk of aspiration.

    3.   A person who has a nasogastric tube should not be placed in the dorsal recumbent position because of the risk of aspiration.

    4.   A person who has a nasogastric tube should not be placed in prone position because of the risk of aspiration.

#30. 2. **The first flap is opened away from the nurse; then the side flaps and finally the last flap are opened toward the nurse. This way the nurse does not have to reach across a sterile field. Reaching across a sterile field contaminates the field, and it is no longer considered sterile.**
 Pl   Sa/2   1

    1.   If the first flap is opened toward the nurse, the last flap will be opened away from the nurse, causing the nurse to reach across the sterile field.

    3.   The first flap is opened away from the nurse; then the side flaps and finally the last flap are opened toward the nurse. This way the nurse does not have to reach across a sterile field. Reaching across a sterile field contaminates the field, and it is no longer considered sterile.

    4.   The first flap is opened away from the nurse; then the side flaps and finally the last flap are opened toward the nurse. This way the nurse does not have to reach across a sterile field. Reaching across a sterile field contaminates the field, and it is no longer considered sterile.

#31. 2. **Neuropathy, as evidenced by pain in the legs, is characteristic of pernicious anemia. Vitamin B₁₂ is necessary for neurological function.**

   Dc   Ph/9   1

1. Easy bruising would be seen in a clotting disorder such as hemophilia, in leukemia, or in bone marrow depression.
3. Rash is not seen in pernicious anemia.
4. Pruritus is characteristic of Hodgkin's disease.

#32. 2. **The client is given radioactive Vitamin B₁₂ orally and a 24-hour urine is collected to see if Vitamin B₁₂ is absorbed from the GI tract into the blood stream and excreted in the urine. The nurse should collect a 24-hour urine.**

   Dc   Ph/9   1

1. There are no blood samples to be collected in a Schilling test.
3. The Schilling test does not involve X-rays.
4. No enema is administered before or during a Schilling test.

#33. 4. **Penicillin is usually prescribed for streptococcal infection. Penicillin allergy is fairly common. The nurse should ask the client about allergic reactions to penicillin.**

   Dc   Ph/8   5

1. Sulfa drugs are not usually prescribed for streptococcal infections.
2. Vitamins are not a contraindication for penicillin therapy.
3. Alcoholic beverages do not cause adverse reactions when taken with penicillin. Alcohol will cause an Antabuse-like reaction when taken with metronidazole (Flagyl).

#34. 3. **A sore throat is probably symptomatic of immunosuppression as a result of taking immunosuppressants.**

   Dc   Ph/8   5

1. Moon face is an expected side effect of prednisone therapy.
2. Acne is an expected side effect of prednisone therapy.
4. Mood swings are an expected side effect of prednisone therapy.

#35. 4. **When walking with a cane, the cane should be held in the nonaffected hand, which in this case is the right hand. This action indicates understanding of his care.**

   Ev   Ph/7   1

1. The client who has had a total hip replacement should keep the hips in extension. Sitting in a soft, over-stuffed easy chair causes hip flexion and indicates the client does not understand his care.
2. The client who has had a total hip replacement should keep the hips in extension. Bending over to pat his cat causes hip flexion and indicates the client does not understand his care.
3. The client who has had a total hip replacement should keep the hips abducted. Crossing the legs causes adduction, which may cause the hip to move out of the socket. Crossing his legs indicates the client does not understand his care.

#36. 1. **Initial responses should open communication and let him express his feelings.**   Im   Ps/5   2

    2.   This response is not therapeutic in that it argues with the client and encourages denial of illness.

    3.   This response denies the client's feelings.

    4.   This response is not an appropriate initial response. Telling the client about successful people who also share his condition may be appropriate later on.

#37. 1. **Phenytoin and phenobarbital are prescribed to prevent seizures.**   Dc   Ph/8   5

    2.   These drugs do have a sedating effect. However, that is a side effect and not the purpose for which they are given to this client.

    3.   These drugs do not prevent clotting. Heparin followed by coumadin might be given to stop clots from forming.

    4.   These drugs do not stop bleeding.

#38. 4. **Clay-colored stools mean bile is not getting through to the duodenum. The bile duct is obstructed so bile backs up into the bloodstream, causing jaundice.**   Dc   Ph/10   1

    1.   An obstruction in the pancreatic duct might cause fatty stools but would not block bile and therefore would not cause clay-colored stools and jaundice.

    2.   Gallstones in the gallbladder would cause pain but would not cause clay-colored stools and jaundice unless they blocked the common bile duct.

    3.   Bile is not produced in the gallbladder. The liver produces bile, and the gallbladder stores it.

#39. 4. **350 ml in 24 hours after surgery is a normal amount of bile drainage.**   Im   Ph/9   1

    1.   There is no need to notify the physician, because the normal T tube drainage in the immediate post-operative period is 350–500 ml.

    2.   Raising the level of the drainage bag might cause reflux of bile. There is no need to do anything, as this amount of drainage is normal.

    3.   The drainage is normal. The LPN/LVN should not readjust the IV drip rate unless there is an obvious problem or emergency.

#40. 1. Hoarseness may occur after thyroidectomy if the laryngeal nerve is damaged.   Pl   Ph/9   1

    2. The nurse should observe the post-thyroidectomy client for signs of hypocalcemia, which may occur if the parathyroids were damaged or removed. Signs of hypocalcemia are tetany and Trousseau's or Chvostek's sign.

    3. The nurse should observe the post-thyroidectomy client for hyperreflexia, not loss of reflexes. Hyperreflexia can be determined by assessing for Trousseau's or Chvostek's sign.

    4. Mental confusion is not a sign of the usual post-thyroidectomy complications.

#41. 1. A person who has diabetic neuropathy has altered sensation in the extremities and should not use a hot water bottle. This answer indicates a need for further instruction.   Ev   Ph/9   1

    2. A person who has diabetes needs meticulous foot care. This response indicates the client understands her care.

    3. A person who has diabetes and especially one with diabetic neuropathy should have professional assistance with cutting toenails. This response indicates the client understands her care.

    4. Tegretol is a drug frequently given to persons who have diabetic neuropathy. It is an anticonvulsant and blocks painful nerve impulses, reducing the pain of neuropathies.

#42. 3. Crackles are an indication that fluid is beginning to collect in the alveoli and the client needs to take deep breaths to expand the alveoli.   Dc   Ph/9   1

    1. Crackles in the lung fields are not normal findings.

    2. Crackles are an early sign that the alveoli are not well-expanded and that fluid is collecting. Crackles are not suggestive of an immediately life-threatening condition.

    4. Crackles are an early sign that the alveoli are not well-expanded and that fluid is collecting. The client who has crackles needs to take deep breaths and cough. Crackles do not indicate the client needs oxygen.

#43. 1. The nurse should auscultate the lung fields before doing hygienic care. If the client should have crackles and need additional deep-breathing and coughing exercises, the nurse can incorporate these into the hygienic care.   Pl   Ph/7   1

    2. Hygienic care should be done after assessing the client's breath sounds so corrective actions can be incorporated into the care if necessary.

    3. Assessing lung fields should be done before ambulating.

    4. Range-of-motion exercises can be incorporated into hygienic care.

#44. 2. **A productive cough could indicate an immediate infectious process and is of most immediate concern.**   Dc   He/3   1

    1. Forgetfulness could be a sign of chronic brain disease. It is not an inevitable sign of aging. However, it is not as immediate a concern as a productive cough.

    3. Ambulating slowly can be a normal part of the aging process or could indicate a condition such as arthritis or even visual deficits. It is a concern, but not as immediate as a productive cough.

    4. Difficulty reading at close range (presbyopia) is a normal part of aging. The nurse will want to recommend to the client that a prescription for reading glasses may easily correct the problem. However, this is not as immediate a concern as a productive cough.

#45. 1. **The client who had surgery earlier today may be in acute pain and should be assessed immediately for pain and the administration of ordered pain medication.**   Pl   Ph/9   1

    2. Changing the dressing of a post-operative client can safely be delayed until the nurse has assessed the pain of the fresh post-op client.

    3. Assisting a client with ambulation can safely be delayed until the nurse has assessed the client who is in pain.

    4. Administering an enema can safely be delayed until the nurse has assessed the client who is in pain.

#46. 2. **The client should talk with the physician if the questions are about specific details regarding the surgery. The nurse might be able to answer general questions. The client should talk with the physician before being medicated.**   Im   Sa/1   1

    1. The question states that the client wants to know specific details of the surgery. These are questions the physician should answer, not the nurse. The nurse can answer general questions about pre-operative and post-operative care, etc.

    3. The client has specific questions about the details of the surgery. The nurse should not ignore these questions by reassuring the client.

    4. The nurse is about to medicate the client for surgery. The client will be under the influence of medications when she is in the operating room.

ANSWER   RATIONALE

#47. 3. **Baked chicken is lower in both salt and fat than beef. Wild rice and broccoli are low in fat and sodium. This choice indicates understanding of his diet.**

   1. Spinach is high in sodium and meat loaf is high in sodium and fat. This choice indicates the client does not understand his diet.

   2. Swordfish, like all ocean fish, is high in sodium. Hollandaise sauce is high in sodium and fat. Carrots are naturally high in sodium. This choice indicates the client does not understand his diet.

   4. Roast beef is higher in sodium and fat than chicken. Gravy is high in sodium and fat. Sour cream is high in sodium and fat and creamed peas contain fat. This choice indicates the client does not understand his diet.

#48. 4. **Sudden hoarseness following a thyroidectomy may indicate damage to the laryngeal nerve. This should be reported to the charge nurse or physician immediately.**

   1. A sore throat is normal following a thyroidectomy. Most people who have a general anesthetic and are intubated complain of a sore throat.

   2. Pain at the surgical site on the day of surgery is a normal finding.

   3. A low-grade temperature on the day of surgery may well indicate mild dehydration and is quite normal.

#49. 2. **Asking questions about procedures indicates a readiness to learn more about it.**

   1. Asking "why" a problem happened indicates the client has not yet accepted the condition. It is typical of the anger stage of reaction to an illness or problem.

   3. Asking, "When will I get rid of this thing?" in reference to a colostomy indicates the client has not accepted the condition and is probably not ready to learn more about it.

   4. Saying, "The doctor didn't really do a colostomy" indicates the client is in denial and not ready to learn about her colostomy.

#50. 2. **The client should void prior to a paracentesis. If the client has a full bladder, the needle could puncture the bladder rather than remove fluid from the abdominal cavity.**

   1. There is no need to insert an indwelling catheter. Having the client void prior to the procedure will empty the bladder.

   3. There is no need to keep the client NPO prior to a paracentesis. This is performed at the bedside with a local anesthetic in the skin.

   4. There is no need to administer an enema prior to the procedure. During a paracentesis, fluid is removed from the peritoneal cavity.

#	NP	CN	SA
#47	Ev	Ph/7	6
#48	Ev	Ph/10	1
#49	Ev	Ps/5	1
#50	Pl	Ph/9	1

#51. 1.   Deep-breathing and coughing help to prevent atelectasis.   Pl   Ph/9   1

2.   Flexing and extending the feet will help to prevent thrombophlebitis
and are appropriate for a client on bed rest, but do not prevent
atelectasis.

3.   Antiembolism stockings may be ordered for a client on bed rest.
However, they help to prevent thrombophlebitis. They do not prevent
atelectasis.

4.   Range-of-motion exercises are appropriate for someone who is on
prolonged bed rest, but they do not prevent atelectasis.

#52. 1.   A tuberculin skin test is an intradermal test and is administered   Im   He/4   1
at a 10- to 15-degree angle.

2.   A tuberculin skin test is an intradermal test and is administered at a
10- to 15-degree angle.

3.   A tuberculin skin test is an intradermal test and is administered at a
10- to 15-degree angle. A subcutaneous injection is administered at a
60-degree angle.

4.   A tuberculin skin test is an intradermal test and is administered at a
10- to 15-degree angle. An intramuscular injection is administered at
a 90-degree angle.

#53. 3.   Walking is one of the best forms of exercise. Walking daily is   Ev   He/4   1
good for the heart and helps keep weight under control. This
statement indicates the client does not understand the teaching.

1.   Smoking is thought to be a factor in the development of heart disease
and several types of cancer. This statement indicates the client
understands the teaching.

2.   A high fat intake increases the risk of heart disease. This statement
indicates the client understands the teaching.

4.   A diet that is high in fruits and vegetables is thought to reduce the
risk of heart disease and several types of cancer. This statement
indicates the client understands the teaching.

#54. 3.   **The last Hemophilous (HIB) immunization is usually given at**   Im   He/4   4
       12-15 months. Varicella or chickenpox vaccine is recommended
       at 12 months.

1.   Measles, Mumps, Rubella (MMR) is given at 12–15 months. The child
      does not develop adequate antibody levels when MMR is given before
      12 months. Diphtheria, Tetanus, and Pertussis (DTP) is usually given
      at two, four, and six months with a booster at 18 months and another
      booster when the child starts school.

2.   Hepatitis B is given at birth and at one month and six months. Polio
      vaccine is given at two months and four months and a booster at 18
      months, with another booster when the child starts school.

4.   Most well children do not receive pneumonia vaccine. Tetanus is part
      of the DTP and is usually given at two, four, and six months with
      boosters at 18 months and when the child starts school.

#55. 4.   **Bruises and areas that look like cigarette burns on the back are**   Dc   Ps/6   1
       not likely to be due to bumping into things. These findings
       suggest abuse and should be reported so they can be investigated.

1.   Taking some of the client's Social Security money for food and
      medicine does not indicate abuse.

2.   Elderly clients bruise easily. While the nurse should carefully assess
      these bruises, they do not necessarily suggest abuse. Bruises on the
      back and those that look like cigarette burns are much more
      suggestive of abuse.

3.   Hiring a sitter when the family is not at home is an indication of
      concern about the client's safety, not an indication of abuse.

#56. 3.   **The nurse should first inspect the abdomen. Then the abdomen**   Dc   He/4   1
       can be auscultated, followed by percussion and palpation.

1.   The nurse inspects the abdomen before auscultating.

2.   The nurse should first inspect the abdomen. Percussing may affect the
      bowel sounds so auscultation should be done prior to percussing.

4.   The nurse should first inspect the abdomen. Palpation may change
      the bowel sounds so auscultation should be done prior to palpation.

#57. 4.   The woman should use either a circular or an up-and-down pattern to assess every part of both breasts in both an upright and a supine position. This statement indicates the client understands the teaching.   Ev   He/4   3

   1.   The client should examine her breasts every month following her menstrual period. This statement indicates the client does not understand the teaching.

   2.   The woman can do a self breast exam. There is no need to see a physician for a breast exam every six months. This statement indicates the client does not understand the teaching.

   3.   While the incidence of breast cancer increases with age, breast cancer can occur at any age, even in teens. This statement indicates the client does not understand the teaching.

#58. 2.   DPT stands for diphtheria, pertussis (whooping cough), and tetanus.   Im   He/4   4

   1.   DPT stands for diphtheria, pertussis (whooping cough), and tetanus.

   3.   DPT stands for diphtheria, pertussis (whooping cough), and tetanus.

   4.   DPT stands for diphtheria, pertussis (whooping cough), and tetanus.

#59. 3.   Hand-washing is the best way to prevent transmission of infection. The nurse should teach the family proper hand-washing technique.   Pl   Sa/2   1

   1.   There is no need to isolate the client from the rest of the family. Good hand-washing technique should prevent the spread of infection.

   2.   Good hand-washing technique should prevent transmission of infection.

   4.   There is no need to restrict visitors. Good hand-washing technique should prevent the spread of infection.

#60. 3.   Permission can be revoked. The client does have a right to change her mind. The nurse should call the physician and have her talk with the client.   Im   Sa/1   1

   1.   Permission can be revoked. The client does have a right to change her mind.

   2.   The nurse should not medicate the client for two reasons. First, the client said she did not want surgery. Second, the client should be alert when talking with the physician.

   4.   This response does not address the client's statement that she had changed her mind about having the surgery. This is not the appropriate response at this time.

| ANSWER | RATIONALE | | NP | CN | SA |

#61. 2. **The nurse should teach the family to check the restrained extremities at least every two hours for circulation. The restraints should also be removed periodically, usually one at a time, to perform range-of-motion.** — Pl — Sa/2 — 1

  1. The restraints should be removed periodically, usually every two hours, for range-of- motion exercises. They should be removed one at a time.

  3. Removing the restraints whenever someone is with the client may not be feasible. If the caregiver is busy, the client could remove the catheter.

  4. The restraints should be periodically removed, when it is safe to do so. The nurse does not need to be present when the restraints are removed.

#62. 2. **The person who has Parkinson's Disease shuffles when he walks. Smooth-soled shoes allow him to walk without tripping and falling.** — Ev — Sa/2 — 1

  1. The person who has Parkinson's Disease shuffles when he walks. Rubber-soled shoes do not allow the client to shuffle without tripping.

  3. The person who has Parkinson's Disease shuffles when he walks. Elevated shoes would tend to make him unstable.

  4. The person who has Parkinson's Disease shuffles when he walks. If the client wears open-toed shoes, he is likely to injure his toes when he shuffles.

#63. 1. **The nurse should immediately place the syringe with needle attached into the disposal container. The needle should not be recapped. Recapping needles is one of the most common types of injuries to nurses and a common way to spread HIV infection and hepatitis.** — Im — Sa/2 — 1

  2. The needle should not be recapped. Recapping needles is one of the most common types of injuries to nurses and a common way to spread HIV infection and hepatitis.

  3. The needle and syringe should not be separated before placing in the disposal container. This increases the risk of nurse exposure to blood and to needle sticks.

  4. The needle should not be recapped. Recapping needles is one of the most common types of injuries to nurses and a common way to spread HIV infection and hepatitis. There is no need to cut the syringe before placing in disposal container. This would increase the risk of nurse exposure to client's body fluids and needle sticks.

#64. 3. **Oxygen supports combustion so the nurse should immediately turn off the oxygen and then remove the client from the area. Remember RACE (Remove, Alarm, Contain, Evacuate).**   Im   Sa/2   1

    1. The nurse should assure the client's safety first, then sound the alarm. The nurse should not leave the client in danger.

    2. Asking the visitor to tell someone else might be appropriate, but the nurse should turn off the oxygen and remove the client from danger immediately. If the nurse can also calm the client, that might be appropriate, but is not the initial action.

    4. The client's safety is the nurse's first priority. Remember RACE (Remove, Alarm, Contain, Evacuate). Turning off the oxygen should be done immediately. Oxygen supports combustion.

#65. 2. **Clotting disorders such as thrombophlebitis contraindicate the use of oral contraceptives as they can cause clotting. Other vascular conditions such as migraine headaches and smoking more than half a pack of cigarettes a day also contraindicate the use of oral contraceptives.**   Dc   He/3   5

    1. A history of gonorrhea is not a contraindication for oral contraceptives. The client should be advised to use barriers such as condoms in addition to the oral contraceptive to prevent disease transmission.

    3. A family history of diabetes does not contraindicate the use of oral contraceptives.

    4. Bladder infection does not contraindicate the use of oral contraceptives.

#66. 2. **When a woman is admitted in labor, the nurse should assess the frequency and duration of contractions.**   Dc   He/3   3

    1. Age of the client is "nice-to-know information." It is most critical to know the frequency and duration of contractions. Due date is also important information.

    3. Status of the membranes is important information, but not as critical as frequency and duration of contractions.

    4. Who will be assisting the woman during labor is "nice-to-know" information, but not as important as frequency and duration of contractions.

ANSWER	RATIONALE	NP	CN	SA

#67. 3. Swelling in the upper body is suggestive of pregnancy-induced hypertension. The woman is in the third trimester, when PIH is most apt to occur. — Dc He/3 3

   1. A trace of glucose in the urine is common in pregnant women. The woman will be followed carefully, but this should not cause great alarm.

   2. During the third trimester, the client should gain about a pound a week. This is a normal finding.

   4. Ankle and foot edema in the third trimester is a normal finding. The enlarging uterus decreases venous return from the lower extremities and causes foot and ankle edema.

#68. 4. Ego integrity is the developmental task of the older adult. — Pl He/3 2

   1. Identity is the developmental task of the adolescent.

   2. Intimacy is the developmental task of the young adult.

   3. Generativity is the developmental task of the middle adult.

#69. 3. The best method of contraception is usually the one the couple finds most acceptable. If a method is recommended that the couple will not use, the statistics are of little relevance. — Dc He/3 1

   1. The question states that it is a young couple. The exact age is not very important information.

   2. The sexual history of both partners is less important information than the method of contraception they find most acceptable.

   4. How soon they want to start a family may have some relevance. However, the method of contraception they find most acceptable is the most important information for the nurse to obtain.

#70. 2. The cord stump should be cleaned with alcohol at every diaper change. This finding indicates the mother understands the care. — Ev He/3 4

   1. A soft stool after every feeding is normal for a newborn. There is no need for the mother to be concerned.

   3. The circumcised penis should not be cleaned with alcohol. Vaseline gauze may be on the penis, but not alcohol.

   4. The baby should be nursed every 3–4 hours. It is not likely that an eight-pound baby needs to be nursed every hour.

#71. 4. **Testicular cancer is primarily a young man's disease. It is highly curable when found early. This statement indicates the client does not understand the teaching and needs more instruction.**   Ev   He/4   1

    1.   Self testicular examination should be done every month by every man from puberty onward. This answer indicates an understanding of the teaching.

    2.   The self testicular examination should be performed while the client is in the shower. This answer indicates an understanding of the teaching.

    3.   Lumps should be reported to the physician. This answer indicates an understanding of the teaching.

#72. 3. **When people are facing a painful separation, they often think about prior painful separations. Thinking about his friend who died is evidence of separation anxiety.**   Dc   Ps/5   2

    1.   This statement does not indicate separation anxiety.

    2.   This statement does not indicate separation anxiety.

    4.   This statement does not indicate separation anxiety.

#73. 4. **The client's behavior indicates anxiety. This response will open communication and help the client to verbalize concerns.**   Im   Ps/5   2

    1.   Answering the bell quickly is appropriate but is not likely to help control the behavior. A better response is to open communication.

    2.   This response is very nontherapeutic.

    3.   Asking a person "why" is not likely to be therapeutic because it puts the person on the defensive.

#74. 2. **Daily weights are a good indication of fluid restoration. As the fluid is restored, the weight will increase.**   Ev   Ph/10   1

    1.   Skin turgor assessment will give some idea of fluid balance, but daily weights are a better assessment. The client is elderly, and most elderly clients have poor skin turgor.

    3.   Thirst is a late indicator of fluid loss. By the time a client complains of thirst, there is significant fluid loss. Daily weights give a better indication of the effectiveness of fluid restoration.

    4.   The nurse will record all intake. Recording intake shows what measures were taken to restore fluid balance but does not indicate if the measures were effective.

#75. 3. **The chair should be on the client's unaffected side so the client can stand on the unaffected leg, pivot, and sit in the chair.**   Im   Ph/7   1

  1. The chair should be on the client's unaffected side so the client can stand on the unaffected leg, pivot, and sit in the chair. The client's affected side is the right.

  2. The chair should be on the client's unaffected side so the client can stand on the unaffected leg, pivot, and sit in the chair. The chair should face the foot of the bed.

  4. In this answer, the chair is on the correct side of the bed, but it should face the foot of the bed.

#76. 4. **This correctly describes the three-point gait for someone who is unable to bear weight on the right foot. This gait is correct for this client.**   Ev   Ph/7   1

  1. This describes the four-point gait. The four-point gait is not appropriate for someone who has a broken right ankle and cannot bear weight on one foot. This gait is not correct for this client.

  2. This response describes the two-point gait. The two-point gait is not appropriate for someone who has a broken ankle and cannot bear weight on both feet. This gait is not correct for this client.

  3. This response describes the three-point gait for someone who cannot bear weight on the left foot. The client has a fractured right ankle. This gait is not correct for this client.

#77. 4. **Pulling the client by the shoulders is not appropriate. A better approach would be to use a turning sheet or a pull sheet to pull the client up in bed. Pulling the client by the shoulders can damage the shoulders and also cause friction, which may lead to decubitus ulcer formation.**   Ev   Ph/7   1

  1. Using a pull sheet or a turning sheet is appropriate. This makes it easier for the nursing assistant and reduces skin breakdown in the client.

  2. Asking another nursing assistant to help is appropriate. This makes it easier for both the nursing assistant and the client.

  3. The head of the bed should be lowered before the client is pulled up in bed.

ANSWER	RATIONALE	NP	CN	SA

#78. 1. The nurse should try nonpharmacologic methods to help the client relax and go to sleep before asking for sleeping medication. This is not an appropriate initial action. — Im Ph/7 1

2. A back rub often helps a person relax and makes it easier to go to sleep. This is an appropriate initial action.

3. Asking the client if she is concerned about something is an appropriate initial action. This opens communication and may reduce anxiety.

4. Repositioning the client who is having trouble sleeping may promote relaxation and is appropriate initially.

#79. 3. Antiembolism stockings will do most to help prevent venous stasis. — Pl Ph/7 1

1. The immobilized client should deep-breathe and cough every two hours. However, this is done to prevent atelectasis, not thrombophlebitis.

2. Range-of-motion exercises are performed primarily to prevent joint contractures. They may be a little help in preventing thrombophlebitis. During range-of-motion exercises, the joint is moved.

4. Turning every two hours is done primarily to prevent atelectasis and skin breakdown.

#80. 4. A cool and blanched area around the infusion site suggests the IV may be infiltrated. This should be reported to the charge nurse immediately, because the IV must be discontinued. — Dc Ph/8 1

1. Intravenous solutions are at room temperature and may feel cool to the client as they infuse. This is normal and does not need to be reported to the charge nurse.

2. The infusion site is normally covered with clear tape. This does not need to be reported to the charge nurse.

3. It is safe for clients to ambulate when an IV infusion is running. This does not need to be reported to the charge nurse.

#81. 4 Before administering digoxin, the nurse should always check the client's apical pulse. If the adult client's pulse is below 60/min., the nurse should hold the medication and notify the physician. — Im Ph/8 5

1. There is no need to check the client's temperature before administering digoxin. The nurse should check the client's apical pulse.

2. There is no need to check the client's blood pressure when administering digoxin. The nurse should check the client's apical pulse.

3. There is no need to check the client's respirations before administering digoxin. The nurse should check the client's apical pulse.

#82. 1.   Small doses of aspirin are frequently given to persons with long bone fractures to prevent clots from forming. A fat embolus is a potential complication of a long bone fracture. The tibia is a long bone in the lower leg.   Im   Ph/8   5

2.   Small doses of aspirin are frequently given to persons with long bone fractures to prevent clots from forming. Baby aspirin is not given to an adult to lower body temperature.

3.   Baby aspirin is not given to an adult to control pain. Small doses of aspirin are frequently given to persons with long bone fractures to prevent clots from forming.

4.   Aspirin does have an anti-inflammatory effect. However, this is not the reason it is given to the client with a long bone fracture. Small doses of aspirin are frequently given to persons with long bone fractures to prevent clots from forming.

#83. 2.   Many drugs affect the action of warfarin. Both aspirin and acetaminophen potentiate the action of warfarin and could cause bleeding if taken when warfarin is being administered. Clients should be taught to avoid over-the-counter drugs without first checking with their physician.   Pl   Ph/8   5

1.   There is no need to take warfarin on a full stomach.

3.   Aspirin is an anticoagulant and potentiates warfarin, which is also an anticoagulant. Taking aspirin with warfarin could cause the client to bleed.

4.   There is no need to avoid sun exposure when taking warfarin.

#84. 3.   Spansules are capsules with particles of medication that are coated so they will be absorbed at different times. Spansules should be given at 12-hour intervals.   Pl   Ph/8   5

1.   Spansules should be taken at 12-hour intervals.

2.   A spansule should not be opened up. The little pellets are designed to be absorbed at different rates. The contents of the spansule should not be put in food.

4.   A spansule should not be cut.

ANSWER   RATIONALE

#85. 2. The client's remarks sound suicidal. The nurse should ask the client if she is considering hurting herself. This is a safety issue. The nurse should also record and report the client's remarks.   Im   Ps/5   2

  1. Asking the client "why" questions puts her on the defensive. This is not therapeutic.

  3. The nurse should first assess suicide potential. Telling her that life is precious does not give recognition to what she is expressing. It is almost arguing with her and is not therapeutic.

  4. The nurse should first assess for suicide potential. Helping her see the good things in life does not give recognition to what she is expressing at the moment.

#86. 3. Restating the client's remarks will open communication and allow the client to further express his feelings.   Im   Ps/5   2

  1. Saying "you are not a freak" is not therapeutic. This is arguing with the client and denying his feelings.

  2. Telling the client that lots of people have amputations and live a normal life is a true statement but is not the most therapeutic response. The nurse should initially let the client express his feelings.

  4. Responding by telling the client he shouldn't say what he said is very judgmental and will not open communication.

#87. 1. In order to deal with his anxiety, the client must first recognize that he is anxious.   Dc   Ps/5   2

  2. Identifying the situations that precipitated his anxiety is a later step in the process. The client must first recognize that he is anxious.

  3. Understanding the reason for his anxiety is a later step in the process. The client must first recognize that he is anxious.

  4. Selecting a strategy to cope with his anxiety is a later step in the process. The client must first recognize that he is anxious.

#88. 3. The client is experiencing phantom pain. This is real pain. The nurse should administer the ordered medications first. Later, the nurse can encourage the client to discuss his feelings.   Im   Ps/5   2

  1. Elevating the stump will not relieve the pain. The stump should only be elevated for the first 24–48 hours following an amputation.

  2. The client is experiencing phantom pain. This is real pain. The nurse should administer the ordered medications first.

  4. The client is experiencing phantom pain. This is real pain. The nurse should administer the ordered medications first. After medicating the client, the nurse can encourage the client to express his feelings.

#89. 3. Reminding her an hour before meals that mealtime is coming up will allow her time to complete the washing ritual so she will be able to get to meals.

    1. Interrupting the ritual will increase the client's anxiety and may precipitate a panic attack.

    2. The client needs to learn to function. Bringing meals to her only encourages the ritualistic behavior.

    4. The rituals are so important to the obsessive-compulsive client that if given a choice between the rituals and meals, the rituals will seem more important and the client will not eat.

#90. 1. This comment indicates the mother does not understand the developmental level of an eight-month-old. A child of eight months does not cry just to irritate his parents. Parents who abuse their children often have unrealistic expectations of the developmental level.

    2. This comment is one that most parents would make and indicates concern and a desire to understand what the infant needs. This is not suggestive of child abuse.

    3. This comment indicates the mother is trying to meet the infant's needs. It indicates a need for instruction about infants and needs other than feeding. However, it does not indicate possible child abuse.

    4. This comment indicates a desire to understand what the infant wants. It does not suggest child abuse.

#91. 4. Putting her favorite picture on the door to her room should help her find her room.

    1. Wandering is not an indication for restraints.

    2. Asking a roommate in an acute care setting to take responsibility for another client is not appropriate.

    3. Punishing the client is not appropriate. She is not deliberately misbehaving. The disease process makes her confused.

**#92. 2. The LPN/LVN should notify the charge nurse regarding this   Im   Ps/6   2
information. The client needs referral to a battered women's
shelter. The psychiatric clinical specialist nurse may be called in
to talk with this client. This situation needs referral; it is beyond
the scope of the practical nurse.**

1. The woman who is abused often feels helpless and unable to get out
of the situation. Asking the client why she stays with a man who has
caused her to get hurt may give her more guilt.

3. Asking the client about divorce is premature at this time. The practical
nurse should notify the charge nurse so appropriate referrals for the
client's safety can be made is more appropriate. This situation is
beyond the scope of the practical nurse.

4. Simply telling the client she has rights will not ensure her safety. This
situation is beyond the scope of the practical nurse and should be
referred to the charge nurse.

**#93. 2. The client should avoid persons who are sick because radiation   Im   Ph/10   1
therapy causes bone marrow depression making the client
susceptible to infection.**

1. The person receiving external radiation is not a danger to others.

3. The person receiving external radiation is not a danger to others.

4. The person receiving external radiation is not a danger to others.

**#94. 3. When a person is in shock and has a decreased circulating blood   Dc   Ph/10   1
volume, the urine output decreases.**

1. When a person is in shock, the systolic and diastolic blood pressure
drop. The systolic pressure drops more than the diastolic so the pulse
pressure narrows. Elevated systolic and lowered diastolic pressure
are seen with increasing intracranial pressure.

2. When a person is in shock, the heart rate increases.

4. When a person is in shock, the respiratory rate increases.

**#95. 2. When a person is unresponsive the nurse should initially assess   Dc   Ph/10   1
respirations and pulse.**

1. When a person is unresponsive the nurse should assess before
starting chest compressions.

3. When a person is unresponsive the nurse should assess before
starting CPR. If CPR is necessary, the client should be on a hard
surface.

4. When a person is unresponsive the nurse should assess before
starting mouth-to-mouth breathing.

#96. **2.** **Antihypertensives and vasodilators should not be given before dialysis because the blood pressure drops significantly during the procedure.**   Im   Ph/10   5

    1. Antihypertensives and vasodilators should not be given before dialysis because the blood pressure drops significantly during the procedure.

    3. Antihypertensives and vasodilators should not be given before dialysis because the blood pressure drops significantly during the procedure.

    4. Antihypertensives and vasodilators should not be given before dialysis because the blood pressure drops significantly during the procedure.

#97. **1.** **The nurse should release the suction by opening the vent to stop the pulling action of the suction (take your finger off the hole).**   Im   Ph/10   1

    2. If the suction is pulling the tracheal wall, the nurse should not continue to suction. This causes further damage to the tracheal wall.

    3. The nurse should not increase pressure as this would cause further damage to the tracheal wall.

    4. When the catheter is attaching to the tracheal wall it will be nearly impossible to suction deeper. The nurse should release the suction by taking his or her finger off the hole.

#98. **2.** **When there is no bubbling in the water seal compartment it means either that the lung has re-expanded or that there is an obstruction in the tubing coming from the pleural cavity. It is not very likely that the lung has re-expanded in four hours. It is much more likely that there is an obstruction in the tubing.**   Dc   Ph/9   1

    1. When there is no bubbling in the water seal compartment it means either that the lung has re-expanded or that there is an obstruction in the tubing coming from the pleural cavity. It is not very likely that the lung has re-expanded in four hours. It is much more likely that there is an obstruction in the tubing.

    3. An air leak would cause no bubbling in the suction control chamber.

    4. When the suction is not turned on there is no bubbling in the suction control chamber. There may still be bubbles in the water seal chamber as there will still be gravity drainage.

. **#99. 4.** **Increasing respiratory difficulty indicates that the congestive heart failure is worsening. Before calling the physician, the nurse should raise the head of the bed to ease the client's breathing.**   Im   Ph/10   1

1. Increasing respiratory difficulty indicates that the congestive heart failure is getting worse. Increasing the drip rate will further increase the overload situation and make the client worse. The nurse should decrease the IV drip rate and raise the head of the bed.

2. Increasing respiratory difficulty indicates that the congestive heart failure is getting worse. Placing the client in a supine position will make the symptoms worse. The client should be placed in a semi- to high Fowler's position to make breathing easier.

3. Increasing respiratory difficulty indicates that the congestive heart failure is getting worse. The nurse should take measures to make the client more comfortable. Asking questions that require him to talk waste energy without giving useful information.

#100. 2. **Oxygen is very drying to tissues. Humidifying oxygen helps to prevent drying of tissues.**   Im   Ph/10   1

1. The water doesn't cool the oxygen; it humidifies the oxygen.

3. The water humidifies the oxygen. The purpose of the water is not to prevent fires.

4. The reason for humidifying oxygen is to keep the tissues from drying out. Humidifying oxygen does not prevent infections from developing in the tubing.

Practice Test Two

1. An adult client who had major abdominal surgery is returned to her room on the surgical nursing unit. The post-anesthesia nurse reports that the client is awake and has stable vital signs. She has a nasogastric tube in place that is attached to intermittent suction. The nurse should position the client in which of the following positions?

   1. Supine
   2. Semi-Fowler's
   3. Dorsal recumbent
   4. Prone

2. An adult post-operative client vomits, and his abdominal wound eviscerates. What is the best initial action for the nurse to take?

   1. Cover the exposed coils of intestine with sterile moist towels or dressings.
   2. Pack the intestines back into the abdominal cavity.
   3. Irrigate the exposed coils of intestines with sterile water.
   4. Take the client's vital signs.

3. Thirty-six hours after major surgery a client has a temperature of 100°F. What is the most likely cause of the temperature elevation?

   1. Dehydration
   2. Atelectasis
   3. Wound infection
   4. Bladder infection

4. The nurse is preparing to administer pre-operative medication of meperidine and atropine to an elderly adult who is scheduled for surgery. The client tells the nurse he has glaucoma and wants to take his eye drops before going to the operating room. What is the best action for the nurse to take?

   1. Administer medication as ordered and encourage the client to take his eye drops.
   2. Check with the physician before administering pre-operative medication.
   3. Administer pre-operative medication as ordered and suggest the client not take his eye drops.
   4. Administer the meperidine; withhold atropine and suggest the client take his eye drops.

5. An adult client has been medicated for elective surgery. The operating room nurse discovers that the consent form for surgery has not been signed. What should the nurse do?

   1. Have the client sign the consent form.
   2. Tell the physician that the consent form has not been signed.
   3. Have the client's spouse sign the consent form.
   4. Continue preparation for surgery as the client has given implied consent.

6. An elderly man has just returned from the operating room where he spent several hours in lithotomy position during a perineal prostatectomy. Which assessment should the nurse make because the client was in lithotomy position during surgery?

   1. Lower extremity pulses, paresthesias, and pain
   2. The presence of bowel sounds
   3. Radial pulse, sensation, and movement of the arms
   4. Palpation of the bladder

7. An elderly client is admitted to a skilled nursing care facility. When doing a skin assessment the nurse notes a 3-cm round area of partial-thickness skin loss that looks like a blister on the client's sacrum. The nurse interprets this to be a

   1. Stage I pressure ulcer.
   2. Stage II pressure ulcer.
   3. Stage III pressure ulcer.
   4. Stage IV pressure ulcer.

8. The nurse is caring for a client who has been placed on a hypothermia blanket. What should the nurse include in the care plan?

   1. Take frequent vital signs and perform frequent skin assessments.
   2. Leave the hypothermia blanket on until the client's temperature reaches 98.6°F.
   3. Place the client directly on the blanket.
   4. Apply iced alcohol sponges to the part of the client's trunk not in contact with the blanket.

9. The physician's orders include warm compresses to the left leg three times a day for treatment of an open wound. Which action is appropriate when carrying out these orders?

   1. Use medical aseptic technique.
   2. Leave the wet compress open to the air.

3. Place both a dry covering and waterproof material over the compress.
   4. Remove the compress after five minutes.

10. An adult is on a clear liquid diet. Which food should the nurse offer him?

   1. A milk shake
   2. Fruited gelatin
   3. Sherbet
   4. Apple juice

11. Four clients have signaled with their call bell for the nurse. Whom should the nurse observe first?

   1. An adult who needs assistance walking to the bathroom
   2. A postoperative client who is asking for pain medication
   3. An adult who has just been given penicillin
   4. An elderly client who is in a gerry chair with a restraint vest on

12. The nurse is caring for a client who was in a motor vehicle accident. His blood pressure is dropping rapidly. What should the nurse observe the client for before placing the client in shock position?

   1. Long bone fractures
   2. Air embolus
   3. Head injury
   4. Thrombophlebitis

13. The nurse is teaching family members how to correctly transfer a client who has right hemiplegia from the bed to a wheelchair. Which observation indicates the family understands how to transfer the client?

   1. The wheelchair is placed parallel to the bed on the affected side.

2. The family members lift the client up by having her place her arms around their necks.

3. The wheelchair is placed at a 45-degree angle to the bed on the client's unaffected side.

4. The family members ask for a trapeze bar for the client to use in the transfer.

14. An adult is being discharged from the emergency room with instructions to apply a cold pack to his sprained ankle. The client asks why it is necessary to use a cold pack. The nurse replies that the cold pack will do which of the following?

1. Keep the sprain from becoming a fracture

2. Prevent bruising and ecchymosis from occurring

3. Keep the client from developing a fever

4. Help reduce swelling and pain

15. An adult has received an injection of immunoglobulin. The client asks what this injection will do for him. The nurse's reply includes the information that he will develop which type of immunity as a result of this injection?

1. Active natural immunity

2. Active artificial immunity

3. Passive natural immunity

4. Passive artificial immunity

16. An adult is receiving total parenteral nutrition (TPN). Which assessment is essential for the nurse to make?

1. Number of bowel movements

2. Confirmation that the tube is in the stomach

3. Auscultation of bowel sounds

4. Daily weights

17. An adult is on long-term aspirin therapy and complains of tinnitus. Which interpretation by the nurse is accurate?

1. The aspirin is working as expected.

2. The client ingested more medication than was recommended.

3. The client has an upper GI bleed.

4. The client is experiencing a minor overdose.

18. An adult is to receive a narcotic analgesic via patient-controlled analgesia (PCA). Which statement by the client indicates that the client understands how the PCA works?

1. "When I press this button the machine will always give me more medicine."

2. "I will press the button whenever I begin to experience pain."

3. "I should press this button every hour so the pain doesn't come back."

4. "With this machine I will experience no more pain."

19. The nurse is caring for a client who had knee surgery this morning. Post-operative orders include a narcotic every 3–4 hours as needed for operative-site pain and an ice bag. At 7 P.M. the client asks for pain medication. He was last medicated at 3:30 P.M. What is the best initial nursing action?

1. Administer the prescribed analgesic.

2. Assess the location and nature of the pain.

3. Refill the ice bag as needed.

4. Reposition the client.

20. An adult is receiving external radiation therapy. What should the nurse include in the teaching plan about care of the skin at the radiation site?

    1. Tape a loose dressing to the radiation site.

    2. Shower each evening before therapy.

    3. Apply ice compresses to the site to relieve pain.

    4. Avoid washing the skin in the area being radiated.

21. A client is receiving chemotherapy for cancer and develops thrombocytopenia. What should the nurse include in the client's plan of care because of the thrombocytopenia?

    1. Place the client in a semi-upright position.

    2. Limit the client's intake of fluids.

    3. Administer no injections.

    4. Exercise the client's lower extremities.

22. An adult is admitted with a head injury following an accident. He has a severe headache and asks the nurse why he cannot have something for pain. The nurse understands that the client should not receive a narcotic analgesic for which reason?

    Narcotic analgesics

    1. cause mydriasis, which will raise intracranial pressure.

    2. are not effective for pain caused by brain trauma.

    3. cause vomiting, which would mask a sign of increased intracranial pressure.

    4. may depress respirations, which would cause acidosis and further brain damage.

23. A client is scheduled for a cataract extraction. Pre-operatively 1% atropine is instilled into the client's right eye. The nurse knows this drug would be contraindicated if she also had which of the following conditions?

    1. Bradycardia

    2. Hypothyroidism

    3. Diabetes

    4. Glaucoma

24. An adult is admitted with Guillain-Barré syndrome. On day three of hospitalization, the client's muscle weakness worsens, and he is no longer able to stand with support. He is also having difficulty swallowing and talking. The priority in the nursing care plan at this time is to prevent which problem?

    1. Aspiration pneumonia

    2. Decubitus ulcers

    3. Bladder distention

    4. Hypertensive crisis

25. A young woman is admitted to the hospital complaining of severe fatigue and weakness of one week duration. Her physician suspects a diagnosis of myasthenia gravis. Which additional findings would the nurse expect the client to have?

    1. Ataxia and poor coordination

    2. Diplopia and ptosis of the eyelids

    3. Slurred speech

    4. Headaches and tinnitus

26. The nurse is caring for a client who has a C-6 spinal cord injury. He complains of blurred vision and a severe headache. His blood pressure is 210/140. What action should the nurse take initially?

    1. Check for bladder distention.

    2. Place in Trendelenburg position.

    3. Administer prn pain medication.

    4. Continue to monitor blood pressure.

27. The charge nurse in a long-term care facility is making assignments. When assigning personnel to care for residents, which principle is important?

1. Assignments should be rotated on a daily basis.
2. Clients who are confused often do better with the same caregiver for several days.
3. Female caregivers should not care for male residents.
4. Caregivers should be allowed to select the residents they will care for.

28. The family of a young man who has been declared brain dead following an accident tells the nurse that the doctors said their son would be a good organ donor. They ask the nurse if donating his organs would mean that they could not have a regular funeral. Which response by the nurse is most accurate?

    1. "Donating organs does deface the body, so a closed casket is necessary."
    2. "Ask the physician which organs would be donated."
    3. "Organ donation involves a surgical incision but should not interfere with any type of funeral."
    4. "Donating organs is a wonderful service to humanity."

29. All of the following tasks need to be done. Which one can the LPN/LVN safely delegate to the certified nursing assistant (CNA)?

    1. Tube feeding for a client with a nasogastric tube
    2. Routine vital signs for a group of clients
    3. Blood pressure monitoring for a client who is in congestive heart failure
    4. Wound care for a client with a stage III decubitus ulcer

30. The nurse is new to the resident facility and is administering medications. One of the clients does not have a readable identification band in place. What should the nurse do?

    1. Ask the client what his name is.
    2. Ask the client if he is Mr. _____.

3. Ask the roommate if this is Mr. _____.
4. Check the bed tag for the name.

31. The nurse is caring for all of the following persons. Which one is most in need of restraints?

    1. An elderly man who is sitting in a chair
    2. A confused post-operative client who is picking at his nasal oxygen and NG tube
    3. A confused woman who is in bed with the side rails up
    4. An adult who has just returned to the surgical floor from a post-anesthesia care unit

32. The RN charge nurse hands the LPN/LVN a syringe filled with medication that the RN has just drawn and asks the LPN/LVN to administer this to a client. How should the LPN/LVN respond?

    1. Do as requested by the charge nurse.
    2. Ask the charge nurse what the medication is and then administer it.
    3. Ask the charge nurse what the medication is, check the order and then administer it.
    4. Refuse to administer the medication.

33. An adult client in an acute care facility says to the nurse, "I hope this hospital doesn't have student doctors and nurses. I do not want a student taking care of me." The nurse's response should be based on which of the following understandings?

   1. When a client signs permission for treatment in a hospital, this includes treatment by medical and nursing students.

   2. The client has the right to know if the hospital is affiliated with a medical school and to refuse care by students.

   3. The client may sign a special form that says he refuses to be cared for by medical or nursing students.

   4. The client should be informed if any caregivers are students, but the client does not have the right to refuse to be cared for by students.

34. An adult client in an acute care setting asks the nurse to show him his hospital records. The nurse's response should reflect which understanding?

   1. The client has no right to see his records without a court order.

   2. The client must have the physician's approval before he can see his records.

   3. The client has the right to see his records and to have information explained when necessary.

   4. The client must ask permission to view his records from the medical records department and must appear before a special committee.

35. The LPN/LVN has delegated basic hygienic care of several clients to a certified nursing assistant. Which action by the nurse will ensure that the clients receive the best care?

   1. Observe the nursing assistant during the performance of all care.

   2. Ask the nursing assistant if there were any problems.

   3. Check the nursing assistant's charting.

   4. Observe the clients following administration of care by the nursing assistant.

36. A client who is withdrawing from alcohol says to the nurse, "There are snakes on the wall." Which action should the nurse take initially?

   1. Reassure the client there are no snakes.

   2. Turn the lights on brighter.

   3. Tell the client that while he may see snakes there are really no snakes.

   4. Reassure the client the snakes will not hurt him.

37. The client is scheduled for a myelogram today. The permit has been signed. The client tells the nurse that she has changed her mind and does not want to have the procedure. What should the nurse do?

   1. Tell the client that once permission has been given the procedure has to be done.

   2. Tell the client that the physician will be very upset if she does not have it done.

   3. Suggest to the client that it is in her best interests to have the procedure as scheduled.

   4. Understand that the client has the right to change her mind about procedures.

38. The nurse is caring for a woman who is receiving internal radiation for cancer of the cervix. Which nursing action will do most to reduce the risk of radiation exposure to other clients?

   1. Keep the door to the client's room closed.

   2. Place the client in the bed closest to the outside window.

3. Place the client in a room close to the nurse's station for continuous observation.

4. Place a "do not enter" sign on the door to the client's room.

39. The nurse is caring for a 79-year-old client. Which observation is not normal and should be reported for follow-up?

   1. The client has several brown spots on her cheek and neck.

   2. The client says, "I move slower than I used to."

   3. The client is short of breath when walking down the hall.

   4. The client says, "I have trouble telling the colors of my socks."

40. The nurse is caring for an aging client. Which statement the client makes indicates he is having difficulty with the developmental tasks of aging?

   1. "I like to make toys for my grandchildren."

   2. "I used to be a farmer, now I can't do all that hard work."

   3. "I wish I had changed careers when I really wanted to; now it's too late."

   4. "We don't have as much money now as we did before I retired."

41. A young woman who is at 32 weeks gestation reports to the physician's office for a routine prenatal visit. Which comment by the woman must be reported to the physician?

   1. "I had to stop wearing my rings because my fingers are swollen."

   2. "I seem to be hotter than everyone else."

   3. "My feet tend to swell in the hot weather."

   4. "My breasts are so big and tender."

42. The nurse is caring for an older adult. Which statement made by the client is not typical of normal aging?

   1. "I seem to be more sensitive to the taste of salt than I used to be."

   2. "I have trouble reading the newspaper."

   3. "I don't drive at dusk any more."

   4. "Sometimes I have trouble matching my socks."

43. The nurse is to obtain pedal pulses on a client following a cardiac catheterization. Which is the proper procedure?

   1. Place the fingertips against the wrist bone.

   2. Place the stethoscope over the apex of the heart.

   3. Place the fingertips against the side of the neck.

   4. Place the fingertips on top of the foot.

44. The nurse is to obtain an apical-radial pulse on a client. Which statement is true regarding obtaining an apical-radial pulse?

   1. After taking the apical pulse the nurse immediately takes the radial pulse.

   2. The radial pulse is usually higher than the apical pulse.

   3. One person takes the apical pulse while the second person takes the radial pulse at the same time.

   4. The nurse should take the radial pulse while listening to the apical pulse.

45. The nurse is assessing the client's vital signs and notes that the client is breathing very noisily. The nurse describes this pattern of breathing as

   1. hyperpnea.

   2. Cheyne-Stokes.

   3. orthopnea.

   4. sterterous.

46. The nurse is obtaining a blood pressure on a client who weighs over 300 pounds. The nurse chooses to use a large cuff for which of the following reasons?

 1. A large cuff is more comfortable for the client.

 2. Using a cuff that is too small causes the blood pressure reading to be abnormally high.

 3. When a regular cuff is used on a large person it is difficult to hear the pulse.

 4. A small cuff on a large person causes the systolic pressure to read lower than normal and the diastolic pressure to read higher than normal.

47. A post-operative client is to be discharged today. She will need to change her dressing daily. Which statement she makes indicates she understands the process?

 1. "I will wash my hands before and after I change the dressing."

 2. "I can touch the dressings with my hands if I only touch the edges."

 3. "I should clean the area around the incision by moving the swab toward it."

 4. "I can put the old dressings directly in the waste basket."

48. The nurse is caring for a client who is on bed rest for an extended period of time. When planning care the nurse knows that which nursing action will do most to help prevent muscle atrophy?

 1. Perform passive range-of-motion exercises on the client.

 2. Turn the client at two-hour intervals.

 3. Encourage the client to change positions frequently.

 4. Assist the client in the performance of active exercises.

49. The nurse is caring for a client who has been on bed rest for several weeks. Which problem is least likely to be related to bed rest?

 1. Muscle atrophy

 2. Hypostatic pneumonia

 3. Varicose veins

 4. Thrombophlebitis

50. The nurse is planning care for a client who must remain in bed for several weeks. Which action will do most to prevent the development of pressure ulcers?

 1. Performing range-of-motion exercises

 2. Deep breathing and coughing

 3. Keeping the feet against a footboard

 4. Changing position in bed frequently

51. The nurse is observing a certified nursing assistant move a client. Which action, if observed, indicates that the nursing assistant needs more instruction?

 The assistant

 1. stands with feet spread apart.

 2. bends from the waist.

 3. turns her whole body.

 4. keeps her back straight.

52. An adult client who is ambulating in the corridor with the nurse becomes dizzy and faint. What should the nurse do at this time?

 1. Have her put her head between her legs.

 2. Quickly go to get help.

 3. Guide her to a chair in the corridor and ease her into it.

 4. Encourage the client to walk more quickly.

53. The nurse is caring for a client admitted with a sickle cell crisis. What assessment finding is not consistent with the diagnosis?

 1. Enlarged liver and spleen

 2. Jaundice and icterus

3. Decreased white blood count

4. Abdominal and joint pain

54. The wife of a man who is diagnosed with angina pectoris asks the nurse how she would know if her husband had a heart attack rather than angina. What should the nurse include in the reply?

   1. Crushing chest pain not relieved by nitroglycerine is likely to be a heart attack.

   2. Epigastric pain relieved by antacids is likely to be angina.

   3. Chest pain that does not go down the left arm is usually angina.

   4. Chest pain not associated with activity or excitement is probably angina.

55. The nurse is caring for a man who has recently been diagnosed with angina. Which statement he makes indicates understanding of his condition?

   1. "I should not exercise now that I have angina."

   2. "If I have chest pain I will take a nitroglycerine."

   3. "Sexual activity is likely to cause a heart attack."

   4. "If I have any chest pain, I should immediately call my doctor."

56. The mother of a boy who has recently been diagnosed with sickle cell anemia is pregnant and asks the nurse if her unborn baby will have sickle cell. What information should the nurse include in the answer?

   1. Sickle cell anemia is a contagious disease, but your child should no longer be communicable by the time the baby is born.

   2. When both parents are carriers there is a 25% chance that each child will have sickle cell anemia.

3. Your sons have a 50% chance of having sickle cell, but daughters can only be carriers.

4. The next child should be disease-free, but additional children have a chance of being born with the disease.

57. What nursing action is essential when oxygen is ordered for a client who is living at home?

   1. Assist the client and family in checking all electrical appliances in the vicinity for frayed cords.

   2. Encourage the client and family to purchase fire extinguishers.

   3. Remove electrical devices from the room where oxygen is in use.

   4. Encourage the client and family to carpet the client's room.

58. An adult who has a tracheostomy needs to be suctioned. How should the nurse position the client for this procedure?

   1. Supine

   2. Semi-Fowler's

   3. Sim's

   4. Semi-lateral

59. The client is admitted for a bronchoscopy this morning. Which question is essential for the nurse to ask the client?

   1. "When did you last eat?"

   2. "Did you take the laxative as ordered?"

   3. "What has the doctor told you about your procedure?"

   4. "Have you had conscious sedation before?"

60. The nurse is caring for a client who had thoracic surgery yesterday and has a chest tube attached to water seal drainage. The client's family asks why he has to have a chest tube. What should the nurse include in the response?

The chest tube

1. allows air to enter the thoracic cavity to equalize pressures in the lung.
2. removes air from the pleural cavity and promotes re-expansion of the lung.
3. increases the amount of oxygen available to the lungs.
4. will help the wound heal faster and reduce scarring.

61. The nurse is caring for a client who had a chest tube inserted and attached to Pleurovac® drainage two days ago. There is no bubbling in the water seal chamber. What should the nurse assess initially?

1. Observe the wound for excess drainage.
2. Check the system for air leaks.
3. Auscultate the lungs.
4. See if the suction is turned on.

62. The client is receiving gentamicin IV. Which finding may indicate an adverse response to gentamicin?

1. Decreased urine output
2. Blurred vision
3. Orange sputum
4. Hypertension

63. The nurse is caring for a client who had a cystoscopy earlier in the day. Which data from the client is of greatest concern to the nurse?

1. Complaint of back pain
2. Tea-colored urine
3. Leg cramps
4. Pink-tinged urine

64. A client who is diagnosed with cystitis has been given a prescription for pyridium. She asks the nurse why she has been given this medication. What should the nurse reply?

1. "Pyridium is an antibiotic that will kill the bacteria causing your infection."
2. "Pyridium is an analgesic that will make you less aware of the pain and discomfort."
3. "Pyridium is a urinary tract anesthetic that will kill the pain until the antibiotics have had time to work."
4. "Pyridium will help to prevent kidney damage from the bladder infection."

65. An adult is admitted with suspected urolithiasis. Which nursing diagnosis is of highest priority when planning nursing care for this client immediately after admission?

1. Acute pain
2. Diarrhea
3. Risk of ineffective health maintenance
4. Risk of infection

66. When admitting a client who has acute glomerulonephritis the nurse expects the client will report which information?

1. Recent bladder infection
2. History of previous kidney infections
3. Pharyngitis three weeks ago
4. Multiple sexual partners

67. The nurse is caring for an adult who has kidney stones. Which action is essential for the nurse to take?

1. Take blood pressure frequently.
2. Keep the client on bed rest.
3. Position the client supine.
4. Strain all urine.

68. The client is to be discharged after passing a uric acid kidney stone. This is the third time

the client has been hospitalized for kidney stones. The nurse should teach the client to do which of the following?

1. Eat generous amounts of chicken and organ meats.
2. Drink lots of water.
3. Avoid vigorous activity.
4. Take the ordered allopurinol (Zyloprim) if the symptoms recur.

69. The client has just had a basal cell carcinoma removed in the doctor's office. Which statement the client makes indicates understanding regarding prevention and early detection of basal cell carcinoma?

1. "Moles that are round and brown should be seen immediately by my doctor."
2. "I should wear long sleeves when I am out in the sun."
3. "I should avoid using lotions and powders on my skin."
4. "I can use a tanning booth to get a tan since I can't stay in the sun very long."

70. Which statement made by an adolescent indicates understanding of how to reduce risk of osteoporosis later in life?

1. "I will be careful not to sprain my ankle when I play sports."
2. "I drink a glass of milk with every meal."
3. "As I get older I will reduce the amount of weight-bearing exercise I do."
4. "My favorite beverages are cola drinks."

71. The nurse is caring for a client who has right-sided weakness and has been told to use a cane for walking. Which action by the client indicates he can use a cane correctly?

1. He moves the cane with the right leg when walking.
2. He moves the cane from hand to hand when walking.

3. He carries the cane on his left side and moves it at the same time he moves his right foot.
4. He puts the cane forward, then moves the left foot forward followed by the right foot.

72. An adult has low back pain. Which position is likely to be most comfortable for the client?

1. Prone
2. Supine
3. Side-lying with knees flexed
4. Semi-Fowler's with legs extended

73. One of the campers at summer camp sprains his ankle. What action can the nurse take to help reduce the pain?

1. Encourage the camper to gently exercise the ankle several times every hour.
2. Apply an ice pack to the ankle.
3. Keep the leg down to encourage blood flow.
4. Apply a topical steroid ointment.

74. A home care client says she is having difficulty getting to sleep at night. Which suggestion could the nurse make to help the client?

1. Exercise shortly before going to bed.
2. Drink a cola beverage during the evening.
3. Watch television after going to bed.
4. Drink warm milk before going to bed.

75. The client's blood gas values are:

pH 7.35; CO_2 60; HCO_3 34; pO_2 60.

The nurse correctly interprets these to indicate the client is in which state?

1. Compensated respiratory acidosis
2. Partly compensated metabolic alkalosis
3. Metabolic alkalosis
4. Metabolic acidosis

76. What question should the nurse ask the client who presents for an MRI test?

    1. "Are you allergic to iodine or shellfish?"
    2. "When did you last eat or drink anything?"
    3. "Do you have any metal in your body?"
    4. "Did you take the laxative prep?"

77. The nurse notes all of the following. Which situation needs immediate attention?

    1. Dirty linen has fallen on the floor beside the bed of a bedridden client.
    2. Breakfast dishes remain on the overbed table two hours after mealtime.
    3. An elderly ambulatory client drops a glass of water on the floor beside the bed.
    4. The client's hi-low bed cannot be moved to the high position.

78. While caring for a woman who delivered a healthy term infant six hours ago, the nurse notes the fundus is soft, 2 cm above the umbilicus and off to the left. The lochia is red. The nurse suspects that the client has which problem?

    1. Retained placental fragments
    2. Perineal laceration
    3. Urinary retention
    4. Normal involution

79. The mother of a week-old infant says to the nurse "When will that ugly black cord thing come off?" How should the nurse reply?

    1. "Are you wiping it with alcohol each time you change the baby's diaper?"
    2. "It usually comes off in ten days to three weeks."
    3. "It sounds as if it bothers you. Would you like to talk about it?
    4. "It should be off by now. I'll have the doctor check to be sure there is no problem."

80. A six-month-old infant is being seen in the doctor's office. Which observation by the nurse should be brought to the physician's attention?

    The baby

    1. sits up but needs slight support.
    2. was seven pounds at birth and now weighs ten pounds.
    3. frequently drops objects and looks for them.
    4. smacks her lips and drools.

81. The nurse is to administer a tube feeding to an adult. What action is essential before administering the feeding?

    1. Position the client in a supine position.
    2. Check the position of the feeding tube.
    3. Give the client something to suck on during the feeding.
    4. Check to see when the client last had a bowel movement.

82. An adult who had a mastectomy yesterday says to the nurse, "I guess I'm not a real woman anymore. How could my husband possibly love me now?" What is the best response for the nurse to make?

    1. "You don't feel like a woman now?"
    2. "Has your husband said anything to you?"
    3. "Of course your husband will love you."
    4. "True love is not dependent on breasts."

83. A client who has been waiting for several hours in the clinic waiting room suddenly begins to shout, "I need some attention and I need it now!" How should the nurse respond initially?

    1. Tell the client to be quiet and that she will be seen as soon as possible.
    2. Immediately call security and the police.
    3. Talk with the woman and determine her immediate needs.

4. Explain to the woman how busy the doctors are and that she will be seen soon.

84. The mother of six-month-old twins is in the doctor's office because one of the infants has an ear infection. The mother says to the nurse, "I just don't know if I can handle another problem. It is all so overwhelming." How should the nurse respond initially?

   1. "You're their mother. I'm sure you know what's best for them."

   2. "Have you called social services to see if you qualify for assistance?"

   3. "My sister had twins and she survived. You will too."

   4. "It must be tough to have two little ones. What seems to be the biggest problem?"

85. There have been several clients recently who have fallen in the long-term care facility. The nurse would like to reduce the number of falls. Which action is likely to do the most to help prevent falls?

   1. Ask the nursing assistants to watch the clients more carefully.

   2. Restrain clients who cannot walk independently.

   3. Provide call bells the clients can carry with them when they walk.

   4. Keep beds in the lowest position unless the nurse is performing care for the client.

86. The nurse is observing a nursing assistant providing care. Which action indicates that the nursing assistant understands universal precautions?

   The nursing assistant

   1. washes hands first thing in the morning before giving care to any client and again after all morning care is completed.

   2. wears gloves during all client contact.

   3. wears a gown when changing linen soiled with urine and feces.

4. changes gloves between clients but does not wash hands if gloves have been worn.

87. The nurse is changing a dressing. Which event indicates a break in sterile technique?

   The nurse

   1. opens the sterile dressing set by opening the first flap away from the nurse.

   2. turns around when answering a question asked by the client in the other bed.

   3. opens the dressing set on the overbed table.

   4. pours sterile saline into the container in the dressing set.

88. The nurse is assisting at a disaster shelter set up following a devastating earthquake. What is the most common problem the nurse is likely to see in those who come to the shelter?

   1. Thirst

   2. Traumatic injuries

   3. Stress

   4. Exacerbation of medical problems

89. The nurse is caring for a frail elderly client in her home. Which behavior, if observed or reported, should the nurse report to the supervisor for further evaluation of possible abuse?

   1. The client's daughter is attempting to be declared her mother's legal guardian.

   2. The client is frequently left in bed alone in the house for several hours at a time.

   3. The client has brown spots on her arms.

   4. The client says "My daughter doesn't like me very much. She yells at me."

90. A woman is being seen in the physician's office for a medical complaint. When she is called to see the physician she goes to the restroom and washes her hands over and over, missing her allotted time with the physician. How should the nurse deal with this woman?

1. Send her home without seeing the doctor if she is not available when called.

2. Give her advance warning that she will be seeing the physician and tell her if she needs to wash her hands she should do so.

3. Interrupt her washing ritual and insist she see the physician when it is her turn.

4. Give her a choice of seeing the physician or washing her hands.

91. A woman who was recently widowed says to the nurse, "I just can't believe he's gone. Sometimes I even think I see him standing there." What does this comment indicate about the client?

1. She is in an early stage of normal grief.

2. She may be hallucinating.

3. She is having illusions.

4. She may be in a severe depression.

92. The pre-operative client is from a different country and tells the nurse that his family will be coming for a prayer service. Eighteen persons arrive and start chanting in the client's semi-private room. What is the best response for the nurse?

1. Explain that visitors are limited to two per client.

2. Ask the client's roommate if they object to so many persons in the room.

3. Ignore the large number of people and the chanting.

4. Arrange for the group to go to the conference room or the chapel.

93. An adolescent is to be admitted to the orthopedic floor with several fractures. The client has been taking hallucinogens this evening. What should the nurse expect on admission because the client is using hallucinogens?

1. Severe depression

2. Violent behavior

3. Respiratory distress

4. Convulsions

94. An adult has completed an alcohol detoxification program and is being discharged with disulfiram (Antabuse). Which statement the client makes indicates a need for more teaching?

1. "I have learned my lesson. I won't drink more than two beers."

2. "I will not use mouthwash while I am taking Antabuse."

3. "I should take the Antabuse every day."

4. "If I have to go to the emergency room for any reason I will tell them I take Antabuse."

95. The nurse is caring for a woman who is admitted following a beating by her husband. The woman says, "It wasn't really his fault. Dinner was late." The husband arrives to visit his wife with a large bouquet of flowers and a box of chocolates. The woman later says to the nurse, "He feels so bad about what he did and says it will never happen again." What concept should guide the nurse when replying to the client?

1. Men who abuse their wives and then repent usually do not do it again.

2. The woman is quite perceptive and should be safe when she is discharged.

3. Abuse is often followed by repentance and then again by abuse.

4. Spousal abuse is usually a result of misbehavior on the part of the abused.

96. Which characteristic is most likely to be present in persons who abuse others?

1. Financial security
2. Positive self image
3. Substance abuse
4. Physical illness

97. An adult man believes that someone is poisoning his food. What is the best nursing action in response to this belief?

    1. Explain to him that no one is poisoning his food.
    2. Tell him that the food is prepared in the hospital under secure conditions.
    3. Taste his food to assure him that it is not being poisoned.
    4. Offer him food that is in individual containers.

98. A newly admitted client is exhibiting signs of severe anxiety. She is pacing back and forth and has difficulty concentrating on the nurse's questions. What nursing action is most appropriate at this time?

    1. Tell the client to sit down and get control of herself.
    2. Leave the room until she regains control.
    3. Whisper to her that everything will be all right.
    4. Attend to her behavior and direct her to a quiet area.

99. A two-year-old child is seen in the pediatrician's office. The child screams when the nurse approaches him to give him the ordered IM medication. How should the nurse approach the child?

    1. Tell him to stop screaming and he can have a lollipop after he gets the shot.
    2. Ask him to point to the leg he wants you to use.
    3. Tell him he is a big boy and shots don't hurt big boys.
    4. Explain to him that the shot is important for his health and ask him to watch you.

100. An adult who is admitted for surgery today says to the nurse "I'm so afraid. Do you think the doctor knows what he is doing? Does anyone ever survive this type of operation?" How should the nurse reply?

    1. "People who have this type of surgery almost always survive and get better."
    2. "Don't worry, your doctor is very skilled and has done many operations like yours."
    3. "You seem concerned about the surgery."
    4. "I cared for a woman last week who had the same type of surgery and she did very well."

Answers and Rationales for Practice Test Two

Answer	Rationale	NP	CN	SA

#1. 2. **Semi-Fowler's position will facilitate respirations, take pressure off the abdominal incision, and aid drainage if a drain is in place. Semi-Fowler's position is indicated when a client has a nasogastric tube in place to prevent backflow of gastric juices.**   Im   Ph/9   1

    1. Supine position is lying flat on the back. This position is not recommended when a nasogastric tube is in place as supine position would promote leakage of gastric contents into the esophagus.

    3. Dorsal recumbent is lying on the back and is not recommended when a nasogastric tube is in place as this position would promote leakage of gastric contents into the esophagus.

    4. Prone position is lying on the abdomen and is not recommended when a nasogastric tube is in place. Prone position would promote leakage of gastric contents into the esophagus.

#2. 1. **The first action indicated is to cover the exposed intestines with a sterile towel to prevent infection and moisten it to prevent intestines from drying and sticking.**   Im   Ph/10   1

    2. The intestines will be reinserted into the abdominal cavity by the surgeon under sterile operating room conditions.

    3. The exposed coils of intestines should be covered with a sterile moist towel. Normal saline is the solution of choice. Sterile water might cause fluid and electrolyte imbalances.

    4. Taking the client's vital signs is not the initial nursing action. The first action indicated is to cover the exposed intestines with a sterile towel to prevent infection and moisten it to prevent intestines from drying and sticking.

#3. 2. **Pulmonary complications such as atelectasis usually develop 24 to 48 hours post-operatively.**   Dc   Ph/9   1

    1. A low-grade fever related to dehydration usually occurs in the first 24 hours.

    3. It takes at least 72 hours and often longer for a wound infection to develop and cause a fever.

    4. Fever due to bladder infection is most likely to occur 48 to 72 hours after surgery.

ANSWER	RATIONALE	NP	CN	SA

#4. 2. **Atropine is contraindicated for persons with glaucoma. The nurse**   Im   Ph/8   5
should check with the prescribing physician, who may not know
the client has glaucoma.

   1. Atropine is contraindicated for persons with glaucoma. The nurse
should check with the prescribing physician, who may not know the
client has glaucoma.

   3. Atropine is contraindicated for persons with glaucoma. The nurse
should check with the prescribing physician, who may not know the
client has glaucoma.

   4. Atropine is contraindicated for persons with glaucoma. The nurse
should check with the prescribing physician, who may not know the
client has glaucoma. Meperidine and atropine were ordered as a
pre-operative medication. The nurse should not decide to give one
drug, but not the other. Meperidine is a central nervous system
depressant and decreases vital signs. Atropine is anticholinergic and
will increase the heart rate in addition to slowing peristalsis and
drying secretions.

#5. 2. **The client must sign a consent form before surgery. After a person**   Im   Sa/1   1
has been medicated for surgery they cannot legally sign a consent
form because they have received mind-altering drugs. The
physician must be notified, and surgery will be postponed.

   1. The client must sign a consent form before surgery. After a person
has been medicated for surgery they cannot legally sign a consent
form because they have received mind-altering drugs. The physician
must be notified, and surgery will be postponed.

   3. The client must sign a consent form before surgery. After a person
has been medicated for surgery they cannot legally sign a consent
form because they have received mind-altering drugs. If the person
would have been able to sign the consent form except for the
medication, the spouse cannot sign for them. We must wait until the
medication has worn off and the client can sign the form.

   4. The client must sign a consent form before surgery. After a person
has been medicated for surgery they cannot legally sign a consent
form because they have received mind-altering drugs. Even though
the client has presented for surgery there must be a signed consent
form before surgery can be performed. The only exception to this is a
life-threatening emergency.

#6. 1. **Prolonged lithotomy position may interfere with circulation to the**   Dc   Ph/9   1
lower extremities.

   2. Presence of bowel sounds is not related to lithotomy position.

   3. Lithotomy position should not affect the upper extremities.

   4. The nurse may palpate the client's bladder, but not because he was in
lithotomy position.

#7. 2.   A stage II pressure ulcer may look like a blister, abrasion, or   Dc   Ph/10   1
shallow crater and only involves a partial-thickness skin loss of
the epidermis and/or dermis.

   1.   A stage I pressure ulcer is red and the skin is intact.

   3.   A stage III pressure ulcer is a full-thickness skin loss involving
         damage to or necrosis of subcutaneous tissue that may extend down
         to, but not through, underlying fascia. It generally looks like a deep
         crater.

   4.   A stage IV pressure ulcer is a full-thickness skin loss with extensive
         destruction, tissue necrosis, or damage to muscle, bone, or
         supporting structures.

#8. 1.   The nurse should take vital signs frequently and assess the skin   Pl   Ph/10   1
for signs of frostbite or breakdown.

   2.   The hypothermia blanket is turned off when the client's temperature
         is one to two degrees above the target temperature. The client's
         temperature will usually drift downward after the blanket is turned
         off.

   3.   There should be a sheet between the client and the cooling blanket.

   4.   Direct application of ice is not used as it may stimulate shivering (the
         temperature-raising mechanism) and may cause skin breakdown.

#9. 3.   The layers act as insulators and prevent moisture loss. Some   Im   Ph/10   1
nurses place the waterproof layer next to the compress and then
cover with a dry cover, whereas others reverse the order, putting
the waterproof layer on the outside.

   1.   Surgical asepsis (sterile technique) is indicated. Medical asepsis is
         clean technique.

   2.   The wet compress should be covered with a dry cover and a
         waterproof material. A wet dressing that is left open to the air can
         conduct organisms into the wound. It will also lose heat very quickly.

   4.   Compresses are generally applied for 20 to 30 minutes.

#10. 4.   Apple juice is a clear liquid.   Im   Ph/7   6

   1.   Milk is not a clear liquid.

   2.   Fruited gelatin is not a clear liquid. Gelatin without fruit is allowed on
         a clear liquid diet.

   3.   Sherbert contains milk and is not allowed on a clear liquid diet.

#11. 3. **The client who has just been given penicillin should be checked on first. An adverse drug reaction is possible and could be life-threatening. The other clients all need to be checked but are not in potentially life-threatening situations.**   Im   Sa/1   5

1. This client needs assistance, but the nurse should first observe the client who has been given penicillin and is at risk for a reaction.

2. This client needs to be medicated, but the nurse should first observe the client who has been given penicillin and is at risk for a reaction.

4. This client needs assistance, but the nurse should first observe the client who has been given penicillin and is at risk for a reaction. The client is restrained and not likely to be in immediate danger.

#12. 3. **A client who has a head injury should not be placed in shock position as this would increase intracranial pressure. The other conditions would not be contraindications for shock position.**   Dc   Ph/10   1

1. Long bone fractures will put the client at risk for fat emboli, but this is not a contraindication for putting the client in shock position.

2. Air embolus is a serious condition. The treatment for air embolus would be to place the client's head lower than his chest. The client's head is lowered in shock position.

4. Thrombophlebitis is not a contraindication for shock position. In shock position the legs are elevated. The legs are elevated for a client who has thrombophlebitis.

#13. 3. **The wheelchair should be placed on the unaffected side at a 45-degree angle. This position best allows the client to stand on the unaffected leg and pivot before sitting in the wheelchair. A person who has hemiplegia will have difficulty placing her arms around someone's neck and will not be able to use a trapeze effectively.**   Ev   Ph/7   1

1. The wheelchair should be placed on the unaffected side so the client can pivot on the unaffected foot and sit in the chair.

2. The client has hemiplegia and will not be able to put her arms around the neck of a family member.

4. The client has hemiplegia and will not be able to use a trapeze bar. A trapeze bar would be appropriate for a client who had paraplegia.

#14. 4. **Cold applied to a sprained ankle should help reduce bleeding and swelling in the area. Cold has an anesthetic effect and should reduce pain.**

Im   Ph/10   1

  1. Ice will not keep a sprain from becoming a fracture. Sprains are damage to soft tissue rather than to bone. Sprains do not become fractures.

  2. There will be some bruising and ecchymosis following a sprain. Ice may reduce the amount of bleeding under the skin but will not eliminate it.

  3. Ice applied to a sprain is not given to lower body temperature or to keep fever from developing. Fever is not common following a sprain.

#15. 4. **Passive artificial immunity occurs when antibodies are produced by another person or animal and injected into the recipient. This gives a temporary immunity to protect against this exposure to an organism.**

Im   He/4   1

  1. Active natural immunity occurs when the person's own body produces antibodies in response to an active infection. This takes time to develop, and the person has the disease.

  2. Active artificial immunity is developed when antigens, either vaccine or toxoids, are administered to stimulate antibody response. This takes time to develop.

  3. Passive natural immunity occurs when antibodies are transferred from an immune mother to a baby through the placenta or colostrum. This is usually temporary.

#16. 4. **The nurse must assess daily weights for a client who is receiving total parenteral nutrition (TPN).**

Dc   Ph/8   1

  1. The number of bowel movements should be observed for any client but is not the most essential observation for the client who is receiving TPN. Remember TPN is nutrition given via a central venous line directly into the right atrium. It is not given into the GI tract.

  2. TPN is nutrition given via a central venous line directly into the right atrium. There is no tube in the stomach.

  3. TPN is nutrition given via a central venous line directly into the right atrium. Bowel sounds are not an issue related to TPN.

#17. **4.** **Tinnitus (ringing in the ears) is a sign of aspirin toxicity and is**   Dc   Ph/8   5
consistent with a minor overdose.

1. Tinnitus (ringing in the ears) is a sign of aspirin toxicity and is
    consistent with a minor overdose.

2. Tinnitus (ringing in the ears) is a sign of aspirin toxicity. The client
    does not have to exceed the recommended dosage. Some clients will
    develop toxicity at the recommended dosage.

3. Tinnitus (ringing in the ears) is a sign of aspirin toxicity. There is no
    evidence of an upper GI bleed. An upper GI bleed could occur with
    aspirin toxicity.

#18. **2.** **Patient controlled analgesia (PCA) allows the client to administer**   Ev   Ph/8   1
analgesic before the pain becomes severe, thus allowing better
pain control.

1. The machine will only give the analgesic after a preset time has
    elapsed. This is designed to prevent overdosing. The client can see
    this by the ready light on the machine and the beep that accompanies
    the delivery of the medicine.

3. The client should press the button only when experiencing pain.

4. The client may experience pain when using the PCA pump correctly.
    If this happens the client should notify the nurse.

#19. **2.** **The medication is ordered for operative pain. The client asks for**   Dc   Ph/8   1
pain medication but does not indicate where the pain is. The
nurse should *initially* assess the client. If the pain is in the operative
area, then the nurse can administer the ordered medication.

1. The medication is ordered for operative pain. The client asks for pain
    medication but does not indicate where the pain is. The nurse should
    initially assess the client. If the pain is in the operative area, then the
    nurse can administer the ordered medication.

3. An ice bag will not usually be effective by itself for the relief of pain
    on the day of surgery.

4. Repositioning the client will not likely remove pain on the day of
    surgery.

#20. **4.** **The skin at the radiation site should not be washed. The client**   Pl   Ph/10   1
should not attempt to wash off the purple marks.

1. The skin will be dry so there is no need for a dressing.

2. The client should avoid washing the skin at the radiation site so
    showering is not indicated.

3. Ice should not be applied following radiation therapy. The skin is very
    sensitive and might be damaged from an ice bag.

#21. 3. Thrombocytopenia (low platelet count) makes the client at risk for bleeding. The client should not receive injections. The other choices are not related to thrombocytopenia.   Pl   Ph/10   1

1. Thrombocytopenia is a low platelet count, which places the client at risk for bleeding. A semi-upright position will not reduce the risk of bleeding.

2. Thrombocytopenia is a low platelet count, which places the client at risk for bleeding. Limiting the client's intake of fluids will not reduce the risk of bleeding.

3. Thrombocytopenia is a low platelet count, which places the client at risk for bleeding. Exercising the client's lower extremities will not reduce the risk of bleeding. Exercising the lower extremities will help prevent thrombophlebitis.

#22. 4. Narcotic analgesics are respiratory depressants. Rising intracranial pressure causes respiratory depression. Further respiratory depression would cause acidosis, causing more blood flow to the brain, resulting in more cerebral edema and a further increase in intracranial pressure.   Dc   Ph/10   5

1. Narcotic analgesics cause miosis or constriction of the pupil.

2. Narcotic analgesics would be effective for the pain but would increase intracranial pressure and are thus contraindicated.

3. Narcotic analgesics may cause vomiting. Vomiting can be a sign of increased intracranial pressure. However, this is not the reason they are contraindicated in persons who have head injuries.

#23. 4. The treatment of glaucoma includes constriction of the pupil so the aqueous humor can flow more easily. Atropine is an anticholinergic which causes mydriasis (dilation of pupils).   Dc   Ph/8   5

1. Atropine is an anticholinergic, which causes increased heart rate. Bradycardia is not a contraindication for atropine.

2. Atropine is an anticholinergic, which causes increased heart rate. Hypothyroidism is not a contraindication for atropine.

3. Atropine is an anticholinerigic agent. It is not contraindicated in diabetes.

#24. 1. **The client is having difficulty swallowing. The highest priority is to prevent aspiration pneumonia. Decubitus ulcers may also be a concern, but are not a higher priority than preventing aspiration pneumonia.**   Pl   Ph/9   1

2. Preventing decubitus ulcers is a concern for this client, who is having difficulty moving. However, preventing aspiration pneumonia is a higher priority. Aspiration pneumonia is more immediately life-threatening than decubitus ulcers.

3. Bladder distention could be a concern for this client, who has Guillain-Barré syndrome. Aspiration pneumonia is more immediately life-threatening. If the client develops bladder distention, he is likely to become incontinent, which is not life-threatening.

4. Hypertensive crisis is not likely to occur in the client who has Guillain-Barré syndrome.

#25. 2. **Diplopia and ptosis of the eyelids are characteristic of myasthenia gravis. Upper-body symptoms occur before lower-body symptoms. Symptoms are related to cranial nerves.**   Dc   Ph/9   1

1. Ataxia and poor coordination are lower-body symptoms. Upper-body symptoms occur before lower body symptoms.

3. Slurred speech is not an early sign of myasthenia gravis. The client may have a weak voice, however.

4. Headaches and tinnitus are not characteristic of myasthenia gravis.

#26. 1. **The symptoms suggest autonomic hyperreflexia, which is usually caused by bladder distention. The patient will need to be catheterized and the physician notified. Autonomic hyperreflexia is a medical emergency.**   Im   Ph/10   1

2. The client should be put in semi-Fowler's position, not Trendlenburg.

3. Pain is neither a symptom nor a cause of autonomic hyperreflexia.

4. Autonomic hyperreflexia is a medical emergency. The nurse must notify the charge nurse or the physician immediately. The client is likely to need antihypertensive medication as well as catheterization if a distended bladder is the cause.

#27. 2. **Confused persons will often be more oriented if the same caregiver is assigned for several days in a row.**   Pl   Sa/1   1

1. While some rotation of assignments may be appropriate, residents will often be more oriented and do better if there is consistency in caregivers.

3. Female caregivers frequently will need to care for male residents.

4. It is important to consider any special requests from caregivers. However, the nurse making the assignments has the big picture and should make assignments according to the needs of the unit.

#28. 3. **This answer is accurate. There is a surgical incision to retrieve the organs but it is no more defacing than abdominal surgery and should not interfere with an open casket.** — Im — Sa/1 — 1

    1. This statement is not true. Donating organs does not deface the body and does not make it necessary to have a closed casket.

    2. This response does not answer the client's direct request. The nurse should be able to give the information.

    4. This response is a true statement. However, this does not answer the direct question that was asked. The nurse should not avoid answering the questions.

#29. 2. **The certified nursing assistant should be able to take routine vital signs.** — Pl — Sa/1 — 1

    1. Tube feeding is more appropriately performed by a LPN/LVN. It is beyond the scope of a nursing assistant.

    3. A client who is in congestive heart failure has to be monitored very carefully. The nurse should take the blood pressure for this client, who is not stable.

    4. Wound care is a sterile procedure and should be performed by the nurse.

#30. 1. **The best choice is to ask the client what his name is.** — Im — Sa/2 — 1

    2. Persons who are confused may not answer accurately if asked "Are you Mr. _____?"

    3. Asking the roommate if a client is Mr. _____ may not give accurate information.

    4. Clients may get in the wrong bed. Checking the bed tag is not as accurate as asking the client for his name.

#31. 2. **The client who is confused and picking at his nasal cannula and NG tube is endangering himself and may need restraints.** — Dc — Sa/2 — 1

    1. There is no data in this answer that suggests the client is putting himself at risk. Restraints are indicated for persons who are putting themselves or others at risk.

    3. Side rails are usually sufficient protection for a confused client who is in bed. There is no data to suggest that this is not true.

    4. An adult who has just returned from a post-anesthesia care unit is probably not very alert, but there is no data to suggest that the client is putting himself or others in danger.

#32. 4. **The nurse should not administer medication that has been drawn up by someone else, even if that someone else is the RN charge nurse.**   Im   Ph/8   1

    1.   The nurse should not administer medication that has been drawn up by someone else, even if that someone else is the RN charge nurse.

    2.   The nurse should not administer medication that has been drawn up by someone else, even if that someone else is the RN charge nurse. Asking what the medication is does not assure the nurse that the medication was drawn up accurately.

    3.   The nurse should not administer medication that has been drawn up by someone else, even if that someone else is the RN charge nurse. Asking what the medication is does not assure the nurse that the medication was drawn up accurately.

#33. 2. **According to the Patient's Bill of Rights, the patient has the right to know who is caring for him/her and to know if any persons caring for him/her are students or other trainees. The client has the right to refuse any treatment.**   Im   Sa/1   1

    1.   The client has the right to refuse treatment by students. Signing permission for care does not take away these rights.

    3.   It is not necessary to sign a special form to refuse care by medical and nursing students.

    4.   The client should be informed if caregivers are students. However, the client can refuse to have students caring for him/her.

#34. 3. **According to the Patient's Bill of Rights, the client has the right to see his records and to have information explained and interpreted when necessary.**   Im   Sa/1   1

    1.   According to the Patient's Bill of Rights, the client has the right to see his records and to have information explained and interpreted when necessary. There is no need to obtain a court order.

    2.   According to the Patient's Bill of Rights, the client has the right to see his records and to have information explained and interpreted when necessary. It is not necessary to have the physician's approval to see his records.

    4.   According to the Patient's Bill of Rights, the client has the right to see his records and to have information explained and interpreted when necessary. It is not necessary to appear before a committee. It is the client's right.

#35. 4.   **The nurse should determine that care was administered as**   Pl   Sa/1   1
         delegated. One of the best ways to do this is to observe the clients.
         The nurse must follow up when delegating to other personnel.

   1.   The nurse does not have time to observe the nursing assistant during the
        administration of all care. It is not necessary to observe the nursing
        assistant during all care.

   2.   Asking the nursing assistant if there were any problems is all right,
        but not the best way to determine that care was given as delegated.

   3.   Checking the charting of the nursing assistant does not ensure that
        the clients received the care that was charted.

#36. 2.   **The client is probably having an illusion—a misinterpretation of**   Im   Ps/5   2
         reality. The nurse should turn the lights up brighter so there are
         no shadows to be misinterpreted as snakes.

   1.   The client is probably having an illusion—a misinterpretation of
        reality. The client is not likely to believe the nurse who simply
        reassures him there are no snakes. When dealing with an illusion the
        nurse should change the conditions that support an illusion.

   3.   The client is probably having an illusion—a misinterpretation of
        reality. The nurse should turn the lights up brighter so there are no
        shadows to be misinterpreted as snakes. Telling him there are really
        no snakes is not likely to change his interpretation of the shadows he
        sees.

   4.   The client is probably having an illusion—a misinterpretation of
        reality. The nurse should turn the lights up brighter so there are no
        shadows to be misinterpreted as snakes. Reassuring him the snakes
        will not hurt him confirms for him that there are snakes on the wall.

#37. 4.   **Permission is revocable. Clients have the right to change their**   Im   Sa/1   1
         minds about treatments and procedures and to revoke consent.

   1.   Clients have the right to change their minds about treatments and
        procedures and to revoke consent.

   2.   Trying to coerce the client by telling her the physician will be upset is
        not appropriate. Clients have the right to change their minds about
        treatments and procedures and to revoke consent.

   3.   Clients have the right to change their minds about treatments and
        procedures and to revoke consent. Trying to talk the client into the
        procedure is not appropriate.

#38. 2. Increasing the distance of persons from the client who has internal radiation reduces the amount of exposure to radiation.

Pl   Sa/2   1

1. Keeping the door to the room closed will reduce the exposure only very slightly. Wooden doors do not stop radiation. Heavy metal stops radiation.

3. Placing the client close to the nurse's station where the traffic is high increases the amount of exposure to other clients and personnel.

4. Placing a "Do not enter" sign might be done. However, usually clients do not enter other client's rooms.

#39. 3. An older client should not be short of breath walking down the hall. This is abnormal and should be reported.

Dc   He/3   1

1. Brown spots or age spots are normal in the older adult.

2. Older persons usually move more slowly than they did earlier in life.

4. It is common for older adults to have difficulty with color discrimination.

#40. 3. This answer has a sense of regret for actions not taken in the past. This suggests despair rather than ego integrity. According to Erickson, the developmental task for the aging client is ego integrity versus despair.

Ev   He/3   2

1. Making toys for his grandchildren suggests the client has an interest in life and meaning in life. This indicates ego integrity.

2. This statement gives facts, but does not carry regret, as is obvious in statement number 3.

4. Adjusting to less income is a normal part of aging. This statement does not carry the tone of regret as statement number 3 does.

#41. 1. Edema in the hands and face is suggestive of pregnancy-induced hypertension and should be reported to the physician.

Dc   He/3   1

2. Pregnant women have an increase in metabolic rate and usually feel warmer than those around them. This is a normal finding.

3. Swelling of the feet is normal in pregnant women. The enlarging fetus reduces the venous return and causes swelling of the feet and ankles in latter part of pregnancy. This is a normal finding.

4. The pregnant woman will have enlarged and tender breasts as a result of progesterone stimulation and in preparation for lactation. This is a normal finding.

#42. 1. Most persons lose the sense of salt and sweet as they age.   Dc   He/3   6

2. Most persons develop presbyopia, the farsightedness of aging, as they age. They have trouble focusing on close work.

3. As people age there are pupillary changes with loss of light responsiveness, so they adapt to darkness more slowly and have difficulty seeing in dim light.

4. As people age they often develop decreased color discrimination.

#43. 4. The pedal pulse is felt by placing the fingertips on the top of the foot and gently pressing the artery against the bone.   Dc   He/4   1

1. The radial pulse is obtained by placing the fingertips against the wrist bone.

2. The apical pulse is obtained by placing the stethoscope over the apex of the heart.

3. The carotid pulse is obtained by placing the fingertips against the side of the neck.

#44. 3. An apical-radial pulse is obtained by having one person take the apical pulse while the second person takes the radial pulse at the same time.   Dc   He/4   1

1. An apical-radial pulse is obtained by having one person take the apical pulse while the second person takes the radial pulse at the same time.

2. The radial pulse is never higher than the apical pulse. Ideally both pulses are the same. A pulse deficit exists when the radial pulse is less than the apical pulse.

4. An apical-radial pulse is obtained by having one person take the apical pulse while the second person takes the radial pulse at the same time. It is impossible for the nurse to count two pulses at the same time.

#45. 4. Noisy breathing is best described as sterterous.   Dc   He/4   1

1. Deep respirations are described as hyperpnea.

2. Cheyne-Stokes respirations are periods of apnea alternating with hyperpnea.

3. A person who has orthopnea must sit up to breathe.

#46. 2. **Using a cuff that is too small causes the blood pressure reading to be abnormally high.**   Dc   He/4   1

    1. A large cuff may be more comfortable for the client. However, the reason the nurse uses a large cuff for a large person is that using a cuff that is too small causes the blood pressure reading to be abnormally high.

    3. Using a cuff that is too small causes the blood pressure reading to be abnormally high. It does not make the pulse hard to hear.

    4. Using a cuff that is too small causes both the systolic and diastolic blood pressure readings to be abnormally high.

#47. 1. **Handwashing is the best way to prevent spread of infection. Hands should be washed before and after changing the dressing. This indicates the client understands the procedure.**   Ev   Sa/2   1

    2. Touching the edges of the dressings with bare hands contaminates the dressings. This indicates the client does not understand the procedure.

    3. A wound is cleansed from the wound out. The client should not move a swab from the outside into the wound. This statement indicates the client does not understand the procedure.

    4. The dressings should not be put directly into the wastebasket. They should be placed in a waterproof bag and sealed before being disposed of. This statement indicates the client does not understand the procedure.

#48. 4. **Active exercises prevent muscle atrophy. The other activities do not prevent muscle atrophy.**   Pl   Ph/7   1

    1. Passive range-of-motion exercises help to prevent joint contractures, but do not prevent muscle atrophy. Active exercises are necessary to prevent muscle atrophy.

    2. Turning the client at two-hour intervals will help to prevent respiratory complications and skin breakdown but will not prevent muscle atrophy.

    3. Changing positions frequently will help to prevent skin breakdown and may help in preventing respiratory complications but is not likely to prevent muscle atrophy.

#49. 3. Varicose veins are related to venous stasis, which may be caused by prolonged standing. They are not a result of prolonged bed rest.   Dc   Ph/7   1

   1. Muscle atrophy is a complication of prolonged bed rest.

   2. Hypostatic pneumonia is a complication of prolonged bed rest.

   4. Thrombophlebitis is a complication of prolonged bed rest.

#50. 4. Changing position in bed frequently, thus avoiding prolonged pressure on any one bony prominence, will help to prevent development of pressure ulcers.   Pl   Ph/7   1

   1. Passive range-of-motion exercises help to prevent joint contractures and active range-of-motion exercises help to prevent muscle atrophy. They do not prevent pressure ulcers.

   2. Deep breathing and coughing help to prevent atelectasis and hypostatic pneumonia. Deep breathing and coughing does not prevent pressure ulcers.

   3. Keeping the feet against a footboard helps to prevent foot drop. It does not prevent development of pressure ulcers.

#51. 2. Proper body mechanics involves bending from the hip and knees, not the waist. Bending from the waist indicates the nursing assistant needs more instruction.   Ev   Ph/7   1

   1. The feet should be separated to provide a wide base of support. This action indicates the nursing assistant understands body mechanics.

   3. Turning the whole body rather than twisting the body indicates an understanding of body mechanics.

   4. Keeping the back straight indicates an understanding of proper body mechanics.

#52. 3. Having the client sit down will help to prevent her from falling and keep her safe.   Im   Ph/7   1

   1. Putting her head between her legs is not going to prevent her from falling. In fact, it may cause her to fall.

   2. The nurse should never leave a client who is dizzy and faint.

   4. Encouraging her to walk more quickly is likely to aggravate the client's dizziness and faintness.

#53. 3. A decreased white blood cell count is not typical of sickle cell crisis. The client will have a decreased red blood cell count.   Dc   Ph/10   1

1. Enlarged liver and spleen are often seen in persons who are in sickle cell crisis. The red blood cells live only 1 to 3 weeks rather than the usual 4 months. The spleen and liver are involved with RBC breakdown.

2. In sickle cell crisis RBCs live only 1 to 3 weeks and are rapidly broken down by the spleen. The liver normally converts bilirubin (produced when RBCs are broken down) into bile. The liver cannot keep up with the extra load and jaundice and icterus result.

4. Abdominal and joint pain are common in persons with sickle cell crisis. RBCs are broken down too rapidly and agglutinate and cause clumping in the vessel, blocking the blood supply and causing pain distal to the agglutination.

#54. 1. Crushing chest pain not relieved by nitroglycerine or rest is likely to be a heart attack. Chest pain that is relieved by nitroglycerine or rest is usually angina.   Im   Ph/9   5

2. Epigastric pain relieved by antacids is likely to be gastric in origin and is probably not either angina or a heart attack.

3. Both anginal pain and the pain of a heart attack can radiate down the left arm. Anginal pain is relieved by rest or nitroglycerine; heart attack pain is not.

4. Chest pain due to angina is usually related to excitement, exercise, environment (hot or cold), or eating.

#55. 2. Persons who have angina should take nitroglycerine at five-minute intervals times three when they have chest pain. If not relieved after three doses of nitroglycerine, they should call the physician or go to the emergency room.   Ev   Ph/9   5

1. Persons who have angina should exercise within the limits recommended by the physician. They should not remain completely sedentary.

3. Persons who have angina may have some chest pain with sexual activity. Heart attacks can occur during sexual activity but are not likely. The physician may recommend taking nitroglycerine before sexual activity.

4. If the client with angina has chest pain he should take nitroglycerine at five-minute intervals times three. If the chest pain is not relieved he should immediately call his physician or go to the hospital, as he may be having a heart attack.

#56. 2.   **Sickle cell anemia is an inherited disease transmitted as a**   Im   Ph/10   1
              recessive gene. When both parents are carriers there is a 25%
              chance that each baby will be born with sickle cell, a 50% chance
              that each child will be born with the trait, and a 25% chance that
              each child will be disease- and carrier-free. It is possible to have
              two children in a row with the disease.

    1.   Sickle cell anemia is not contagious. It is an inherited disease
              transmitted as a recessive gene. When both parents are carriers there
              is a 25% chance that each baby will be born with sickle cell, a 50%
              chance that each child will be born with the trait, and a 25% chance
              that each child will be disease- and carrier-free. It is possible to have
              two children in a row with the disease.

    3.   This answer describes the transmission of an x-linked disease such as
              hemophilia or Duchenne's muscular dystrophy. Sickle cell anemia is
              an inherited disease transmitted as a recessive gene. When both
              parents are carriers there is a 25% chance that each baby will be born
              with sickle cell, a 50% chance that each child will be born with the
              trait, and a 25% chance that each child will be disease- and carrier-
              free. It is possible to have two or more children in a row with the
              disease.

    4.   Statistically parents who are both carriers of the sickle cell gene have
              a 25% chance of having a child who is both disease- and carrier-free.
              However, there is no way of knowing which child that will be. It is
              possible to have two or more children in a row with the disease.

#57. 1.   **The home should be assessed for items that might cause an**   Im   Sa/2   1
              electrical spark such as frayed cords.

    2.   It is more important to check for frayed cords than it is to purchase
              fire extinguishers. It is more important to prevent a fire than to treat a
              fire.

    3.   It is not necessary to remove electrical appliances from a room where
              oxygen is in use. It is more important to assess for frayed cords
              because these could start a fire. A well-grounded electrical device
              does not produce sparks.

    4.   The client's room should not be carpeted. Shuffling across a carpet
              can produce static electricity, which can start a fire.

#58. 2. **The client should be positioned in semi-Fowler's position to promote thoracic expansion.**

Im   Ph/10   1

1. Supine position will make it more difficult for the client to breathe and for secretions to be removed.

3. Sim's position (semi-lateral with the lower arm behind the client's back) will make it more difficult for the client to breathe and for secretions to be removed.

4. Semi-lateral position will make it more difficult for the client to breathe and for secretions to be removed.

#59. 1. **The client must remain NPO before a bronchoscopy.**

Dc   Ph/9   1

2. There is no need for the client to take a laxative prior to a bronchoscopy. A rigid tube (bronchoscope) will be passed down the throat into the bronchi. The client will probably have a lidocaine spray to deaden the gag reflex during the procedure.

3. This is "nice-to-know" information, but is not essential information.

4. This is "nice-to-know" information, but is not essential before the procedure.

#60. 2. **Air is in the pleural cavity following thoracic surgery. A chest tube removes air from the pleural cavity thus re-establishing negative pressure and allowing the lung to re-expand.**

Im   Ph/9   1

1. Air in the thoracic cavity causes the lung to collapse. The chest tube removes air from the thoracic cavity so the lung can re-expand.

3. A chest tube does not bring oxygen to the lungs. A chest tube removes air from the pleural cavity, thus re-establishing negative pressure and allowing the lung to re-expand.

4. A chest tube does not help the wound heal faster and reduce scarring. A chest tube removes air from the pleural cavity, thus re-establishing negative pressure and allowing the lung to re-expand.

#61. 3 **The most likely cause for no bubbling in the water seal chamber two days following insertion of a chest tube is re-expansion of the lung. The nurse should auscultate the chest to determine if there are bilateral breath sounds.**   Dc   Ph/9   1

    1. Excessive wound drainage is not a likely cause of absence of bubbling in the water seal chamber when a three-chamber system such as Pleuravac® is being used. The most likely cause for no bubbling in the water seal chamber two days following insertion of a chest tube is re-expansion of the lung. The nurse should auscultate the chest to determine if there are bilateral breath sounds.

    2. Air leaks cause lack of bubbling in the suction control chamber. No bubbling in the water seal chamber is usually due either to obstructions in the tubing or re-expansion of the lungs. Two days following insertion of a chest tube the most likely reason for no bubbling in the water seal chamber is re-expansion of the lung. Tubing obstruction is more likely to occur in the first day or so.

    4. If the suction is not turned on there will be no bubbling in the suction control chamber. The water seal chamber may still bubble if air is leaving the thoracic cavity by gravity drainage even when the suction is not turned on.

#62. 1. **A major toxicity of gentamicin is nephrotoxicity. Diminished urine output indicates damage to the kidneys.**   Dc   Ph/8   5

    2. Blurred vision is not a common adverse response to gentamicin. The major adverse responses are nephrotoxicity (kidneys) and ototoxicity (ears).

    3. Orange sputum is not an adverse response to gentamicin. Orange-colored secretions may occur with rimactane (Rifampin). The major adverse responses to gentamicin are nephrotoxicity (kidneys) and ototoxicity (ears).

    4. Hypertension is not an adverse response to gentamicin. Sometimes it can cause hypotension. The major adverse responses are nephrotoxicity (kidneys) and ototoxicity (ears).

#63. 1. **Back pain following a cystoscopy could indicate kidney damage and should be reported to the charge nurse or the physician.**   Dc   Ph/9   1

    2. Tea-colored urine is a normal finding following a cystoscopy.

    3. Leg cramps are common following a cystoscopy because the client has been in lithotomy position.

    4. Pink-tinged urine is a normal finding following a cystoscopy.

#64. 3. **Pyridium is a urinary tract anesthetic that will kill the pain until the antibiotics have had time to work.** — Im — Ph/8 — 5

    1. Pyridium is not an antibiotic. Pyridium is a urinary tract anesthetic that will kill the pain until the antibiotics have had time to work.

    2. Pyridium is not an analgesic. Pyridium is a urinary tract anesthetic that will kill the pain until the antibiotics have had time to work.

    4. Pyridium does not prevent kidney damage. Pyridium is a urinary tract anesthetic that will kill the pain until the antibiotics have had time to work.

#65. 1. **The client who has a stone in the urinary tract is in severe pain. Acute pain is the priority nursing diagnosis.** — Pl — Ph/10 — 1

    2. Diarrhea often occurs from the pain and irritation caused by the stones. However, the client who has a stone in the urinary tract is in severe pain. Acute pain is the priority nursing diagnosis.

    3. Risk for altered health maintenance related to insufficient knowledge of prevention of recurrence, dietary restrictions, and fluid requirements is an appropriate nursing diagnosis. This diagnosis is most appropriate related to discharge planning. Upon admission the client who has a stone in the urinary tract is in severe pain. Acute pain is the priority nursing diagnosis.

    4. Risk for infection is not likely to be a realistic nursing diagnosis for the client who has a stone in the urinary tract. This client will be in severe pain. Acute pain is the priority nursing diagnosis.

#66. 3. **Pharyngitis or sore throat caused by the beta hemolytic strep organism usually precedes acute glomerulonephritis. Acute glomerulonephritis is an antigen-antibody response to beta hemolytic strep. The antibodies made to attack the microorganism also attack the basement membrane of the glomerulus.** — Dc — Ph/10 — 1

    1. Pyelonephritis is caused by an ascending bladder infection. Acute glomerulonephritis is an antigen-antibody response to beta hemolytic strep.

    2. A person with chronic glomerulonephritis is likely to have a history of previous kidney infections.

    4. Acute glomerulonephritis is not a sexually transmitted disease. Acute glomerulonephritis is an antigen-antibody response to beta hemolytic strep.

#67. 4. The nurse should strain all urine to detect any stones, which the   Im   Ph/10   1
client may pass. If a stone is passed it will be sent to the
laboratory for analysis.

   1. There is no need to take frequent blood pressures for the client with a
      kidney stone. The nurse should strain all urine to detect any stones
      which the client may pass. If a stone is passed it will be sent to the
      laboratory for analysis.

   2. Persons who have kidney stones often prefer to ambulate. Walking
      not only helps the pain but also may help the stone to pass through
      the ureter and urethra.

   3. The client will be uncomfortable in the supine position. Persons who
      have kidney stones often prefer to ambulate. Walking not only helps
      the pain but also may help the stone to pass through the ureter and
      urethra.

#68. 2. The nurse should teach the client to drink generous amounts of   Pl   Ph/9   1
fluids each day to help prevent formation of kidney stones.

   1. The person who has a uric acid kidney stone should be on a low
      purine diet. Chicken and organ meats are high in purines. The client
      should be taught to avoid purine-containing foods.

   3. There is no need for the person who has a history of kidney stones to
      avoid activity. In fact, immobility predisposes to the formation of the
      kidney stone. The client should be active.

   4. Allopurinol (Zyloprim) should be taken daily as ordered. This drug is
      used to promote excretion of uric acid and thus prevent the formation
      of kidney stones.

#69. 2. Exposure to the ultraviolet rays of the sun can cause skin cancer.   Ev   He/4   1
The client should wear a long-sleeved shirt and a hat when
exposed to the sun.

   1. Moles that are round and a single color are usually not malignant.
      Moles that have irregular borders and multiple colors are more apt to
      be malignant and should be seen by the physician.

   3. Lotions and powders do not cause skin cancer. Exposure to the
      ultraviolet rays of the sun cause skin cancer.

   4. Tanning booths expose the person to ultraviolet rays and are a
      significant risk for the development of skin cancer.

#70. 2. Calcium deposits are laid down early in life. The time to prevent   Ev   He/4   1
osteoporosis is in adolescence.

1. Athletic injuries are not risk factors for osteoporosis. They are more apt to be related to osteoarthritis.

3. Physical activity should be continued throughout life. Weight-bearing exercises are important to prevent osteoporosis.

4. Carbonated beverages pull calcium from the bones and increase the risk of osteoporosis.

#71. 3. The cane should be held on the nonaffected side. When walking   Ev   Ph/7   1
with a cane the client should move the cane and the affected foot
at the same time.

1. The cane should be held on the nonaffected side. When walking with a cane the client should move the cane and the affected foot at the same time.

2. The cane should be held on the nonaffected side. When walking with a cane the client should move the cane and the affected foot at the same time. Moving the cane from side to side could increase the risk of tripping over the cane.

4. The cane should be held on the nonaffected side. When walking with a cane the client should move the cane and the affected foot at the same time.

#72. 3. The client with low back pain will be most comfortable in a   Pl   Ph/7   1
position that opens the spaces between the vertebrae, such as
side-lying with knees flexed or semi-Fowler's with knees bent.

1. The client with low back pain will be most comfortable in a position that opens the spaces between the vertebrae, such as side-lying with knees flexed or semi-Fowler's with knees bent.

2. The client with low back pain will be most comfortable in a position that opens the spaces between the vertebrae, such as side-lying with knees flexed or semi-Fowler's with knees bent.

4. The client with low back pain will be most comfortable in a position that opens the spaces between the vertebrae such as side-lying with knees flexed or semi-Fowler's with knees bent.

#73. 2. Ice works in two ways to reduce pain of a sprained ankle. First, it   Im   Ph/7   1
has an anesthetic effect. Second, it helps to prevent swelling.

1. Exercising a sprained ankle several times an hour is likely to increase the pain. The ankle should not be stressed.

3. The leg and ankle should be elevated.

4. Topical steroids help to prevent itching and inflammation. They do not reduce pain.

#74. 4. **Drinking warm milk helps to induce sleep in many people.**   Im   Ph/7   1

1. Exercising increases body metabolism and makes it harder to go to sleep. Exercise should be done several hours before going to bed.

2. Cola beverages contain caffeine, which is a stimulant and keeps many people awake. Cola beverages have a diuretic effect. If the client did get to sleep she is likely to have to get up during the night to urinate.

3. The bed should be for sleeping. Reading and watching television in bed tend to aggravate sleep difficulties.

#75. 1. **The blood gas values indicate compensated respiratory acidosis. The pH is normal on the low or acid side. All the other values are abnormal, so the nurse knows this is compensated. Because the pH is on the acid side, it is compensated acidosis. CO_2 is high. Because CO_2 is acid, it is causing the acid pH. CO_2 is respiratory. The HCO_3 is also high. However, it is alkaline and is not causing the acid pH. It is compensating for the high acid.**   Dc   Ph/9   1

2. The values are not consistent with alkalosis. The blood gas values indicate compensated respiratory acidosis. The pH is normal on the low or acid side. All the other values are abnormal, so the nurse knows this is compensated. Because the pH is on the acid side, it is compensated acidosis. CO_2 is high. Because CO_2 is acid, it is causing the acid pH. CO_2 is respiratory. The HCO_3 is also high. However, it is alkaline and is not causing the acid pH. It is compensating for the high acid.

3. The values are not consistent with alkalosis. The blood gas values indicate compensated respiratory acidosis. The pH is normal on the low or acid side. All the other values are abnormal, so the nurse knows this is compensated. Because the pH is on the acid side, it is compensated acidosis. CO_2 is high. Because CO_2 is acid, it is causing the acid pH. CO_2 is respiratory. The HCO_3 is also high. However, it is alkaline and is not causing the acid pH. It is compensating for the high acid.

4. The values are not consistent with metabolic acidosis. The blood gas values indicate compensated respiratory acidosis. The pH is normal on the low or acid side. All the other values are abnormal, so the nurse knows this is compensated. Because the pH is on the acid side, it is compensated acidosis. CO_2 is high. Because CO_2 is acid, it is causing the acid pH. CO_2 is respiratory. The HCO_3 is also high. However, it is alkaline and is not causing the acid pH. It is compensating for the high acid.

#76. **3.** MRI means magnetic resonance imaging using magnetic fields. Persons who have metal in their bodies such as artificial knees, hips, plates in the skull, or metal fragments from previous injuries such as gunshot wounds should not have that part of the body imaged.   Dc   Ph/9   1

1. No iodine dye is used during magnetic resonance imaging so there is no need to inquire about iodine allergies.

2. There is no need for the client to fast prior to magnetic resonance imaging.

4. A laxative prep is not used prior to magnetic resonance imaging.

#77. **3.** A glass of water dropped on the floor beside the bed of an elderly ambulatory client is a serious safety hazard and needs immediate attention. The other options are not immediate safety hazards.   Im   Sa/2   1

1. Dirty linen on the floor beside the bed of a non-ambulatory client is less of a safety hazard than a glass of water dropped on the floor beside the bed of an elderly ambulatory client.

2. Breakfast dishes on the overbed table two hours after mealtime is unsightly but does not pose a hazard and does not need immediate attention.

4. A bed that cannot go from the low to high position does need attention. This bed is stuck in the low position, which does not present an immediate hazard for the client.

#78. **3.** When the fundus is soft, high above the umbilicus and deviated to the left, the most likely cause is urinary retention. The woman is six hours post-partum. The nurse should encourage her to void and if she is unable to do so, catheterize her as ordered.   Dc   He/3   3

1. Retained placental fragments may cause bleeding and a soft fundus but would not cause the fundus to rise and deviate to one side. These findings are more consistent with a full bladder.

2. A perineal laceration would cause bright red perineal bleeding but would not cause changes in consistency and location of the fundus.

4. At six hours post-partum the fundus should be near the umbilicus but should be firm and there should be no deviation to one side. Red lochia is normal at this time. The findings are not normal; they are consistent with urinary retention.

#79. 2. The cord usually dries up and falls off in ten days to three weeks. Im He/3 4

1. The cord should be wiped with alcohol with each diaper change. However, the client asked for specific information. The nurse should answer the client's question.

3. The client does sound a bit upset about the cord. However, the nurse should give the client the information she asked for.

4. This answer is not correct. It usually takes ten days to three weeks for the cord to dry up and fall off.

#80. 2. The baby should double her birth weight by six months and should now weigh close to 14 pounds. This observation indicates the baby is not gaining weight as expected. Dc He/3 4

1. Infants should sit up with slight support and may lean forward at six months. This is normal and does not need to be brought to the physician's attention.

3. Infants at six months of age often drop objects and will look for them. This is normal and does not need to be brought to the physician's attention.

4. An infant of six months will smack her lips and drool. The infant gets her first tooth around six months of age.

#81. 2. The nurse should determine that the feeding tube is in the stomach. This is essential. Im Ph/7 1

1. The client should be positioned upright in a semi-Fowler's position.

3. There is no need to give the client something to suck on during the feeding.

4. It is not essential to check when the client last had a bowel movement.

#82. 1. Reflecting the client's feelings helps to create a rapport with the client and should open communication and allow the client to further express her feelings regarding the loss of her breast. Im Ps/5 2

2. This response focuses on the husband and not on the woman. It is not therapeutic.

3. This response does not let the client express her feelings, focuses on the husband, and is a false reassurance. It is not therapeutic.

4. Responding with a cliché type answer is not therapeutic. It does not allow the client to express her feelings.

#83. 3. **The nurse should initially talk with the woman and determine what her immediate needs are.**   Im   Ps/5   2

1. Telling the client to be quiet is not the best approach. The nurse should determine if the client has any immediate needs.

2. The data given are not sufficient to warrant calling security and the police. After talking with the client the nurse might determine the client was potentially violent and call security.

4. Simply telling the woman everyone is busy is not attending to the client's needs. This response is not therapeutic.

#84. 4. **The nurse should initially empathize and clarify the problem.**   Im   Ps/5   2

1. This response is not therapeutic. It does not allow the mother to express her feelings, and it will probably make her feel guilty that she doesn't feel as though she can cope.

2. The nurse should initially respond with empathy and help to clarify the problem. If the use of social services is indicated the nurse should suggest this after determining the mother's needs and coping skills.

3. This response will probably make the mother feel guilty about her feelings of frustration. The nurse should initially respond with empathy and help to clarify the problem.

#85. 4. **Keeping the beds in the lowest position except when the nurse is performing care for the client is likely to reduce the number of falls. Many falls occur when persons are getting out of bed.**   Pl   Sa/2   1

1. Asking nursing assistants to watch the clients more carefully is very nonspecific. The nurse should give more specific directions.

2. The nurse should not restrain persons just because they cannot walk well independently.

3. Providing traveling call bells might help the clients to call the nurse for help quickly if they did fall, but is not likely to prevent falls. It is also a costly choice. Keeping beds in the lowest position costs nothing and should reduce the number of falls.

#86. 3. If linens are soiled with urine and feces the nursing assistant should wear a gown to prevent soiling of uniform with body secretions. This behavior indicates understanding of universal precautions.   Ev   Sa/2   1

   1. The nursing assistant should wash hands before and after each and every client contact. This behavior indicates the nursing assistant does not understand universal precautions.

   2. Gloves should be worn when the client does not have intact skin or when mucous membranes are being touched. The nursing assistant does not need to wear gloves for all client contact. This action indicates the nursing assistant does not understand universal precautions.

   4. Hands should be washed before and after each and every client contact even if gloves have been worn. This action indicates the nursing assistant does not understand universal precautions.

#87. 2. The nurse should never turn her back on a sterile field, and all sterile objects should be within view. Turning around to answer a question does not maintain sterile technique.   Ev   Sa/2   1

   1. The first flap of a sterile dressing set or package should be opened away from the nurse. This allows the last flap to be opened toward the nurse avoiding the need to reach across the sterile field. This behavior maintains sterile technique.

   3. Sterile objects should sit about waist high. The overbed table is an appropriate place to open the dressing set. This behavior helps to maintain sterile technique.

   4. Pouring sterile saline into a container in the dressing set is appropriate providing the nurse does not spill any liquid on the sterile field. The behavior as described is consistent with sterile technique.

#88. 3. Although all of the problems could be seen, the most common problem seen in a disaster shelter is stress.   Pl   Sa/2   2

   1. Thirst can be a problem, and the disaster shelter should have water available. The most common problem seen in a disaster shelter is stress.

   2. Traumatic injuries may be present. The most common problem seen in a disaster shelter is stress.

   4. There may be persons who have exacerbation of medical problems. The most common problem seen in a disaster shelter is stress.

#89. 2. **Leaving a frail elderly client in bed alone in the house for several hours at a time may well constitute abuse. This should be reported to the supervisor for further evaluation.**   Ev   Ps/6   1

    1. Asking to be a legal guardian for a frail elderly mother is not in any way indicative of abuse and does not need to be reported to the supervisor.

    3. Brown spots or even petecchiae on the body of an elderly adult are normal and not suggestive of abuse.

    4. Before reporting that the daughter yells at her mother the nurse should check out the complaint, checking especially for hearing loss in the mother.

#90. 2. **The client appears to have an obsessive-compulsive disorder. The nurse should give her advance warning that her turn is coming so she can perform her washing ritual to reduce her anxiety level.**   Im   Ps/6   2

    1. Sending her home without seeing the doctor is a punitive response and not appropriate.

    3. Persons with an obsessive-compulsive disorder perform rituals to decrease anxiety. If the nurse interrupts the ritual the client may develop severe anxiety.

    4. Given a choice of performing the ritual or seeing the doctor, the obsessive-compulsive client will usually choose the ritual.

#91. 1. **Saying, "I just can't believe he's gone" is indicative of the denial stage of grief. People who have lost someone close to them often think they see the person standing there.**   Dc   Ps/5   2

    2. It is common for a recently bereaved person to think they see the loved one. This does not indicate hallucinations.

    3. Illusions are a misinterpretation of reality. Thinking you see a recently deceased loved one standing there is not an illusion. It is a common part of the grief process.

    4. Her behavior is indicative of early grief, not severe depression.

#92. 4. **The nurse should arrange for the group to meet in a conference room or the hospital chapel. The client has a right to practice his religion. The nurse also has the responsibility to protect the rights of the other clients in the hospital.**   Im   Ps/5   2

    1. Rather than simply explaining the rules, the nurse should attempt to help the client meet his spiritual needs.

    2. The nurse should not put the roommate on the spot. The nurse knows that 18 people are too many in a semi-private room and should help the client make alternate arrangements.

    3. The nurse has a responsibility to the rest of the clients in the unit to maintain a therapeutic environment and cannot ignore the large number of people and the chanting.

#93. **2.** **Persons who are taking hallucinogens are apt to be violent. They**   Pl   Ps/6   5
       may think they can fly and react with violence when forced to
       remain in bed.

     1.   Severe depression is not a characteristic manifestation of
        hallucinogen use. The client who is withdrawing from cocaine will get
        severely depressed.

     3.   Respiratory distress is not characteristic of persons who are taking
        hallucinogens. Persons who are taking cocaine may develop sudden
        cardiac arrest.

     4.   Convulsions are not typical of hallucinogen use. Persons who are
        withdrawing from heroin may develop convulsions.

#94. **1.** **Drinking any alcohol when taking Antabuse will cause a severe**   Ev   Ps/6   5
       gastrointestinal upset and severe headache. The client should take
       no alcohol in any form. This statement indicates the client does
       not understand his treatment.

     2.   Mouthwash contains alcohol and can cause an Antabuse reaction.
        The client should not have alcohol in any form when taking Antabuse.
        This statement indicates the client understands his therapy.

     3.   The client should take the Antabuse daily. It stays in the system for up
        to three weeks so the client cannot decide he wants to drink in the
        evening and skip a dose. This statement indicates the client
        understands his treatment.

     4.   The client should tell emergency room personnel he is taking
        Antabuse. Many drugs including preps for intravenous and
        intramuscular injections contain alcohol. This statement indicates the
        client understands his treatment.

#95. **3.** **Abusers often feel remorse after the episode and seek forgiveness.**   Pl   Ps/6   2
       However, the next time they are frustrated, tired, or angry they
       are likely to strike out again and repeat the cycle.

     1.   Abusers often feel remorse after the episode and seek forgiveness.
        However, the next time they are frustrated, tired, or angry they are
        likely to strike out again and repeat the cycle.

     2.   Abusers often feel remorse after the episode and seek forgiveness.
        However, the next time they are frustrated, tired, or angry they are
        likely to strike out again and repeat the cycle.

     4.   Spousal abuse is not caused by misbehavior on the part of the victim.
        The abuser does not know how to deal with his feelings. The victim
        often takes the blame and has poor self-esteem.

#96. 3. **Persons who are violent and abuse others frequently have a substance abuse problem, which contributes to the problem.**   Dc   Ps/6   2

1. Abuse often happens in times of financial distress.

2. Abusers usually have a negative self-image.

4. Physical illness is not associated with the abuser. The abused is apt to suffer from numerous physical illnesses related to the abuse.

#97. 4. **A person who has the delusion that his food is being poisoned will not be talked out of it. The nurse should offer him food in individually wrapped containers.**   Im   Ps/6   2

1. Delusions come from the unconscious mind and cannot be reasoned with. Logic is useless when a person is delusional.

2. Delusions come from the unconscious mind and cannot be reasoned with. Logic is useless when a person is delusional.

3. The nurse should not serve as the client's taster. If the client should eat the food the nurse has tasted, what will he do when the nurse is off-duty?

#98. 4. **By attending to the client's behavior the nurse is sending a message to the client that she is concerned and that she is in control. Having the client go to a quiet area will decrease environmental stimuli. Extremely anxious persons respond to environmental stimuli.**   Im   Ps/5   2

1. Telling the client to do something is apt to increase the client's anxiety. At this time the client is so anxious that she has minimal voluntary control over her behavior. She is not likely to be able to get control of herself.

2. Leaving the room when the client is severely anxious is likely to increase the client's anxiety level.

3. The client may well not hear a whisper. Telling the client at this point that everything is going to be all right is false reassurance and something the client is not likely to believe.

#99. 2. **Giving the child some control over what is happening to him is likely to reduce his fear.**   Im   Ps/5   4

1. The nurse should not bribe the child with candy.

3. Telling him that shots don't hurt big boys is not truthful. When the shot does hurt he will feel betrayed, lose trust in the nurse and believe that he is not a big boy.

4. A two-year-old is not able to respond to reason. A two-year-old will probably not do well watching the nurse give him a shot.

ANSWER	RATIONALE	NP	CN	SA

#100. **3.** **The client is expressing rather severe anxiety and fear. The nurse should respond with empathy and encourage her to vocalize her concerns.** Im Ps/5 2

1. The nurse should respond to the client's anxious feeling rather than giving her facts. This statement implies that sometimes people do not get better. This response would likely increase the client's anxiety.

2. The nurse should respond to the client's anxious feelings rather than giving her reassurance about her doctor. The doctor's competence is not the real issue.

4. The nurse should respond to the client's anxious feelings rather than sharing the story of another patient with her.

Practice Test Three

1. A client has fludrocortisone acetate (Florinef) prescribed. What blood tests would the nurse monitor when administering this drug?

   1. Liver function tests
   2. Renal function tests
   3. Serum electrolytes
   4. Complete blood count

2. A 40-year-old woman is admitted in labor with high blood pressure, edema, and proteinuria. She is started on magnesium sulfate. The nurse caring for her should be sure to keep which drug at the bedside?

   1. Calcium gluconate
   2. Narcan
   3. Ritodrine
   4. Glucose

3. A woman who is in labor is being treated for pre-eclampsia. How will the nurse know if the client develops eclampsia?

   1. The client has albuminuria.
   2. The client has a seizure.
   3. The client's face and hands are edematous.
   4. There are no fetal heart tones.

4. A two-month-old infant is admitted with pyloric stenosis and will be going to surgery. What toy should the nurse provide for this infant?

   1. A stuffed teddy bear with a large colorful bow
   2. A "busy box"
   3. A mobile with large shapes and a music box
   4. Spoons for each hand so he can bang them together

5. A four-year-old child with Down syndrome is admitted to the hospital with pneumonia. She has a heart murmur and appears to be in respiratory distress. Her mother asks why her child has a heart murmur. What is the best nursing response?

   1. "Because she has pneumonia, her heart is working harder and causes the murmur."
   2. "Heart murmurs come and go in children. It is not a great concern."
   3. "Because of the pneumonia, her ductus arteriosus is functioning again."
   4. "Heart defects are common in children with Down syndrome. Her illness may make the murmur louder."

6. A seven-year-old boy is in the hospital with Reye's syndrome. He has been ill for two weeks with the flu. He ran high fevers and was treated with four baby aspirin alternating with 325 mg chewable Tylenol and sponge baths to control the fever. He also had a rash on his body that was itchy and his mother used lotion and Benadryl to control the itching. Which factors in his history are associated with development of Reye's syndrome? History of the flu and

   1. the use of Benadryl.
   2. the use of Tylenol.
   3. aspirin treatment.
   4. the presence of a rash.

7. A 15-month-old child with Hirschsprung's disease comes for a checkup. The mother reports all of the following. Which indicates a need for more instruction?

   1. The mother limits the child's physical activity to preserve calories.
   2. The child receives daily saline enemas.
   3. The child eats a low-residue diet.
   4. The mother gives the child daily stool softeners.

8. A mother noticed a large abdominal mass when helping her three-year-old child bathe. The child is taken to the physician and admitted to the hospital after an IVP confirms the diagnosis of Wilm's tumor. Which nursing action is essential to include in the nursing care plan?

   1. Strain all urine and save for analysis.
   2. Avoid palpating the abdomen.
   3. Prepare the child for permanent dialysis.
   4. Help the family understand the poor prognosis.

9. A woman who is pregnant for the first time asks the nurse when during pregnancy is the best time to take Lamaze classes. What should the nurse respond?

   1. During the first trimester
   2. During the second trimester
   3. During the third trimester
   4. Whatever fits into your schedule

10. A woman who comes in for prenatal care has a history of herpes with outbreaks that occur every six months to a year. She asks if this means she will have a cesarean delivery. How should the nurse respond?

    1. "If you have active lesions when you go into labor, you will need a cesarean section."
    2. "Cesarean delivery is the only way to protect your baby from herpes."

3. "Cesarean delivery is no longer recommended for persons with herpes."
4. "Your obstetrician will decide at the time of delivery which is best for you."

11. The nurse is discussing health concerns with a group of adolescent girls. When discussing genital warts caused by condyloma acuminata (HPV), the nurse should emphasize that the organism increases the risk of which condition?

    1. Infertility
    2. Congenital anomalies
    3. Cervical cancer
    4. Uterine prolapse

12. The nurse caring for newborns observes for jaundice. Which type of jaundice is likely to be most serious?

    1. Jaundice that occurs during the first day of life.
    2. Jaundice occurring after 48 hours of life.
    3. Jaundice occurring 7–10 days after birth.
    4. Any jaundice is potentially life-threatening.

13. The mother of a newborn asks why the nurse is checking the baby's nose. The nurse replies that it is important to check nasal patency because the newborn:

    1. Does not have the ability to sneeze.
    2. Must breathe through his nose.
    3. Is subject to periods of apnea.
    4. Has rapid respirations.

14. The nurse is caring for a 31-year old gravida 2, para 1 woman who is in labor. The woman calls the nurse and says "My water has broken and I feel something between my legs." The nurse looks and sees a loop of umbilical cord at the vaginal outlet. After signaling for help, what should the nurse do?

1. Try to replace the cord with a sterile gloved hand.

2. Place the mother in knee chest position.

3. Quickly apply manual pressure on the fundus.

4. Expect a rapid vaginal delivery.

15. A laboring woman prefers to lie in the supine position during labor. The nurse teaches her that this is not a good position for which reason?

    1. It will cause more back pressure.

    2. Her baby will not come down well into the pelvis.

    3. Her blood pressure may drop and cause the baby's heart rate to drop.

    4. Contractions will be too close together, not giving her a rest.

16. All of the following clients are on the unit. Which one is most likely to have an order for catheterization for residual?

    1. A woman who had a modified radical mastectomy yesterday.

    2. A man who had an abdominal cholecystectomy this morning.

    3. A woman who had an abdominal hysterectomy yesterday.

    4. A man who had surgery for a ruptured appendix.

17. A client who had a total knee replacement is to be discharged today. Which statement the client makes indicates a need for further instruction?

    1. "When I am walking, I will wear that ugly immobilizer."

    2. "I will sit with my leg elevated."

    3. "I think I understand how to use the continuous passive motion machine."

    4. "I won't put any weight at all on my affected leg."

18. An adult is receiving cancer chemotherapy. Metoclopramide (Reglan) is also prescribed. The client asks why she is getting Reglan. How should the nurse respond?

    1. "Reglan helps to prevent bleeding that may occur as a side effect of your other medications."

    2. "Reglan helps to prevent any nausea and vomiting that may occur as a side effect of your other medications."

    3. "Reglan increases the effectiveness of the cancer chemotherapeutic agents."

    4. "Reglan helps to control pain associated with your disease."

19. A very tall, heavy-set man is admitted. The nurse is taking vital signs. Which statement is correct about taking the blood pressure?

    1. 10 mm should be added to each reading to compensate for the cuff size.

    2. 15 mm should be subtracted from the systolic reading and 10 mm from the diastolic reading.

    3. An extra-large cuff is needed to obtain an accurate measurement.

    4. The client should lie down before the blood pressure is taken.

20. The nurse is auscultating the lungs in a post-operative client and hears something that sounds like a cellophane bag being wrinkled when the client takes in a breath. How should the nurse record this finding?

    1. Crackles

    2. Stridor

    3. Stertor

    4. Wheezes

21. The client who is scheduled for a knee replacement asks the nurse why she should donate her own blood before surgery. How should the nurse respond?

    1. "The blood bank is very short of blood."
    2. "Your own blood is the correct type for you."
    3. "It eliminates the chance of blood-borne diseases such as hepatitis and HIV."
    4. "Your own blood increases your energy level after surgery."

22. The client who is receiving hydantoin (Dilantin) tells the nurse his urine is pink-colored. What action should the nurse take?

    1. Report this serious side effect immediately to the physician.
    2. Reassure the client that this occurs often in persons taking Dilantin.
    3. Ask the client if he drank cranberry juice or ate red gelatin recently.
    4. Strain the client's urine for possible urinary tract stones.

23. A woman who was recently diagnosed with multiple myeloma says to the nurse, "Why did this happen to me? I've always been a good person. What did I do to deserve this?" What should the nurse do initially?

    1. Remind the client that she is not dying now and has some time left.
    2. Call the chaplain to discuss why it happened to her.
    3. Respond by recognizing how difficult this situation must be.
    4. Tell her she didn't do anything to deserve it.

24. A client asks the home care nurse to look at the bruises on her arms and legs. The woman also tells the nurse that her gums bleed when she uses dental floss or brushes her teeth. The client is taking all of the following medications. Which is most likely related to the client's symptoms?

    1. Metformin (Glucophage)
    2. Estrogen (Premarin)
    3. Atenolol (Tenormin)
    4. Ibuprofen (Motrin)

25. The client is taking streptomycin, isoniazid, and rimactane. Which data indicates toxicity to isoniazid?

    1. My ears ring all the time.
    2. I have sharp pains in my legs.
    3. My urine is orange-colored.
    4. I'm having trouble at traffic lights.

26. The nurse observes the certified nursing assistant doing all of the following. Which action needs correction?

    1. Changing the dressing of a client with an abdominal wound
    2. Asking a standing client to sit down while vital signs are taken
    3. Emptying a urine drainage bag from the tube at the bottom
    4. Changing water in the middle of a bed bath

27. A man who has diabetes complains of hunger and is pale, shaky, perspiring, and has cool skin. What is the most appropriate initial action for the nurse?

    1. Call the physician for orders.
    2. Give the client cola to drink.
    3. Have the client lie down.
    4. Administer the next dose of insulin.

28. A client who had a total thyroidectomy this morning returns to the nursing care unit. How should the nurse position the client?

    1. Semi-Fowler's
    2. Supine

3. Prone

4. Sims

29. All of the following clients need care. Whom should the nurse see first?

   1. A diabetic whose blood sugar is 40

   2. A post-operative client who is complaining of severe pain

   3. A person with terminal cancer who is complaining of pain

   4. A client with an indwelling catheter who is complaining of bladder pain

30. The nurse is working with a person who was just diagnosed with diabetes mellitus Type II. What should the nurse teach the client first?

   1. How to self-inject insulin

   2. How to follow a diabetic diet

   3. Signs and symptoms of insulin reaction

   4. Complications of diabetes

31. The nurse is caring for a person admitted with myasthenia gravis. What should be included in the nursing care plan for this person?

   1. Have the client bathe late in the day.

   2. Check swallowing reflexes before feeding.

   3. Have the client void every hour.

   4. Observe for signs of neuropathy.

32. Which of the following clients should be cared for first?

   1. An elderly woman who has been incontinent in bed

   2. An elderly man who has had fecal incontinence

   3. A man who has been up in the chair for two hours and wants to go back to bed

   4. A woman who needs to be turned every two hours and was last turned two hours ago

33. The nurse is caring for a person who is admitted with progressive amyotrophic lateral sclerosis. What nursing care measures should the nurse expect to be ordered for this client?

   1. Change dressing daily.

   2. Monitor IV fluids.

   3. Insert indwelling catheter.

   4. Chest physical therapy qid

34. All of the following need to be done. Which should the nurse delegate to the certified nursing assistant?

   1. Administering prn acetaminophen to a person who has arthritis

   2. Hygienic care to a person who had a CVA

   3. Catheterizing a client who is scheduled for surgery today

   4. Changing the dressing on a client who has a Stage III decubitus ulcer

35. The nurse is assessing a 78-year-old woman. The woman says she has some bladder discomfort and urinary frequency. She also says "I mind the cold so, but I don't seem to shiver. I don't have much energy these days." Her temperature is 98.9°F, pulse is 76, respirations 20, and blood pressure is 140/88. Which findings are of most concern to the nurse and need to be further evaluated?

   1. Temperature, pulse, respirations

   2. Blood pressure and temperature

   3. Bladder symptoms and fatigue

   4. Inability to shiver and cold sensitivity

36. All of the following individuals live at home with their families. Which of the following persons is least at risk for abuse?

   1. An 82-year-old woman who is incontinent and bosses people around
   2. An 80-year-old man who is ambulatory with help following a brain attack
   3. A 78-year-old woman who asks for help with all of her activities of daily living
   4. A 75-year-old man who wanders at night and frequently yells out

37. Triazolam (Halcion) 0.25 mg is ordered for a client at h.s. When the nurse goes to give the medication, the client asks the nurse to leave it at the bedside because she wants to finish reading a book. What is the best action for the nurse to take?

   1. Leave the medication at the bedside as requested.
   2. Return in one hour and offer the medication again.
   3. Tell the client to call when she is ready for the medication.
   4. Explain to the client that this is the time medications are given, and she should take it now.

38. The family of a frail elderly man who is bedridden asks the nurse what they can do to prevent bedsores. Which response by the nurse is best?

   1. "Get him out of bed at least once a day."
   2. "Turn him every two hours."
   3. "Rub his buttocks and apply lotion several times a day."
   4. "Change the sheets every day."

39. After returning from the post-anesthesia care unit, a man who had abdominal surgery is ordered to be in semi-Fowler's position. What is the primary reason for this position for this client?

   1. To prevent venous stasis
   2. To promote circulation
   3. To reduce tension on the incision
   4. To prevent respiratory distress

40. A woman who has been hospitalized for several days says she is having trouble getting to sleep. What is the best initial nursing intervention?

   1. Offer her a back rub.
   2. Ask her what she is worrying about.
   3. Give the ordered prn sedative.
   4. Notify the physician.

41. The nurse is observing a nursing assistant move a client from bed to chair. Which action by the nursing assistant indicates a lack of understanding about transfer techniques?

   1. Bending from the waist when moving the person
   2. Keeping the feet separated when lifting and moving the person
   3. Turning the whole body when moving the person to the chair
   4. Asking for help in moving the person from bed to chair

42. A woman is scheduled for an electromyography procedure (EMG) in the outpatient department. What should the nurse say to the woman?

   1. "Do not eat or drink anything after midnight the night before the procedure."
   2. "Are you allergic to shellfish or iodine?"
   3. "Do not eat or drink anything that contains caffeine for 2–3 days before the procedure."
   4. "There is no special preparation for this procedure."

43. The nurse checks the lab values of a newly admitted client.

RBC 4.0 million/mm³

WBC 1500/mm³

Platelets 40,000/mm³

What nursing actions are indicated because of these lab values?

1. Keep the client on bed rest and protective isolation.

2. Plan for protective isolation and do not give injections.

3. Keep the client on bed rest and avoid trauma.

4. There are no special nursing actions indicated.

44. The nurse is caring for a client who is receiving an intravenous infusion. Which finding would indicate the client's IV has infiltrated?

1. The client's arm is red and warm to the touch.

2. The IV is running faster than the desired rate.

3. The area around the infusion site is pale and cool to the touch.

4. The client complains of severe pain up and down the arm.

45. The nurse has been teaching a woman who has iron deficiency anemia. Which menu, if selected, indicates the woman understands her dietary instructions?

1. Applesauce, green beans, bread, and butter

2. Peanut butter and jelly sandwich, carrots, and milk

3. Broccoli, spinach salad with tomatoes, and orange juice

4. Macaroni and cheese, pickles, and hot chocolate

46. A client is admitted with pernicious anemia. The client reports all of the following. Which

is most likely related to the admitting diagnosis?

1. "I often have diarrhea."

2. "My tongue is more red and thick than usual."

3. "I have little bruise-like spots on my arms and legs."

4. "I have been running a fever for the last two days."

47. A man who had a right below-the-knee amputation is placed in the prone position for one hour three times a day. The nurse explains to the man that this is done to prevent which problem?

1. Atelectasis

2. Thrombophlebitis

3. Hip flexion contractures

4. Wound infection

48. The client has contact dermatitis from poison ivy. Which statement, if made by the client, indicates he understands how to care for his condition?

1. "A hot bath should make the itching go away."

2. "I will use a good strong soap when I wash the affected areas."

3. "A cool wet cloth to the area should help."

4. "Wearing wool socks will help my itchy feet."

49. The nurse is caring for a client who has psoriasis. Which observation by the nurse is most consistent with the diagnosis?

1. The client has thick, yellow toenails.

2. The client has open, weeping lesions.

3. The skin lesions are multicolored.

4. The pain follows a nerve root.

50. The nurse is caring for a man who has severe burns and had a skin graft. What nursing care measures are appropriate at the graft site the day of the graft?

   1. Leave the graft site open to the air.
   2. Elevate the recipient site.
   3. Encourage range-of-motion exercises.
   4. Change the dressing twice a day.

51. The nurse is to make several home visits today. All of the visits are within a five-mile radius. All of the following persons need to be seen. Which person should the nurse visit first?

   1. An older adult who has diabetes, peripheral vascular disease, and leg ulcers and needs hygienic care and wound care
   2. An adult who has multiple myeloma and needs her weekly injection of Interferon
   3. A woman with multiple sclerosis that needs hygienic care
   4. An elderly woman who is recovering from a cerebral vascular accident and needs hygienic care and ROM exercises

52. The nurse is caring for a client who was admitted following a motor vehicle accident. The client's blood pressure one hour ago was 118/76, pulse was 80; now the blood pressure is 90/60, pulse is 98. What action should the nurse take initially?

   1. Continue to monitor the blood pressure.
   2. Ask another nurse to check the blood pressure reading.
   3. Elevate the client's legs.
   4. Call the physician.

53. The nurse is caring for a person who has a nasogastric tube attached to drainage. Which complaint by the client needs to be reported to the charge nurse?

   1. Dry mouth
   2. Weak muscles

3. Sore throat
4. Irritated nose

54. A cooling blanket is ordered for an adult client who has a temperature of 106°F. What nursing action is essential because the client has a cooling blanket?

   1. Keep a padded tongue blade at the bedside.
   2. Turn every two hours.
   3. Apply ice to the groin area.
   4. Cover with a sheet and blanket.

55. The nurse is to suction a client. What action is essential prior to inserting the suction catheter?

   1. Clear the mouth and throat of secretions.
   2. Lower the head of the bed.
   3. Oxygenate the client.
   4. Check the suction pressure.

56. The nurse is caring for a man who has chronic emphysema and is receiving oxygen at 2 liters per minute. The nurse enters the room to find his wife has turned the oxygen up to 10 liters per minute because her husband is having increasing difficulty breathing. What is the best immediate action for the nurse?

   1. Explain to the wife that his oxygen was ordered at 2 liters per minute, and it should stay there until the physician orders something else.
   2. Turn the oxygen setting back to 2 liters per minute.
   3. Tell the wife that 10 liters per minute is too high and turn it back to 5 liters per minute.
   4. Assure her that 10 liters per minute will ease her husband's breathing.

57. The nurse discovers that a client is not breathing and has no pulse. After calling for help, what should the nurse do next?

1. Give the client two breaths.

2. Administer five chest compressions.

3. Go get the emergency cart.

4. Defibrillate the client.

58. The nurse is caring for a man who has radiation pellets in his mouth for mouth cancer. The nurse discovers one of the pellets in the sheets. What should the nurse do initially?

    1. Check the client's mouth for other loose pellets.

    2. Using long-handled forceps, put the pellet in a lead-lined container.

    3. Ask the client to hold the pellet until the radiologist arrives.

    4. Call the radiation safety officer.

59. The physician has ordered crutches and specified the client use a four-point gait. Which action by the client indicates an understanding of the four-point gait?

    The client moves:

    1. The left foot, then the left crutch, followed by the right foot and the right crutch

    2. The left foot, then the right foot, followed by the left crutch and the right crutch

    3. The left foot and the right crutch together followed by the right foot and the left crutch

    4. The left foot, then the right crutch, followed by the right foot and the left crutch

60. A man is a client in a semi-private room. When a new person is admitted to his room he says to the nurse, "What is wrong with the man in the other bed?" How should the nurse respond?

    1. Tell the man he should ask him himself.

    2. Tell the man in general terms the new client's diagnosis.

3. Ask the man why he wants to know.

4. Tell him that all clients' diagnoses are confidential.

61. An adult is to go to surgery this morning. When the nurse goes to medicate the client she notes that she has a ring with several shiny stones in it on her left ring finger. There are no relatives present. What is the best nursing action?

    1. Tape the ring before medicating the client.

    2. Ask the client to put the ring in the bedside drawer.

    3. Label the ring and place in an envelope in the hospital safe.

    4. Have the client sign a waiver regarding responsibility for the ring.

62. The nurse is providing home care for a client who has Parkinson's disease and is ambulatory. Which activity will help to prevent slipping and falling?

    1. Encourage the client to wear smooth-soled shoes.

    2. Leave the bed rails up at all times.

    3. Have the client spend several hours daily sitting in a chair.

    4. Place a scatter rug beside his bed.

63. The LPN/LVN in a long-term care facility sees and hears a nursing assistant give a resident a hard slap. What initial action should the LPN/LVN take?

    1. Be alert to further incidences of a similar nature.

    2. Report the incident to the supervisor.

    3. Write an incident report.

    4. Report the incident to the police.

64. The nurse is giving pre-operative medication to an adult who is scheduled for surgery. The client says to the nurse that she does not want to have a transfusion during surgery because it is against her religion. The client has signed a consent form for surgery. How should the nurse respond?

1. Explain that she has signed a consent form for surgery and that includes the use of transfusions if necessary.
2. Explain that the surgeon will probably not perform surgery if she won't have a transfusion.
3. Have the client sign an addendum to the operative permit excluding transfusions.
4. Withhold the medication and notify the physician.

65. The daughter of a 78-year-old woman asks the nurse why her mother is giving away some of her belongings to her children and grandchildren. What should the nurse include when responding?

1. Older adults usually become more generous.
2. It is normal for older adults to think about and prepare for their own death.
3. Her mother probably does not trust her children to divide her things appropriately.
4. Her mother is probably thinking about suicide.

66. The nurse in a residence facility for older adults is planning for the year. During which month should the influenza vaccine be offered to the residents?

1. May
2. July
3. September
4. November

67. The nurse is giving instructions to a group of women about self breast examination. Which statement indicates the client needs more instruction about the procedure?

1. "I will perform the exam every month after my period."
2. "I should do the exam both standing and lying down."
3. "Some ridges are normal in my breast."
4. "I will do the self breast exam every month until menopause."

68. The nurse is teaching a group of women about health issues. Today's topic is food poisoning. Which statement indicates a need for further instruction?

1. "I always wash my hands after I put raw meat in to cook."
2. "I should put foods away in the refrigerator immediately after meals."
3. "I will wash my kitchen counters with a bleach solution after preparing raw meat."
4. "Rare meat is okay to eat as long as it is eaten immediately after cooking."

69. The nurse is to administer a tuberculin skin test. What is the correct procedure?

1. Give it subcutaneously in the inner aspect of the forearm.
2. Use a 21-gauge needle and administer in the forearm.
3. Give it at a 10-degree angle in the volar surface of the arm.
4. Administer intradermal in the upper arm.

70. The nurse is planning care for a client who has a hearing impairment. Which action will likely help the most with communication?

1. Repeat everything twice
2. Speak loudly
3. Speak slowly and clearly
4. Use gestures

71. An 80-year-old woman has been hospitalized for three days with pneumonia. She is now able to sit in a chair for the first time. How should the nurse plan care for today?

    1. Give her a bed bath and then get her up and make her bed while she is in the chair.

    2. Get her up in the chair and have her give herself a bath while the nurse makes the bed.

    3. Give her a bed bath and come back later to get her up in the chair. Make the bed while she is up in the chair.

    4. Give her a bed bath and immediately get her up in the chair so the bed can be made.

72. The nurse is to administer a tube feeding to a client. Before administering the feeding, what is essential for the nurse to do?

    1. Ask the client if she feels full.

    2. Aspirate the nasogastric tube and check for acid.

    3. Change the tubing.

    4. Feel over the end of the tube and do not administer if air is felt.

73. The nurse is planning an approach to decrease urinary incontinence in an elderly client. Which activity will do the most to help prevent incontinence?

    1. Restrict fluids until continence has been achieved and then hydrate well.

    2. Offer the bedpan at two-hour intervals during the day and every four hours at night.

    3. Encourage the client to ambulate frequently and have the client do deep-breathing exercises.

    4. Encourage fluids during the day and offer the bedpan every two hours.

74. A woman in a residence facility is having difficulty sleeping at night. Which action by the nurse is most appropriate initially?

    1. Ask the physician for a sleeping medication.

    2. Offer the woman a back rub and warm milk.

    3. Suggest to the woman that she take a walk around the unit.

    4. Offer the woman a cup of hot tea.

75. A post-operative client is having difficulty voiding. Palpation of the bladder indicates the bladder is full. What should the nurse do initially?

    1. Ask the physician for a catheterization order.

    2. Pour water over the client's perineum.

    3. Encourage the client to take deep breaths.

    4. Administer pain medication.

76. The physician has recommended that the client increase the amount of dietary iron. The nurse knows the client understands the recommendations when the client selects which foods?

    1. Orange juice, scrambled eggs, and toast

    2. Hot dog and roll, French fries, and cola

    3. Roast beef, carrots, and rice

    4. Baked chicken, peas, and noodles

77. The nurse is to start oxygen therapy via nasal cannula. Which action is correct?

    1. Set the oxygen at 12 liters per minute.

    2. Lubricate the cannula with petrolatum before inserting.

    3. Give 100% oxygen by mask before inserting the cannula.

    4. Insert the cannula 1 cm into the nostrils.

78. A woman calls the physician's office stating that her 16-year-old daughter took 20 or 30 sleeping pills. The mother tells the nurse that her daughter is awake and says, "Leave me alone. I just want to die." How should the nurse respond?

   1. "Ask her why she wants to die."

   2. "Try to convince her she wants to live."

   3. "Give her a glass of milk to bind the medication."

   4. "Do you have syrup of Ipecac in the house?"

79. A wet-to-dry dressing is ordered for a client who has a decubitus ulcer. Which technique is appropriate?

   1. Irrigate the wound, then apply a dry dressing and cover with a wet compress.

   2. Apply a wet dressing for two hours followed by a dry dressing for 2 hours.

   3. Apply a wet dressing and cover with a dry dressing.

   4. Apply a wet dressing above the wound and a dry dressing below the wound.

80. The nurse is providing home care to a confused older adult. The family members have tied the client in a chair with a large leather belt. They say the client wanders if he isn't restrained. What initial nursing action is most appropriate?

   1. Report the family to family protective services.

   2. Congratulate the family on solving the problem.

   3. Help the family think of ways to make the environment safer for the client.

   4. Tell the family that you are not allowed to restrain the client with a leather belt.

81. The nurse is assessing the nursing care unit in a long-term facility for fire hazards. Which finding is the greatest fire hazard?

   1. Some of the nurses and nursing assistants smoke in the restroom.

   2. There are several cardboard boxes and cleaning supplies stored in the room with the emergency oxygen supply.

   3. Several residents have dust under their beds.

   4. Two of the residents have closets that are stuffed full of photo albums and sewing supplies.

82. A woman who recently had a simple mastectomy is about to be discharged. She seems very concerned about such things as where to find the best prosthesis, suitable underwear, and swimsuits, and adjusting to life with only one breast. Which resource is appropriate for the nurse to recommend?

   1. A psychologist or psychiatrist

   2. Reach for Recovery

   3. Pastoral counseling

   4. Her physician

83. A man who had a cerebral vascular accident has expressive aphasia. Which approach will help communication the most?

   1. The nurse should write to the client and the client should write back.

   2. The nurse should anticipate the client's needs as much as possible.

   3. The nurse should encourage the client to speak as much as possible.

   4. A family member should stay with the client and express the client's needs to the nurse.

84. An upset client says to the nurse, "Where did you learn to be a nurse? You don't know anything." How should the nurse respond?

   1. "I'm sorry you feel that way."

   2. "I went to a fine nursing school."

   3. "You sound upset."

   4. "Please don't speak to me that way."

85. A terminally ill client says to the nurse, "Do you believe in heaven?" How should the nurse respond?

1. "Yes, I believe in heaven and hell."
2. "My personal belief is private."
3. "Do you believe in heaven?"
4. "Do you want to see your clergyman?"

86. The nurse is assessing a child admitted who has a fractured humerus. The family says the child fell. Which piece of data would cause the nurse to suspect child abuse?

1. The child has been to the emergency room twice in the last month.
2. The child also has several bruises on the arms and legs.
3. The child has small round burned areas on the abdomen and back.
4. The child is holding his mother's hand.

87. Which comment, if made by the client, indicates adjustment to the diagnosis of insulin-dependent diabetes mellitus?

1. "Will it ever get easier to give myself a shot?"
2. "This can't be happening to me?"
3. "When I get over this, I'm going to eat chocolate cake every day."
4. "At least no one at work will know what they say I have."

88. An adult who is admitted to the hospital for a colostomy says to the nurse, "I'm so scared. Do you think I'll make it?" What is the nurse's best initial response?

1. "Of course you'll make it."
2. "Why are you so scared?"
3. "You're not likely to die."
4. "You sound scared."

89. The wife of a man who is comatose following a head injury asks the nurse if she should visit since he is unresponsive. How should the nurse reply initially?

1. Explain that since he is unresponsive there is no need for her to be here.
2. Tell her that the nurse will call if there is any change.
3. Suggest her presence is important even though he seems unaware.
4. Recommend that she ask his coworkers to visit.

90. A 14-year-old girl is brought to the emergency room because she is difficult to arouse. She is 5 feet, 8 inches tall and weighs 80 pounds. What additional findings would the nurse expect to be present?

1. Tachycardia
2. Amenorrhea
3. Wheezing
4. Acne

91. An adult is admitted to a detoxification unit for withdrawal from alcohol. Which medication does the nurse expect will be ordered for the client upon admission?

1. Thiamin
2. Antabuse
3. Ascorbic acid
4. Dilantin

92. The nurse is discussing dementia with the families of older adults. All of the following behaviors are reported. Which behavior is most suggestive of dementia?

1. The woman can't remember what year each of her six children was born.
2. A woman walked to the store and got lost on the way home.
3. A woman forgot where she put her purse.
4. A man is wearing one green sock and one red sock and doesn't see the difference.

93. A behavior modification program is planned for an adolescent who exhibits disruptive behavior. Which action by the nurse is most consistent with a behavior modification program?

1. Punish the client if she becomes disruptive.
2. Give the client extra privileges when she is not disruptive for a day.
3. Remind the client what she is supposed to do at regular intervals.
4. Ask the client what she sees as good behavior.

94. A client on the psychiatric unit does not get to the dining room to eat because she is continually washing her hands and doesn't finish until after lunch. What should be included in the nursing care plan?

1. Give the client a choice between eating lunch and performing her ritual.
2. Tell the client an hour before lunch so she can perform her ritual before lunch.
3. Discuss the problem with the client and ask her why she washes her hands so long.
4. Tell the client she cannot wash her hands at all if she is going to be late for lunch.

95. The nurse has been assigned a client who is thought to be suicidal. All of the following are in the client's room. Which is safe to leave in the room?

1. Paper cup
2. Leather belt
3. Razor
4. Pillow

96. The nurse has just completed a dressing change on an elderly client who is allowed bathroom privileges. Which action is most essential for the nurse to take before leaving the client's bedside?

1. Wash hands.
2. Lower the bed.
3. Toilet the client.
4. Assess for pain.

97. The nurse is caring for a woman who has internal radiation for cancer of the cervix. Which of the following situations poses the greatest risk for others?

1. The client's daughter spends several hours sitting next to the client's bed.
2. The client's husband kisses her and visits for five minutes before leaving.
3. The nurse brings the client her lunch tray and sets it up on the overbed table for her.
4. The cleaning lady damp mops the room.

98. An infant is to be admitted with severe diarrhea. Which room assignment is best for this infant?

1. A private room
2. A room close to the nurse's station
3. A room with a two-year-old child who has a broken leg
4. A room with another infant with severe diarrhea

99. A client who is blind is admitted to the hospital for surgery tomorrow. The client is able to get out of bed and eat until midnight. Which nursing action is most appropriate?

1. Describe the surroundings and the objects in the room to the client.
2. Put up the siderails and have the client ask for help when getting out of bed for any reason.
3. Describe the voices of the personnel to the client.
4. Remove objects such as water pitchers and glasses from the immediate vicinity.

100. The nurse is providing care in the home to a person who has AIDS. Which behavior, if observed by the nurse, indicates a need for further instruction?

   1. The client uses the same dishes as the rest of the family.

   2. The client shares a bathroom with the rest of the family.

   3. The client and his brother use the same razor.

   4. The client often cooks for the family.

Answers and Rationales for Practice Test Three

Answer	Rationale	NP	CN	SA

#1. 3. Florinef is given to clients whose adrenal cortex is not functioning adequately or to clients who have had an adrenalectomy. It acts like aldosterone to cause sodium and water retention and potassium excretion. Serum electrolytes are important to monitor to determine sodium and potassium levels. The client may need potassium supplements.　　Dc　Ph/8　5

  1. Fludrocortisone acetate does not primarily affect liver function. Liver toxicity is not a common side effect of this drug.

  2. Renal toxicity is not a common side effect of this drug.

  4. This drug does not commonly affect the blood count.

#2. 1. Calcium gluconate is the antidote for magnesium toxicity and must be available immediately for the respiratory depression that occurs when magnesium levels are too high.　　Pl　Ph/8　5

  2. Narcan is a narcotic antagonist and is used to treat respiratory depression caused by narcotic overdose.

  3. Ritodrine is used to treat pre-term labor.

  4. Glucose is used to treat hypoglycemia.

#3. 2. Eclampsia means that the client has seizures.　　Dc　Ph/10　3

  1. Albuminuria is a classic symptom of pre-eclampsia.

  3. Edema of the hands and face is a classic symptom of pre-eclampsia.

  4. Absence of fetal heart tones is suggestive of fetal death and could be associated with severe eclampsia but is not definitive of eclampsia. Eclampsia means the client has developed seizures.

#4. 3. This choice is most age-appropriate. The infant can focus on the large shapes and listen to the music box.　　Im　He/3　4

  1. The teddy bear will not hold the attention of a two-month-old for long. The bow can present a choking hazard unless it is very well attached.

  2. A two-month-old infant does not have the dexterity to play with a "busy box."

  4. A two-month-old infant cannot bang spoons together.

#5. **4.** **Heart disease is very common in children with Down syndrome.** **The strain on her system from pneumonia may increase blood** **flow through the defect making the murmur louder.**   Im   Ph/10   4

1. It is true that pneumonia may make the heart work harder and may intensify a murmur. However, it does not cause the murmur. Heart defects are very common in children with Down syndrome.

2. This is not correct information. Heart murmurs do not come and go in children.

3. The ductus arteriosus should have closed at birth unless it was kept open by the defect. Pneumonia does not cause the ductus arteriosus to reopen.

#6. **3.** **Reye's syndrome is associated with the use of aspirin in children** **who have a viral infection. Aspirin is not recommended for** **children.**   Dc   Ph/10   4

1. Benadryl use is not associated with the incidence of Reye's syndrome.

2. Reye's syndrome is not associated with the use of Tylenol.

4. Reye's syndrome is not associated with a rash.

#7. **1.** **There is no reason to limit activity in a child who has** **Hirschsprung's disease. This indicates the mother needs more** **teaching.**   Ev   Ph/9   4

2. Daily saline enemas are part of the recommended treatment for a child with Hirschsprung's disease.

3. A low-residue diet is part of the recommended treatment for a child with Hirschsprung's disease.

4. Stool softeners daily are part of the recommended treatment for a child with Hirschsprung's disease.

#8. **2.** **A Wilm's tumor is an encapsulated tumor. If palpated excessively** **it may rupture and spread cancer cells throughout the abdomen.** **It is essential that it not be palpated.**   Pl   Ph/9   4

1. There is no need to strain and save urine. Straining urine is appropriate for kidney stones.

3. Following surgery the child will still have one kidney and will not need dialysis.

4. The prognosis for recovery from Wilm's tumor is good if it is caught early when it is confined to the kidney.

#9. **3.** **Taking Lamaze classes closer to delivery is ideal. The mother is thinking about labor and she is more likely to practice and keep up conditioning.**   Im   He/3   3

1. Taking Lamaze classes closer to delivery is ideal. The mother is thinking about labor and she is more likely to practice and keep up conditioning.

2. Taking Lamaze classes closer to delivery is ideal. The mother is thinking about labor and she is more likely to practice and keep up conditioning.

4. Taking Lamaze classes closer to delivery is ideal. The mother is thinking about labor and she is more likely to practice and keep up conditioning.

#10. **1.** **Cesarean section delivery is only necessary if there are active lesions at the time of delivery. If active lesions are present at delivery, the baby could become severely ill or die.**   Im   Ph/9   3

2. Cesarean section delivery is only necessary if there are active lesions at the time of delivery. If active lesions are present at delivery, the baby could become severely ill or die.

3. Cesarean section delivery is only necessary if there are active lesions at the time of delivery. If active lesions are present at delivery, the baby could become severely ill or die.

4. Cesarean section delivery is only necessary if there are active lesions at the time of delivery. If active lesions are present at delivery, the baby could become severely ill or die.

#11. **3.** **HPV infections are associated with an increased risk of cervical cancer.**   Im   He/4   3

1. HPV infection is not associated with infertility. Pelvic inflammatory disease increases the risk of infertility.

2. Genital warts do not cause congenital anomalies. Diseases such as rubella and syphilis can cause congenital anomalies.

4. Uterine prolapse is not caused by genital warts.

#12. **1.** **Jaundice occurring in the first 24 hours of life is called pathological jaundice and is most serious because it is often related to blood incompatibilities.**   Dc   Ph/9   4

2. Jaundice occurring after 48 hours is called physiologic jaundice and is related to an immature liver that cannot keep up with the breakdown of red blood cells.

3. Jaundice that occurs 7–10 days after birth is usually breast milk jaundice and is usually of little concern.

4. Jaundice occurring after 48 hours and at 7–10 days is usually of little concern and is certainly not life-threatening.

#13. 2. **The newborn is an obligate nose breather and can only breathe through his mouth when he is crying. When he becomes fatigued, he falls asleep and turns blue if he cannot breathe through his nose.**

Dc   He/3   4

1. Newborns sneeze easily.

3. Newborns do have periods of apnea but this has nothing to do with being a nose breather.

4. Newborns have rapid respirations but this is not related to being a nose breather.

#14. 2. **The nurse should attempt to relieve pressure on the cord by putting the mother in knee-chest position. This lets gravity help to relieve pressure on the cord.**

Im   He/4   3

1. The nurse should not attempt to replace the cord. If the nurse discovers a prolapsed cord during a sterile vaginal exam, the hand may be left in the vagina to help relieve pressure on the cord.

3. The nurse should not apply manual pressure on the fundus.

4. The baby will be delivered by c-section as rapidly as possible.

#15. 3. **Supine hypotension may occur as the weight of the uterus presses on the vena cava. This may cause the baby's heart rate to drop.**

Im   He/3   3

1. The major problem with supine position is not back pressure but supine hypotension, which may occur as the weight of the uterus presses on the vena cava, causing the mother's blood pressure to drop and the baby's heart rate to drop.

2. The supine position may or may not hinder descent. The major problem with supine position is supine hypotension, which may occur as the weight of the uterus presses on the vena cava, causing the mother's blood pressure to drop and the baby's heart rate to drop.

4. Contractions usually slow down in the supine position.

#16. 3. Catheterization for residual urine is usually done for persons who   Pl   Ph/7   1
      have been catheterized for a long period of time or persons who
      have had pelvic area surgery. It is frequently ordered for women
      who have had gynecological surgery. Surgery in the pelvic area
      often makes it difficult to regain bladder tone.

1. A mastectomy does not affect bladder tone. It would be unusual for
    the woman who had a modified radical mastectomy to have an order
    to be catheterized for residual urine.

2. The client who had an abdominal cholecystectomy might or might not
    have an indwelling catheter for a few hours. A cholecystectomy does
    not affect bladder tone. It would be unusual for the client who had an
    abdominal cholecystectomy to have an order to be catheterized for
    residual urine.

4. It would be unusual for the client who had surgery for a ruptured
    appendix to have an order to be catheterized for residual urine.

#17. 4. The client should be gradually increasing weight-bearing on the   Ev   Ph/9   1
      affected leg. This answer indicates a need for further instruction.

1. The immobilizer should be worn when the client is walking. This
    answer indicates an understanding of instructions.

2. The client should sit with leg elevated. This answer indicates an
    understanding of instructions.

3. The client will use the continuous passive motion (CPM) machine at
    home. This answer indicates an understanding of instructions.

#18. 2. Cancer chemotherapeutic agents frequently cause nausea and   Im   Ph/8   5
      vomiting. Reglan is an antiemetic given to help control nausea
      and vomiting.

1. Reglan does not control bleeding. Cancer chemotherapeutic agents
    frequently cause nausea and vomiting. Reglan is an antiemetic given
    to help control nausea and vomiting.

3. Reglan does not increase the effectiveness of cancer
    chemotherapeutic agents. Cancer chemotherapeutic agents
    frequently cause nausea and vomiting. Reglan is an antiemetic given
    to help control nausea and vomiting.

4. Reglan is not an analgesic. Cancer chemotherapeutic agents
    frequently cause nausea and vomiting. Reglan is an antiemetic given
    to help control nausea and vomiting.

#19. 3. **When the client's arm is long or larger around than average, a wide cuff should be used. If the regular cuff is used, the blood pressure reading will be higher than it actually is.**   Im   He/4   1

     1. When the client's arm is long or larger around than average, a wide cuff should be used. If the regular cuff is used, the blood pressure reading will be higher than it actually is. The nurse should not add numbers to the reading.

     2. When the client's arm is long or larger around than average, a wide cuff should be used. If the regular cuff is used, the blood pressure reading will be higher than it actually is. The nurse should use a larger cuff, not subtract numbers from the reading.

     4. When the client's arm is long or larger around than average, a wide cuff should be used. If the regular cuff is used, the blood pressure reading will be higher than it actually is. Lying down usually raises blood pressure.

#20. 1. **The sounds described are crackles and are abnormal.**   Dc   He/4   1

     2. Stridor is a shrill, harsh sound heard during inspiration in laryngeal obstruction.

     3. Stertor describes a breathing pattern that is noisy and caused by a partial obstruction of the upper airway.

     4. A wheeze is a high-pitched respiratory sound common in asthma.

#21. 3. **The reason persons who are having elective surgery are often encouraged to donate their own blood is to reduce the risk of blood-borne diseases such as hepatitis and HIV, which can be contracted when donor blood is used. There is often significant blood loss with a knee replacement.**   Im   Ph/9   1

     1. It may well be true that the blood bank is short of blood. However, that is not the primary reason elective surgical clients are asked to donate their own blood.

     2. Donor blood of the correct type can be given to the client. This is not the reason clients who are scheduled for elective surgery are asked to donate their own blood.

     4. Blood transfusions are not given primarily to increase energy level following surgery, although that may be one effect. There would be no difference in effect on energy between donor blood and autologous transfusion.

#22. 2.   Pink-colored urine occurs frequently in persons taking hydantoin (Dilantin). Im   Ph/8   5

   1.   Pink-colored urine occurs frequently in persons taking hydantoin (Dilantin). It is not a serious side effect. The nurse should record the information.

   3.   Cranberry juice and red gelatin do not turn the urine pink. Pink-colored urine occurs frequently in persons taking hydantoin (Dilantin).

   4.   Pink-colored urine occurs frequently in persons taking hydantoin (Dilantin). It does not suggest kidney stones in this client.

#23. 3.   The initial response should open communication. Responding with empathy or reflection is most appropriate. Im   Ps/5   2

   1.   This response is not therapeutic and will only serve to close communication. The goal of initial communication is to open communication.

   2.   Initially the nurse should open communication by responding with empathy or reflection. Later, the nurse might ask the client if she would like to talk with the chaplain. This is not appropriate initially.

   4.   Telling the client she didn't do anything to deserve it may be appropriate at some point in the discussion, but is not appropriate initially. Initially the nurse should open communication and let the client express her feelings.

#24. 4.   Ibuprofen is apt to cause bleeding as a side effect. None of the other drugs do. Dc   Ph/8   5

   1.   Metformin is a drug used for Type II diabetics to lower blood sugar. Hypoglycemia and renal problems might be adverse effects. It does not cause bleeding as a side effect.

   2.   Estrogen is a female hormone. It is more apt to cause clotting as an adverse effect. It does not cause bleeding as a side effect.

   3.   Atenolol is an antihypertensive. An adverse effect would be slow pulse or hypotension. It does not cause bleeding.

#25. 2.   Peripheral neuropathy is a major side effect of isoniazid. Peripheral neuropathy is characterized by sharp pains in legs. Dc   Ph/8   5

   1.   Ototoxicity is a toxicity of streptomycin.

   3.   Orange-colored urine is a side effect of rimactane.

   4.   Color blindness is a side effect of ethambutol.

#26. **1.** **A nursing assistant should not be changing a sterile dressing. That action is not within the scope of practice.**   Dc   Sa/1   1

    2. Asking a standing client to sit down while vital signs are being taken is an appropriate action and does not need correction.

    3. Emptying a urine drainage bag from the tube at the bottom is an appropriate action and does not need correction.

    4. Changing water in the middle of a bed bath is an appropriate action and does not need correction.

#27. **2.** **The diabetic client has the classic signs of hypoglycemia. The treatment is to administer sugar. Cola has sugar. The nurse could also do a glucose check but that is not one of the options.**   Im   Ph/10   1

    1. Initially the nurse should recognize the symptoms as those of hypoglycemia and give the client something with sugar in it to eat or drink. Calling the physician is not the initial action. The nurse should be able to handle the initial episode and then notify the physician if necessary.

    3. Having the client lie down will not help with hypoglycemia. The client needs sugar.

    4. The symptoms suggest hypoglycemia. Insulin is not what is needed for hypoglycemia. The client needs sugar in some form.

#28. **1.** **Semi-Fowler's position is the appropriate position to reduce edema and keep the airway open.**   Im   Ph/9   1

    2. Supine is not the appropriate position. This position would promote edema and predispose to airway problems.

    3. Prone is not the appropriate position. This position would promote edema and predispose to airway problems.

    4. Sims is not the appropriate position. This position would promote edema and predispose to airway problems.

#29. **1.** **The nurse should attend to the client whose blood sugar is dangerously low. This client will soon lose consciousness. The nurse should give the person sugar in some form.**   Pl   Sa/1   1

    2. The post-operative client who is in pain needs pain medication, but the pain is probably not life-threatening.

    3. The person with cancer needs pain medication, but the pain is probably not life-threatening.

    4. The person with an indwelling catheter who is complaining of bladder pain should be seen soon, but the potential problem is not as immediately serious as the hypoglycemic client.

#30. 2. **The key to controlling Type II diabetes mellitus is usually following a diet and losing weight. The client might also be on oral medication.**   Pl   Ph/9   1

   1. Most Type II diabetics do not need to self-inject insulin. Most Type II diabetics are controlled with diet and oral hypoglycemic agents.

   3. Most Type II diabetics do not receive insulin on a regular basis and do not need to know the signs and symptoms of insulin reaction. They might need to know about hypoglycemia if they are taking oral hypoglycemic agents, but it would not be referred to as an insulin reaction.

   4. The nurse will teach the client about the complications of diabetes, but not initially. First, the nurse should teach the client what they need to know to help control the disease. Later, the nurse can teach about the complications.

#31. 2. **The person with myasthenia gravis has upper body weakness. The major symptoms include difficulty swallowing, double vision, and ptosis of the eyes. The nurse should check the swallowing and gag reflexes before feeding the person.**   Pl   Ph/9   1

   1. The client is usually strongest early in the day with the weakness getting worse as the day progresses. The client should bathe early in the day.

   3. There is no need for the person with myasthenia gravis to void every hour.

   4. Myasthenia gravis is not a neuropathy. There is no need to observe for this.

#32. 4. **The person who needs turning should be attended to first. This will help to prevent skin breakdown and respiratory complications. Turning usually can be done fairly quickly, and the nurse can get on to the others who need attention.**   Pl   Sa/1   1

   1. This person needs attention but not first. It will probably take longer to change this person's bed than it will to turn the other client.

   2. This person needs attention but not first. The person who only needs turning can be done quickly and then this client can be cleaned and changed. This client will take several minutes to clean up.

   3. This person should be tended to but not first. There is nothing in the data that suggests that this client is in any immediate need to go back to bed.

ANSWER	RATIONALE	NP	CN	SA

#33. 4. The person who has ALS will need chest PT at least qid. ALS is a motor neuron disease that results in progressive loss of function. Respiratory congestion is usually what kills persons with ALS.   Pl   Ph/9   1

1. The person with ALS is not likely to have dressings that need changing unless they develop a decubitus ulcer, which is possible. This question does not give that data.

2. The person who has ALS is not likely to have an IV running unless there is an additional problem such as an infection requiring IV antibiotics. The question does not give that information.

3. The person who has ALS might possibly need an indwelling catheter. That information is not given in the question.

#34. 2. A nursing assistant is well qualified to give hygienic care. This act can safely be delegated.   Pl   Sa/1   1

1. The nurse should not delegate administration of medications to a nursing assistant. It doesn't matter what type of medication.

3. A nursing assistant is not qualified to perform a catheterization.

4. Changing the dressing on a Stage III decubitus ulcer is a sterile procedure. The nurse should not delegate this to the nursing assistant.

#35. 3. The bladder symptoms suggest a bladder infection. In older people, temperature is not a very reliable indicator of infection. Other symptoms should be evaluated.   Dc   He/3   1

1. The vital signs are essentially normal.

2. The blood pressure is borderline but not a cause for alarm in a 78-year-old.

4. As people age they usually become more sensitive to the cold and often are less able to shiver. These are normal findings in a 78-year-old.

#36. 2. This client has few risk factors for abuse.   Dc   Ps/6   2

1. Incontinence and being bossy are risk factors for elder abuse.

3. Dependence is a risk factor for elder abuse.

4. Wandering and yelling out are risk factors for elder abuse.

#37. 3. Triazolam (Halcion) is a sleeping medication. If the client is not ready to go to sleep the nurse should have her call when she is ready for the medication.

1. The nurse should not leave medication (with the exception of nitroglycerine) at the bedside. Leaving sedatives at the bedside creates a risk of the client hoarding the medication and making a suicide attempt.

2. It is better for the client to call the nurse. The client may not be ready for the medication in one hour.

4. This response is very rigid. The nurse should be more flexible and give the client the medication at the client's hour of sleep.

#38. 2. The best way to prevent decubitus ulcers (bedsores) is to take the pressure off the pressure points by turning every two hours.

1. Getting him out of bed each day may well be a good thing. However, it is not the best way to prevent decubitus ulcers (bedsores).

3. Rubbing the skin on his buttocks may wear away the delicate skin and actually predispose him to skin breakdown. Sometimes gentle massage near the area is recommended to improve circulation.

4. Changing the sheets several times a day will not prevent pressure ulcers (bedsores). Straightening out the sheets to remove wrinkles is more important than changing the sheets each day, unless they are soiled or wet.

#39. 3. The primary reason for placing a client who has had abdominal surgery in semi-Fowler's position is to reduce tension on the suture line.

1. Elevating the legs and leg exercises are done to help prevent venous stasis. Semi-Fowler's position does not help to prevent venous stasis.

2. Semi-Fowler's position does not particularly promote circulation.

4. Semi-Fowler's position does help to promote thoracic expansion. It does not prevent respiratory distress. However, that is not the primary reason the client who has had abdominal surgery is placed in semi-Fowler's position.

#40. 1. **The nurse should first try nonpharmacologic methods to induce sleep.**   Im   Ph/7   1

   2. The nurse could open communication, but asking her what she is worrying about is making an assumption that worry is the cause of her sleeplessness.

   3. Before giving the ordered prn sedative, the nurse should try nonpharmacologic methods.

   4. There is no need to notify the physician initially. The nurse should try nonpharmacologic methods to induce sleep and, if these are not successful, give the ordered sedative. If these efforts fail, the nurse should notify the physician.

#41. 1. **The nursing assistant should keep the back straight when lifting and moving clients. This action indicates a lack of understanding about transfer techniques and body mechanics.**   Ev   Ph/7   1

   2. The nursing assistant should keep the feet separated when moving and lifting persons. This action indicates understanding of transfer techniques.

   3. The nursing assistant should turn the whole body when moving the person from bed to the chair. This action indicates understanding of transfer techniques.

   4. The nursing assistant should ask for help when necessary. This indicates an understanding of principles related to transfer techniques.

#42. 4. **There is no special preparation for an electromyography procedure (EMG). There is no anesthesia given and no dyes are used. Needle electrodes are inserted into the muscle, and the nerve conduction to the muscles is measured.**   Im   Ph/9   1

   1. No anesthesia is used during an EMG, and no dyes are used so there is no need for the client to be NPO.

   2. No dyes are used during an EMG, so there is no need to ask the question about iodine allergy.

   3. There is no need to limit caffeine before an EMG. Caffeine is restricted before an electroencephalogram (EEG).

ANSWER	RATIONALE	NP	CN	SA

#43. 2. **The WBC and platelet counts are low. The client should be on protective isolation because of the low white blood cell count and the resulting inability to fight infection. The client should also not receive any injections because of the low platelet count and the resulting inability to clot.**
  Pl Ph/9 1

  1. The client's RBC count is normal so there is no need to keep the client on bed rest. The client should be on protective isolation because of the low white blood cell count and the resulting inability to fight infection.

  3. The client's RBC count is normal so there is no need to keep the client on bed rest. The client should not receive any injections because of the low platelet count and the resulting inability to clot.

  4. This answer is not correct. There are special nursing actions indicated. The WBC and platelet counts are low. The client should be on protective isolation because of the low white blood cell count and the resulting inability to fight infection. The client should also not receive any injections, because of the low platelet count and the resulting inability to clot.

#44. 3. **When an IV infiltrates it means the IV needle is out of the vein and the IV fluid goes into the tissue outside the vein. This makes the area cool and pale.**
  Dc Ph/8 1

  1. A red and warm arm when an IV is infusing suggests phlebitis-inflammation of the vein.

  2. An infiltrated IV runs slower than the desired rate.

  4. Usually the discomfort is localized with an infiltration. There would not be pain up and down the entire arm.

#45. 3. **Broccoli and spinach both contain iron. Tomatoes and orange juice are vitamin C sources. When a person eats iron sources, they should also have a vitamin C source to increase absorption of iron.**
  Ev Ph/7 6

  1. None of these food choices contains a significant amount of iron.

  2. None of these food sources contains a significant amount of iron. Milk has protein but no iron.

  4. None of these food sources contains a significant amount of iron. Milk and milk products contain no iron.

#46. 2. **A beefy red tongue is usually seen in pernicious anemia.**
  Dc Ph/9 1

  1. Diarrhea is not a symptom of pernicious anemia.

  3. Ecchymotic areas are not usually seen in pernicious anemia.

  4. A fever is not usually seen in pernicious anemia.

ANSWER	RATIONALE	NP	CN	SA

#47. 3. **Prone position puts the hip in extension and helps to prevent the development of hip flexion contractures, which is a common complication following lower extremity amputation.**　Im　Ph/9　1

  1. Atelectasis is prevented by deep-breathing and coughing.

  2. Leg exercises and antiembolism stockings prevent thrombophlebitis.

  4. Hand washing and good technique will help to prevent wound infection.

#48. 3. **Cool moist compresses help with the itching of contact dermatitis.**　Ev　Ph/10　1

  1. A hot bath will most likely make the itching worse.

  2. The client with contact dermatitis should avoid strong soaps and detergents. They usually make the itching worse.

  4. Wool, nylon, and fur clothing should be avoided, as they tend to make the itching worse.

#49. 1. **The person who has psoriasis usually has thick, yellow toenails. Psoriasis is a chronic type of dermatitis that involves a turnover rate of the epidermal cells that is seven times the normal rate.**　Dc　Ph/10　1

  2. Psoriasis is not characterized by open, weeping lesions. Contact dermatitis caused by poison ivy would have open, weeping lesions. Psoriasis is characterized by sharply circumscribed bright red macules, papules, or patches covered with silvery scales.

  3. Psoriasis is characterized by sharply circumscribed bright red macules, papules, or patches covered with silvery scales. Multicolored skin lesions are typical of skin cancer.

  4. Skin eruptions and pain along a nerve root suggest herpes zoster, which is also called shingles.

#50. 2. **Whenever possible the recipient site should be elevated to prevent edema formation.**　Im　Ph/10　1

  1. Warm compresses will probably be applied to the graft site.

  3. The client should not do range-of-motion exercises as this might separate the graft from the area.

  4. The nurse will not change the dressing twice a day. The nurse should apply sterile warm compresses if ordered.

#51. 2. **The person who has multiple myeloma is immunocompromised. Multiple myeloma is cancer of the bone marrow and the bone. Interferon is an immunosuppressant. This person should be cared for before the client who has an open wound. This is also a short visit.**   Pl   Sa/1   1

    1. The client with leg ulcers has an open wound. The person who is immunocompromised should be cared for first.

    3. This visit will take a long time. There is no reason to care for this person first.

    4. This visit is also a lengthy one. There is no reason to care for this person first.

#52. 3. **The vital signs suggest the client is in shock. The client's legs should first be elevated and then the nurse should notify the charge nurse or the physician.**   Im   Ph 10   1

    1. The blood pressure change is so significant that continuing to monitor the blood pressure is not sufficient.

    2. The nurse should have confidence in his/her own actions and act on the basis of the results obtained.

    4. The nurse will call the physician after elevating the client's legs. The question asked for the initial action.

#53. 2. **Weak muscles may indicate hypokalemia. A nasogastric tube attached to drainage depletes potassium and sodium.**   Dc   Ph/10   1

    1. Most people who have a nasogastric tube in place complain of a dry mouth. This is not a serious problem.

    3. Most people who have a nasogastric tube in place complain of a sore throat.

    4. Most people who have a nasogastric tube in place complain of an irritated nose.

#54. 2. **A person who is on a cooling blanket should be turned every two hours to prevent skin breakdown and to promote effective cooling.**   Im   Ph/10   1

    1. It is possible that the client who has a high fever might have seizures. However, a padded tongue blade is not used during a seizure.

    3. A cool compress may be applied to the groin area and to the axilla. Ice is not used because it may stimulate shivering, which raises body temperature.

    4. The client should be covered with a sheet but not with a blanket. A blanket will promote temperature increase.

#55. 3. Before inserting the suction catheter the nurse should oxygenate the client.   Im   Ph/10 1

   1. The purpose of the suction catheter is to clear the mouth and throat of secretions.

   2. The head of the bed should be raised, not lowered.

   4. The wall suction is usually not regulated.

#56. 2. The stimulus to breathe in a person who has chronic emphysema is a low oxygen level. Ten liters of oxygen per minute will depress the respiratory drive, and the person will die. The nurse must immediately put the oxygen level back to two liters per minute.   Im   Ph/10 1

   1. After turning the oxygen back to a safe level the nurse can discuss the reason with the woman. This explanation is not sufficient. Simply stating it is the doctor's order is not adequate. The implication in this response is that the physician might order higher concentrations of oxygen. This is highly unlikely. The nurse should explain the reason to the woman so she does not try to do it again.

   3. Five liters is too high. The nurse should immediately turn the oxygen flow rate back to two liters per minute.

   4. The woman's actions are not appropriate and are putting her husband's life in danger.

#57. 1. The nurse should initially administer two breaths.   Im   Ph/10 1

   2. The nurse should first give two breaths when starting CPR.

   3. The nurse should stay with the client, not leave the client to get the emergency cart.

   4. The LPN should not initially defibrillate the client.

#58. 2. The nurse should use long-handled forceps to pick up the pellet and place it in a lead-lined container.   Im   Ph/10 1

   1. The initial action is to prevent radiation damage to the client, the nurse, and others. Checking the client's mouth for other loose pellets would be a later action.

   3. The client should not hold the pellet. The pellet will cause radiation burns.

   4. The nurse should call the radiation safety officer after safely putting the pellet in a lead-lined container.

#59. 4. This describes a four-point gait. In a four-point gait, the client moves one foot and then the opposite crutch, followed by the other foot and the opposite crutch.

   1. This is not the four-point gait. Walking as described in this response would be very hazardous.

   2. This is not the four-point gait. This gait would be very difficult to do and very hazardous.

   3. This is not the four-point gait. The gait described is the two-point gait.

Ev   Ph/7   1

#60. 4. The nurse should not discuss one client's diagnosis with another client.

   1. This answer sounds rude. There is some truth to the fact that if one client wishes to discuss his illness with another he may do so.

   2. This response might violate the client's right to confidentiality.

   3. This answer is poor communication.

Im   Sa/1   1

#61. 3. The nurse should identify the ring and place it in an envelope in the hospital safe.

   1. The nurse may tape a ring without a stone. Taping a ring with a stone may cause the stone to become loose and even dislodge.

   2. The ring needs to be placed in a secure place.

   4. The client should not be asked to sign a waiver.

Im   Sa/1   1

#62. 1. The client should wear smooth-soled shoes. Persons with Parkinson's disease shuffle when they walk. Smooth-soled shoes allow him to shuffle.

   2. Leaving the bedrails up at all times may make it more hazardous for the client to get out of bed. It is better to put the bed in the low position.

   3. A person who has Parkinson's disease will get very stiff while sitting in a chair for hours at a time. He should ambulate several times. "The longer he sits, the stiffer he gets."

   4. Scatter rugs would increase the likelihood of falling.

Pl   Sa/2   1

#63. 2. The LPN/LVN should report the incident to the supervisor.

   1. The nurse will continue to be alert to other incidents. However, the nurse should initially report this incident.

   3. This is not the type of event for which an incident report is made.

   4. The LPN/LVN should first report the incident to the supervisor. The supervisor will make the determination as to any other action to be taken.

Im   Sa/1   1

#64. 4. **The nurse should not medicate the client because the client will need to talk with the physician. The client has the right to refuse a transfusion. However, the surgeon may feel that surgery is not safe if a blood transfusion cannot be given if needed.**   Im   Sa/1   1

1. The client has the right to refuse a transfusion and the right to rescind permission. The nurse must notify the physician immediately because the client is scheduled for immediate surgery.

2. This may be a true statement. However, answer #4 is a better response. This response sounds as if the nurse is trying to talk the client into having a transfusion. The nurse should not do that.

3. This is not the best response. The nurse should withhold pre-operative medication and notify the surgeon.

#65. 2. **It is a normal part of aging to think about one's own death and to prepare for it. This often includes giving belongings to the persons they want to have them. Unless this behavior becomes obsessive, it is normal.**   Im   He/3   2

1. The basic personality type usually continues into older adulthood.

3. There is no data to suggest this response.

4. There is no data to suggest this response. If a younger person started giving away personal items it might be a sign of suicide. It could be a sign of suicide in the older adult if it is accompanied by other suicidal behavior.

#66. 4. **The best time to give influenza vaccine is November. This allows the antibody levels to rise for protection during the winter months when the incidence of influenza is highest.**   Pl   He/4   5

1. The best time to give influenza vaccine is November.

2. The best time to give influenza vaccine is November.

3. The best time to give influenza vaccine is November.

#67. 4. **The woman should continue to do self-breast exams on a monthly basis as long as she is able. The incidence of breast cancer increases with age. This statement indicates the client does not understand and needs more instruction.**   Ev   He/4   3

1. This statement is correct and indicates the client understands the teaching.

2. This statement is correct and indicates the client understands the teaching.

3. This statement is correct and indicates the client understands the teaching.

#68. 4. **Meat should be cooked to 160° Fahrenheit. Rare meat can cause food poisoning. This answer indicates the person does not understand how to prevent food poisoning and needs more instruction.**   Ev   He/4   6

1. Hands should be washed after handling raw meat. This answer indicates the person understands how to prevent food poisoning.

2. Food should be placed in the refrigerator as soon as possible after eating to prevent the growth of microorganisms. This answer indicates the person understands how to prevent food poisoning.

3. Kitchen counters should be washed with bleach after raw meat has been handled on them. This answer indicates the person understands how to prevent food poisoning.

#69. 3. **A tuberculin skin test is given intradermal in the volar surface of the forearm. This answer is the correct procedure.**   Im   He/4   5

1. This is not the correct procedure. A tuberculin skin test is given intradermal in the volar surface of the forearm.

2. This is not the correct procedure. A tuberculin skin test is given intradermal in the volar surface of the forearm.

4. This is not the correct procedure. A tuberculin skin test is given intradermal in the volar surface of the forearm.

#70. 3. **Speaking slowly and distinctly will do the most to help with communication.**   Pl   Ps/5   1

1. Speaking slowly and distinctly is better than repeating everything twice.

2. Speaking loudly is usually not as effective as speaking slowly and clearly. When speaking loudly, the individual usually raises the pitch of the voice and makes it even harder to hear.

4. Speaking slowly and distinctly is better than using gestures.

#71. 3. **This is the approach that will allow the client to rest between activities.**   Pl   Ph/7   1

1. This approach does not allow the client to rest between activities.

2. This approach does not allow the client to rest between activities.

4. This approach does not allow the client to rest between activities.

#72. 2. **The nurse should always check for residual and check to be sure that the aspirate is acid, which indicates that it is in the stomach.**   Im   Ph/7   1

1. It is essential to test for placement of the tube. Asking the client if she feels full is not the best way to assess that the tube is in the proper place.

3. It is not necessary to change the tubing before giving a tube feeding. It is essential to test for placement of the tube.

4. It is essential to test for placement of the tube. Feeling over the end of the tube for air is not an appropriate or accurate way to test that the tube is in the stomach.

#73. 4. **The best way to achieve urinary continence is to encourage fluids during the day and offer the bedpan every two hours.**   Pl   Ph/7   1

1. This approach will not help to achieve urinary continence. You cannot bladder train an empty bladder.

2. Offering the bedpan at two-hour intervals during the day is appropriate. The nurse should restrict fluids after 6 P.M. so the client does not need to use the bedpan during the night.

3. Ambulation and deep-breathing exercises are not the protocol for promoting urinary continence.

#74. 2. **The nurse should try nonpharmacologic methods first. A back rub should help the woman relax and encourages sleep. Warm milk has a sleep-inducing effect.**   Im   Ph/7   1

1. The nurse should try nonpharmacologic methods of inducing sleep before asking for sleeping medication.

3. Exercise usually wakes people up. It does not induce sleep.

4. Tea contains caffeine, which is a stimulant. Caffeine sources should not be consumed late in the day if the client has trouble sleeping.

#75. 2. **The nurse should try a noninvasive method to encourage voiding such as running water or pouring water over the client's perineum.**   Im   Ph/7   1

1. The nurse might have to do this eventually. The nurse should try noninvasive methods first, such as running water or pouring water over the client's perineum.

3. Taking deep breaths does not promote voiding.

4. Narcotic pain medication makes it harder for the client to open the urinary sphincter.

#76. 1.   **The best food choices when an increase in iron is recommended**   Ev   Ph/7   6
       contain iron (eggs) and vitamin C (orange juice) to increase the
       absorption of iron.

    2.   There is very little iron and very little vitamin C in this choice.

    3.   Roast beef has iron, but there is not vitamin C in this choice. Vitamin
       C increases absorption of iron.

    4.   Baked chicken contains some iron, but there is no vitamin C in this
       selection. Vitamin C increases the absorption of iron.

#77. 4.   **The cannula should be inserted 1 cm into the nostrils. The other**   Im   Ph/10   1
       responses are incorrect.

    1.   Twelve liters per minute is too high a setting for oxygen.

    2.   The cannula does not need to be lubricated. The nurse should not use
       petrolatum substances near oxygen.

    3.   The nurse does not give 100% oxygen before inserting the cannula.

#78. 4.   **Syrup of Ipecac should be given to induce vomiting, since the**   Im   Ph/10   1
       child is awake and talking.

    1.   This answer is not correct for two reasons. First, this is not the time to
       talk. After the sleeping pills are removed from her system and she is
       physiologically stable, then the nurse may do further inquiry as to
       what happened. Second, asking a person why they want to kill
       themselves is poor communication.

    2.   There is a physiologic emergency. Until the client is stable
       physiologically, neither the nurse nor the parent should start trying to
       convince her she wants to live. It would be poor communication
       technique to try to convince her she wants to live initially. Initially the
       nurse and the parent should recognize the client's distress.

    3.   Milk is not the antidote for sleeping pills. Milk is given in acute lead
       poisoning.

#79. 3.   **When a wet to dry dressing is applied, the nurse first applies a**   Im   Ph/10   1
       wet dressing to the wound and then covers with a dry dressing.

    1.   This is not the appropriate technique.

    2.   This is not the appropriate technique.

    4.   This is not the appropriate technique.

#80. 3. **This approach helps the family to solve the problem and use a better, less restrictive way to keep the client safe.**   Im   Sa/2   2

    1. The nurse should work with the family to provide for the safety of the client. If the family refuses to work with the nurse, there might be a reason for notifying family protective services.

    2. Restraining the client with a leather belt is not appropriate. The nurse should not congratulate the family.

    4. This answer does not help the family learn how to keep the client safe.

#81. 2. **Storing flammable liquids (cleaning supplies) and flammable boxes near the emergency oxygen supply is fire hazard.**   Ev   Sa/2   1

    1. Smoking in the restroom is unhealthy unless it is properly ventilated. However, it is not as great a fire hazard as mixing cleaning supplies, boxes, and oxygen.

    3. Dust under the beds is not sanitary and may spread infection and cause allergies. However, it is not a significant fire hazard.

    4. Stuffed closets can be a safety hazard and could be a fire hazard if a flame was close at hand. This choice is not as great a fire hazard as oxygen and flammable materials.

#82. 2. **Reach for Recovery is a self-help group for persons who have had mastectomies. The types of concerns the client has would be best addressed by Reach for Recovery.**   Pl   Ps/5   2

    1. The concerns this woman has would be better addressed by a support group such as Reach for Recovery.

    3. The concerns this woman has would be better addressed by a support group such as Reach for Recovery.

    4 The concerns this woman has would be better addressed by a support group such as Reach for Recovery.

#83. 3. **The nurse should encourage the client to speak as much as possible.**   Pl   Ps/5   1

    1. The nurse can speak verbally to this client. The data indicates the client has expressive aphasia, meaning she cannot speak. There is no need for the nurse to write communication. Expressive aphasia may be only verbal communication, or it could be verbal and written. The nurse needs to assess this further before asking the client to communicate in writing.

    2. Anticipating the client's needs does not encourage the client to attempt to speak or use other means of communication. It keeps the client dependent.

    4. The nurse and the client should develop some type of communication system. This approach creates dependence on family members.

ANSWER	RATIONALE	NP	CN	SA

#84. **3.** **The nurse should reflect on the tone of the client's feelings and not be defensive.** — Im — Ps/5 — 2

   1. This response does not focus on the client's feelings.

   2. This is a defensive response and not therapeutic.

   4. This does not focus on the client's feelings.

#85. **3.** **This response is most likely to open communication and allow the client to express his/her concerns.** — Im — Ps/5 — 2

   1. Introducing the concept of hell to a dying person is not likely to be therapeutic.

   2. This answer puts the client off and is nontherapeutic.

   4. While it may be appropriate to ask the client at some point if they want to see their clergyman, this answer avoids the question.

#86. **3.** **Small round burned areas on the abdomen and back are not consistent with a fall. This is more consistent with cigarette burns, which would be abuse.** — Dc — Ps/6 — 4

   1. Two visits in a month are not especially indicative of child abuse. This could be a normal pattern. It is also consistent with child abuse.

   2. A fall would cause bruises on the arms and legs.

   4. A child who is abused may not be affectionate and trusting to the parent, especially if the parent is the abuser.

#87. **1.** **This response indicates that the client is performing self-injection of insulin. This is the best indicator of acceptance of the diagnosis.** — Ev — Ps/5 — 2

   2. This comment indicates denial of the diagnosis.

   3. This comment indicates the client expects to get over IDDM. Since IDDM is not a condition from which a person recovers, this comment indicates the client has not accepted the diagnosis.

   4. This comment indicates the client has not accepted the diagnosis.

#88. **4.** **This response opens communication. Initially, the nurse should open communication.** — Im — Ps/5 — 2

   1. This response does not open communication.

   2. Asking "why" puts the client on the defensive.

   3. This response, while true, does not open communication and let the client express feelings.

#89. **3.** **Persons who are apparently unconscious may be aware when family members are present. Her presence is important for the client and for herself. Notice that the nurse suggests and doesn't tell.** — Im — Ps/5 — 1

    1. This statement is not true.

    2. The nurse should call if there is any change. However, the client asked if she should visit. The nurse should encourage her to be present.

    4. This response ignores the woman's question completely and is nontherapeutic.

#90. **2.** **Persons who have anorexia and do not eat are in a starvation state and usually have scanty or absent menstruation.** — Dc — Ps/6 — 1

    1. The person who has anorexia nervosa has a slow metabolic rate and usually has bradycardia, not tachycardia.

    3. Wheezing is not typical of anorexia nervosa.

    4. Acne is not typical of anorexia nervosa.

#91. **1.** **Thiamin deficiency is common in alcoholism. Thiamin is frequently ordered.** — Pl — Ps/6 — 5

    2. Antabuse is not likely to be ordered upon admission. Antabuse helps the client abstain from alcohol and is usually ordered close to discharge.

    3. Ascorbic acid (vitamin C) is not usually ordered for persons who abuse alcohol.

    4. Dilantin is an antiseizure medication. The client may be given a drug such as Valium or Ativan to prevent seizures during withdrawal.

#92. **2.** **Getting lost in familiar territory is a sign of dementia. The other symptoms are not.** — Dc — Ps/6 — 2

    1. Being unable to remember dates from the past is not a sign of dementia.

    3. Not being able to find a purse is not necessarily a sign of dementia.

    4. Not being able to tell the difference between red and green is not a sign of dementia. It is a sign of color blindness.

#93. **2.** **Behavior modification is based on rewarding desired behavior.** — Pl — Ps/6 — 2

    1. Behavior modification is based on rewarding desired behavior, not punishing undesirable behavior.

    3. Reminding the client is not behavior modification.

    4. Asking the client what she sees as good behavior is not behavior modification.

**#94. 2. The client cannot help her need to wash her hands compulsively.
The nurse should remind her that lunch is coming soon so the
ritual can be performed and she can still make it to the dining
room.**   Pl   Ps/6   2

1. It is not appropriate to give the client a choice between ritual and
    eating. The compulsion to perform the ritual is very strong and comes
    from the unconscious mind.

3. A compulsion is thought to come from the unconscious mind and is
    not subject to rational thought and control. The client does not know
    why she washes her hands so often. She probably recognizes that her
    behavior is not rational, but she cannot help it.

4. Prohibiting the client from performing her ritual is likely to put the
    client into an anxiety attack.

**#95. 1. A paper cup is not a hazard and cannot be used to injure one's
self.**   Pl   Sa/2   2

2. A leather belt can be used to hang one's self.

3. A razor can be used to harm one's self.

4. A pillow can be used to smother one's self.

**#96. 2. The client is allowed out of bed. It is essential that the nurse
lower the bed so the client can safely get out of bed. This must be
done before leaving the bedside.**   Im   Sa/2   1

1. The nurse should wash hands before leaving the room, but not before
    leaving the bedside.

3. It is not essential to toilet the client. Lowering the bed is more
    important.

4. Assessing for pain is not the highest priority.

**#97. 1. Several hours is too long to have close contact with someone
who has internal radiation. Limiting time with the client and
increasing distance from the client reduce radiation exposure.**   Ev   Sa/2   1

2. Kissing her is close contact but the time is brief. There is risk but not
    as much as occurs in response #1. Limiting time with the client and
    increasing distance from the client reduce radiation exposure.

3. The time period of exposure is brief. Limiting time with the client and
    increasing distance from the client reduce radiation exposure.

4. The time period of exposure is brief, and the cleaning lady is not too
    close to the client. Limiting time with the client and increasing
    distance from the client reduce radiation exposure.

#98. 1. **An infant who is admitted with severe diarrhea should be in isolation until the cause of the diarrhea has been determined. Many causes of diarrhea are very infectious.**

    2. The most important criterion is that the child be in a private room for isolation until the cause of the diarrhea is determined.

    3. The most important criterion is that the child be in a private room for isolation until the cause of the diarrhea is determined.

    4. The other infant's diarrhea might not be caused by the same thing this child's is. This would put both infants at risk. The most important criterion is that the child be in a private room for isolation until the cause of the diarrhea is determined.

Pl   Sa/2   4

#99. 1. **The nurse should describe the room and the furnishings. The nurse might also have the client walk to the bathroom describing landmarks so the client will feel comfortable ambulating alone.**

    2. Putting up the siderails is not appropriate unless the client is also confused or unable to get out of bed. The nurse should make the environment safe for the client.

    3. Describing the voices of the personnel might be helpful. However, describing the surroundings does more to promote safety.

    4. The nurse should place the water pitcher and glass in a position convenient to the client so the client does not have to search for them.

Im   Sa/2   1

#100. 3. **AIDS is caused by HIV. HIV is spread by body secretions. The razor could come in contact with the client's blood and infect his brother.**

    1. Using the same dishes poses no risk of infection.

    2. Using the same bathroom as the rest of the family poses no risk of infection.

    4. Cooking for the family poses no risk of infection for the rest of the family.

Ev   Sa/2   1

Practice Test Four

1. Which nursing diagnosis is most appropriate for a client who has Cushing's syndrome?

    1. Risk for injury related to osteoporosis
    2. Pain related to cold intolerance
    3. Risk for deficient fluid volume related to excessive loss of sodium and water secondary to polyuria
    4. Risk for injury related to postural hypotension

2. A woman comes into the labor suite stating her water has broken and she is in labor. Which symptoms point to the possible presence of placenta previa?

    1. Sudden knife-like pain in the lower abdomen accompanied by profuse vaginal bleeding
    2. Dark red vaginal discharge that started after she saw the physician this morning
    3. Bright red painless vaginal bleeding
    4. A tender rigid uterine wall and abdomen with no vaginal bleeding evident

3. A 13-month-old is admitted to the pediatric unit with diarrhea and vomiting. The mother tells the nurse that she is worried because her son does not yet walk. She says her other children walked at eight and nine months and asks what could be wrong with this child. How should the nurse respond?

    1. "All babies are different. It is not abnormal that the baby is not yet walking."
    2. "The baby should be walking. I'll let the doctor know he is behind developmentally."
    3. "Your son is probably enjoying being the baby and is not eager to grow up and walk."
    4. "Walking requires complex coordination. Your son is prabably just a little slow to develop this. Don't worry."

4. A woman brings her six-month-old daughter to a clinic for a check-up and immunizations. The mother tells the nurse her infant is cranky, has a bad cold, and has not eaten well the last few days. She asks if the baby will still be able to get her shots. How should the nurse respond?

    1. "There is no problem in giving the shots just because your baby has a cold."
    2. "Your baby will have her check-up, but we will wait until her cold is better before giving her shots."
    3. "The shots often make them a little irritable, so we might as well get it all over with at one time."
    4. "I'm not sure why you came today. We need to reschedule the whole appointment for another day when your baby has no symptoms of a cold."

5. The mother of a two-month-old asks the nurse when she should start her son on solids. He is taking about 30 ounces of formula per day. How should the nurse respond?

    1. "This is a good time to begin."
    2. "When he is taking a quart per day."
    3. "Babies usually are ready for solids between four and six months of age."
    4. "Each baby is different. Some are ready sooner than others."

6. An infant is suspected of having coarctation of the aorta. Which assessment finding is most related to coarctation of the aorta?

    1. Respirations are 70 per minute.
    2. Blood pressure is higher in the upper extremities than in the lower.
    3. There is a heart murmur.
    4. Heart rate is 150 per minute.

7. A young child with a history of grand mal seizures is in public school. He is on phenobarbital and hydantoin (Dilantin) to control the seizures. His teacher tells the nurse that he has not had any seizures, but he does keep falling asleep in class. What should the nurse include when discussing his drowsiness with the teacher?

   1. It is common in children who take barbiturates.
   2. It usually occurs after seizures; let him sleep.
   3. It is probably not related to his seizure disorder or treatment.
   4. It is probably a warning sign that he is about to have a seizure.

8. The nurse is teaching a woman the normal changes of pregnancy. Which statement by the woman indicates correct understanding?

   1. "There is decreased oxygen consumption during pregnancy."
   2. "There is an increased rate of peristalsis in the GI tract."
   3. "I will have a 50% increase in blood volume."
   4. "My metabolic rate will decrease."

9. A prenatal client tests positive for chlamydia in her ninth month. She asks why she should be treated since she does not have symptoms. The nurse should tell the client that if she is not treated before delivery there is a risk of which problem?

   1. Transplacental infection of the fetus
   2. Neonatal ophthalmia
   3. Pregnancy-induced hypertension
   4. Congenital anomalies

10. A baby is delivered following a pregnancy complicated by gestational diabetes. What should the nurse observe the baby for?

    1. Infection

    2. Hyperglycemia
    3. Acidosis
    4. Hypoglycemia

11. A laboring woman who has dystocia is receiving oxytocin. The nurse observes a contraction lasting 90 seconds. What should the nurse do first?

    1. Slow down the rate of the oxytocin.
    2. Turn the woman on her left side.
    3. Give the woman oxygen.
    4. Stop the oxytocin.

12. A laboring woman says to the LPN/LVN "My baby is coming! My baby is coming!" She was last checked 15 minutes ago and was 5 cm dilated. What should the LPN/LVN do initially?

    1. Have her checked to see if she has progressed.
    2. Reassure her she cannot be that far along.
    3. Reposition her to begin pushing.
    4. Request medication to help her relax.

13. A baby boy is delivered after a rapid labor of three hours. The mother wants him to stay with her for as long as possible before he goes to the nursery. What nursing action takes priority in the immediate newborn period?

    1. Suctioning with a bulb syringe.
    2. Wrapping the baby in warm blankets.
    3. Applying identification bracelets and taking footprints.
    4. Assigning an APGAR score.

14. The nurse is talking with a group of young people who are preparing to spend a weekend camping in the woods. Which information is essential to include in the discussion?

    1. Wear long pants and long sleeves to prevent tick bites.
    2. Sunscreen is not necessary because you will be moving and perspiring.
    3. Bring salt tablets to take in case you perspire a lot.
    4. Poison ivy is not likely to be contracted unless you have prolonged contact with the plants.

15. The client who is receiving cancer chemotherapy asks why the physician recommended she take it in the evening. The nurse's response should include which information?

    1. It is best to have one set time to take it. It really doesn't matter what time.
    2. Taking it in the evening means that any nausea that may occur will be during the night when you are asleep and not during meal times.
    3. One of the side effects of cancer chemotherapeutic agents is drowsiness. This is less troublesome during the night than during the day.
    4. The medication is more effective if you are not active immediately after taking it.

16. The nurse is auscultating the lungs in a post-operative client and hears something that sounds like a cellophane bag being wrinkled when the client takes in a breath. What nursing care is essential because of the finding?

    1. Start emergency oxygen and notify the physician.
    2. Have the client take several deep breaths and cough every two hours.
    3. Notify the physician and prepare the client for a tracheostomy.
    4. Carefully observe the client for cyanosis.

17. A client who had a total thyroidectomy this morning is to be admitted to the surgical floor. What should the nurse have at the bedside when the client arrives?

    1. Tracheostomy set
    2. Catheterization tray
    3. Sterile dressing set
    4. Ventilator

18. Iron drops were ordered for a toddler who has iron deficiency anemia. What observation of the child by the nurse indicates the child is receiving the medication?

    1. The child is pale and lethargic.
    2. The child's skin has brown spots.
    3. The child's urine is dark colored.
    4. The child has black stools.

19. Which statement made by the parents of a child who has sickle cell anemia indicate understanding of how to reduce the incidence of crises?

    1. "I should not let my child play outdoors."
    2. "My child should drink lots of fluids every day."
    3. "If my child has a fever I should administer aspirin immediately."
    4. "We should fly in an airplane rather than taking the child for a long car ride."

20. A person who has psoriasis is seen in the clinic. The lesions are covered with coal tar. Which instruction should the nurse give the client?

    1. "Call if you have nausea and vomiting."
    2. "Protect the area from sunlight for 24 hours."
    3. "Wash off the solution after 6–8 hours."
    4. "Call if your skin looks dark during the treatment."

21. The nurse is to observe the client for shock. The client's admitting vital signs are BP 116/70, P 86, R 24. Which finding, if observed, would be most suggestive of shock?

    1. BP 140/60
    2. Pulse 100
    3. BP 114/68
    4. Pulse 60

22. A nursing assistant comes to the LPN/LVN and complains that she has more residents to care for than another nursing assistant (NA). She has one more resident assigned to her than the other NA. However, the other NA has more total care residents than the complaining nurse assistant. How should the LPN/LVN handle this situation?

    1. Tell the complaining NA that this is the assignment.
    2. Promise to give her an easier assignment tomorrow.
    3. Discuss with her the needs of her assignment and help her organize her care.
    4. Tell her that the other NA will help her as needed.

23. An adult who is being admitted to the medical floor with a bleeding ulcer exhibits all of the following. Which finding suggests the client may be experiencing alcohol withdrawal symptoms?

    1. BP 90/60
    2. Dizziness
    3. Tremors
    4. Pallor

24. The client has a prolonged prothrombin time. What question is important to ask the client when interpreting this data?

    1. How often do you eat meat?
    2. How much alcohol do you drink?
    3. Do you take heparin?

4. Have you had a recent injury?

25. The nurse is caring for a newly admitted man who has kidney stones. The man asks if he can get up and take a walk. How should the nurse respond?

    1. "It is better for you to remain in bed until the stones pass."
    2. "Stay in bed until I check with your physician."
    3. "Walking is good for you. Let me help you up."
    4. "It is safe for you to ambulate once a day."

26. The nurse is discussing preventive health care with a group of women. Which woman should the nurse advise to have a mammogram?

    1. A 20-year-old who says her breasts hurt before her period
    2. A 25-year-old who was hit in the breast area by a ball
    3. A 32-year-old who has been breastfeeding for 12 months
    4. A 52-year-old who has no breast symptoms

27. A 79-year-old asks the nurse if she needs any shots. She reports having had "all the usual shots when I was younger." Which immunization is most important for this person to receive?

    1. DPT
    2. MMR
    3. Pneumovax
    4. HIB

28. The LPN/LVN is to assist the school nurse in scoliosis screening. What instructions should be given to the students?

    1. Wear a bathing suit under your clothes on the examination day.

    2. Bring a urine sample to school.

    3. Do not wash your hair the night before the exam.

    4. Wash your feet well the morning of the exam.

29. A woman who had a tuberculosis test three days ago reports to the nurse to have the test read. Which finding, if present, indicates a positive result and a need for referral and follow-up?

    1. A red area 12 mm in diameter

    2. A raised area 10 mm in diameter

    3. Itching at the injection site

    4. A rash on the arm near the test site

30. The nurse is to administer a tuberculin skin test. At what angle should the nurse insert the needle?

    1. A 10-degree angle

    2. A 30-degree angle

    3. A 60-degree angle

    4. A 90-degree angle

31. The nurse is discussing child safety with a group of mothers of toddlers. Which statement indicates a need for more instruction?

    1. "My child should be in the back seat in a front-facing car seat."

    2. "My little one needs constant supervision."

    3. "I should keep syrup of ipecac in the house."

    4. "I should put my medicines on a high shelf."

32. Which statement, if made by the client, indicates a possible problem?

    1. "I have a bowel movement every other day."

    2. "My stools recently are black."

    3. "Sometimes I have to strain when I go to the bathroom."

    4. "I usually have three stools a day."

33. The client has recently had a colostomy. The nurse is providing home care and is teaching the client about care of his colostomy. Which comment by the client indicates understanding of the care of his colostomy?

    1. "I will use hot water to irrigate the colostomy."

    2. "If my skin gets red, I will put alcohol on it."

    3. "I will irrigate the colostomy at the same time each day."

    4. "I should do the irrigation while lying in bed."

34. The nurse is doing a pain assessment on the client who has chronic back pain. Which assessment is of greatest value?

    1. Observe the client for grimaces, flinching, and other signs of pain.

    2. Monitor the client's blood pressure.

    3. Ask the client to rate his pain on a scale of one to ten.

    4. Monitor the client's pulse and respirations.

35. An 80-year-old woman is hospitalized with severe pneumonia. She has been on complete bed rest for several days and receiving complete care. Today she is to be allowed out of bed for the first time. How should the nurse plan the morning care?

    1. Give her a bed bath and then get her out of bed while the nurse makes the bed.

2. Get her up in a chair and allow her to give herself a bath while the nurse makes the bed.

3. Give her a bed bath and allow her to rest. Later get her up in the chair while the nurse makes the bed.

4. Encourage her to give herself a bath while in bed, then get her up in the chair and make the bed.

36. The nurse is caring for a client who had a total gastrectomy performed this morning. When the client returns to the nursing care unit the drainage from the nasogastric tube is red. What is the nurse's best response to this?

1. Report it immediately to the charge nurse or the physician.

2. Record the finding and continue to observe.

3. Immediately apply pressure to the operative site.

4. Place the client in Trendelenburg's position.

37. The nurse is to administer a nasogastric tube feeding to a client. Which action is essential prior to administering the feeding?

1. Position the client in supine position.

2. Aspirate contents from the nasogastric tube and check the pH.

3. Check the client's vital signs.

4. Ask the client if she feels full.

38. The nurse is assisting a client with deep breathing and coughing exercises following abdominal surgery. What instruction is most appropriate for the nurse to give the client?

1. Hold your breath for several seconds and then breathe out forcefully.

2. Splint your incision while taking in deep breaths and coughing.

3. Take deep breaths when you are moving in bed.

4. Deep breathing exercises should be done when you are out of bed.

39. The nurse is caring for all of the following clients. Which is probably at greatest risk for skin breakdown and will need special nursing care measures?

1. A 75-year-old who is admitted with a broken hip

2. An 80-year-old who is admitted with angina

3. An 85-year-old who is admitted for diagnostic tests

4. A 78-year-old who is admitted with asthma

40. The nurse is to perform a routine blood glucose check on a diabetic client before administering insulin. Which action is correct?

1. Puncture the end of the thumb in the middle of the fleshy part.

2. Puncture the end of the finger on the side.

3. Draw blood from the antecubital vein in the arm.

4. Puncture the finger and collect the blood in a vial.

41. A woman is in the clinic complaining of urinary frequency, urgency, and pain on urination. Orders include a urine for culture and administration of Gantrisin and pyridium. Which action should the nurse take first?

1. Obtain a clean catch urine from the client.

2. Ask the client if she is allergic to sulfa drugs.

3. Administer the Gantrisin.

4. Administer the pyridium.

42. An eight-year-old has just had a fiberglass cast applied to his right lower leg following a fractured ankle. The nurse is discussing care of the cast with the parents. Which instruction should be included?

1. Since water does not dissolve a fiberglass cast, your child may take a bath.

2. Check the toes on the right leg to be sure they are warm.

3. Do not cover the cast for two days to allow it time to dry.

4. Keep the casted leg down for the next two days to promote circulation.

43. The nurse is caring for a woman admitted with thrombocytopenia. Which instruction should the nurse give the client?

1. Call me when you need to go to the bathroom.

2. Do not use dental floss or a firm toothbrush.

3. Wear a mask when you leave the room.

4. Be sure everyone washes their hands before touching you.

44. At 10:30 A.M., a young woman who has diabetes calls the nurse and says she feels "funny." The nurse notes she is cool to the touch but her skin is moist. When the nurse asks her if she is hungry she responds in an irritable manner that she is hungry. Which initial nursing action is appropriate?

1. Administer her noon dose of insulin early.

2. Call the lab to draw a blood glucose.

3. Have her drink a glass of cola.

4. Encourage her to drink lots of water.

45. A newborn is to receive phototherapy for hyperbilirubinemia. Which nursing action is essential?

1. Keep the infant NPO for two hours before the treatment.

2. Ask the mother to stay away from the infant during the treatment.

3. Monitor the client's pulse rate very carefully.

4. Cover the baby's eyes during the treatment.

46. A child at school trips on a shoe lace and falls. Her ankle swells immediately, and the child is in a great deal of pain. What is the best initial action for the nurse to take?

1. Keep the foot down.

2. Apply a warm compress.

3. Elevate the foot and apply an ice pack.

4. Ask the child to try to move her ankle.

47. Oxygen has been ordered for a client who was admitted to the hospital with congestive heart failure. Which assessment finding indicates the oxygen has been effective?

1. The client no longer complains of pain.

2. The client's respiratory rate has decreased from 36 to 24.

3. The client has voided 600 ml of urine in the last three hours.

4. The client has less ankle edema than was present when admitted.

48. An adult is admitted with meningitis. During the acute phase of the illness, which measure should the nurse include in the nursing care plan to reduce the chance of seizures?

1. Play the client's favorite music.

2. Stimulate the client every two hours.

3. Keep a padded tongue blade at the bedside.

4. Darken the client's room.

49. The evening nurse caring for an adult who had a partial gastrectomy this morning notes the drainage from the nasogastric tube is bright red. What action should the nurse take?

1. Chart the drainage amount and color.
2. Report the findings immediately to the charge nurse.
3. Disconnect the drainage system.
4. Immediately apply pressure to the wound.

50. The nurse is caring for a man who had a transphenoidal hypophysectomy earlier today. He says he has to spit a lot. What nursing action is essential?

    1. Ask him to blow his nose.
    2. Do a glucose test on his mouth secretions.
    3. Have him rinse his mouth with water.
    4. Ask him if he needs an antiemetic.

51. A client is admitted with a possible gastric ulcer. Suddenly he calls to the nurse and says, "It hurts so bad." The client is pale and diaphoretic. What should the nurse do initially?

    1. Call the physician.
    2. Palpate the abdomen.
    3. Obtain a stool for guaiac.
    4. Place the client in a supine position.

52. A blood transfusion has just been started on an adult. Which assessment is most essential during the first hour?

    1. Temperature
    2. Blood pressure
    3. Respirations
    4. Pulse

53. An adult is admitted in severe hypovolemic shock following an auto accident. A transfusion is ordered. What type of blood is given when the client's blood type is not known?

    1. O positive
    2. O negative
    3. AB positive
    4. AB negative

54. The client has been vomiting for several days. Which blood gas values is he likely to have?

    1. pH 7.32; CO_2 60; HCO_3 30
    2. pH 7.32; CO_2 33; HCO_3 18
    3. pH 7.54; CO_2 28; HCO_3 22
    4. pH 7.54; CO_2 32; HCO_3 34

55. The nurse is caring for an elderly woman who had surgery on her right foot yesterday. The woman had a broken left arm three months ago and has osteo-arthritis. Which type of assistive device will probably be most appropriate for this client?

    1. Quad cane
    2. Crutches
    3. Walker
    4. Tripod cane

56. The nurse administers CPR to an adult male who is found unconscious, has no pulse, and is not breathing. What is the ratio of chest compressions to respirations for one person rescue?

    1. Five chest compressions to one breath
    2. Five chest compressions to two breaths
    3. Fifteen chest compressions to one breath
    4. Fifteen chest compressions to two breaths

57. The nurse is caring for a client who had a portable water seal chest drainage system inserted today. Which observation indicates the client's drainage system is working properly?

    1. There are no bubbles in the water seal bottle.
    2. The suction control chamber has continuous bubbles.
    3. There are bubbles in the drainage chamber.
    4. There is no fluctuation in the fluid in the water seal chamber.

58. What should the nurse do when ambulating a client who has a portable wound drainage system?

    1. Remove the drain during ambulation.

    2. Fasten the collection device below the wound.

    3. Completely empty the collection device before ambulating.

    4. Disconnect the suction apparatus before ambulating.

59. The nurse is discussing positioning with the family of a client who is at home following a total hip replacement a week ago. Which should be included in the discussion?

    1. Keep the client on his unaffected side most of the time.

    2. Position the client to maintain hip flexion.

    3. Keep a pillow between his legs when turning him.

    4. Position the client so the hip is adducted.

60. An 80-year-old woman is having diffculty sleeping. Which nursing action is most appropriate initially?

    1. Ask the physician for an order for a sleeping medication.

    2. Encourage the client to do mild exercises a half hour before going to bed.

    3. Suggest to the client that she not nap during the day.

    4. Recommend the client drink coffee in the evening.

61. The nurse is providing home care to an elderly woman who had a CVA and has right-sided hemiplegia. She is living with her daughter. Which observation indicates that the family needs more instruction?

    1. The client's arms and legs are exercised every day.

    2. The daughter gets her mother out of bed several times a day.

    3. The client is given a shower every other day.

    4. The daughter puts the chair on the right side of the bed when getting her mother out of bed.

62. The family of a 48-year-old woman who has multiple sclerosis and spends most of her time in bed or in a chair asks the nurse why they have been told they should have her take deep breaths and cough frequently. What should the nurse include in the reply?

    1. Deep breathing and coughing will help her to move her secretions so she will not develop pneumonia.

    2. Deep breathing and coughing help to prevent clots from developing in the lung.

    3. When she coughs she increases the amount of oxygen going to the brain, preventing confusion.

    4. Deep breathing increases blood flow to the brain and helps to keep her from getting depressed.

63. An adult is admitted with gastroenteritis. The physician has ordered prochlorperazine (Compazine) 10 mg po tid prn or prochlorperazine (Compazine) 5 mg suppository every 6 hours prn and loperamide (Imodium) 2 mg po prn. The client has an episode of dairrhea and complains of nausea. What should the nurse administer?

    1. Prochlorperazine (Compazine) by mouth

    2. Loperamide (Imodium)

    3. Prochlorperazine (Compazine) po and Loperamide (Imodium)

    4. Prochlorperazine (Compazine) via suppository

64. A clear liquid diet is ordered for an adult following surgery. All of the following are on the client's tray. Which should be removed by the nurse?

1. Ice cream

2. Beef broth

3. Apple juice

4. Iced tea

65. The nurse is administering digoxin to a six-month-old infant. Which finding would cause the nurse to withhold the medication and notify the charge nurse or the physician?

   1. Apical heart rate of 85

   2. Appears lethargic

   3. Circumoral cyanosis

   4. Respiratory rate of 38

66. The nurse is teaching a client how to care for a colostomy. Which factor indicates the client needs more instruction?

   1. The client says, "I will change the bag as soon as it gets full."

   2. The client is observed irrigating the colostomy while sitting on the toilet.

   3. The client positions the irrigating solution container at shoulder level.

   4. The client places a chlorophyll tablet in the drainage bag.

67. The nurse is caring for a client who has dentures. Which action by the nurse is not appropriate?

   1. Place a washcloth in the bottom of the sink before cleaning the dentures.

   2. Brush the dentures with toothpaste.

   3. Rinse the dentures with hydrogen peroxide.

   4. Remove the dentures from the mouth for cleaning.

68. The LPN/LVN is making assignments in a long-term care facility. Staff on duty include another LPN and a new certified nursing assistant.

Which client can most safely be assigned to the nursing assistant?

   1. Ms. A., 92 years old, has dementia and advancing congestive heart failure.

   2. Ms. B., 83 years old, has Alzheimer's and Parkinson's and is ambulatory with assistance.

   3. Mr. C., 76 years old, has just been transferred from an acute care facility where he had a total hip replacement four days ago.

   4. Mr. D., 29 years old, had a closed head injury and is in a semi-vegetative state with a tracheostomy and a gastrostomy.

69. The nurse is caring for a client who is terminally ill. Upon admission the client signed advance directives indicating she does not wish to have any resuscitative measures. The client is now in and out of consciousness. Her daughter comes to the nurse and says "I want everything done for my mother if she stops breathing." How should the nurse respond?

   1. Remove the "Do Not Resuscitate" order from the chart.

   2. Discuss the client's advance directives with the daughter.

   3. Have the daughter sign a consent form since her mother is in and out of consciousness.

   4. When the client is conscious ask her again what her wishes are.

70. When explaining Universal Precautions to a client, the nurse should explain that the primary purpose of Universal Precautions is to

   1. protect the client with a weak immune system.

   2. prevent the spread of AIDS.

   3. prevent nosocomial infections.

   4. reduce the spread of disease.

71. Upon entering a client's room the nurse sees and smells smoke and flames. What is the best initial nursing action?

    1. Attempt to fight the fire.
    2. Move the client out of the room.
    3. Close the door to the room.
    4. Evacuate everyone from the unit.

72. An adult who has liver disease secondary to alcohol abuse has just been told that alcohol is causing his health problems. The nurse expects that the client's initial response will most likely be which of the following?

    1. "I don't drink enough to hurt my health."
    2. "How could this happen to me? I've always been a good person."
    3. "Where can I get help to stop drinking so much?"
    4. "I've known for a long time that I drink too much. I guess I really have to stop now."

73. The client is receiving chemotherapy for cancer. Which statement, if made by the client, would indicate that she has accepted the diagnosis and treatment?

    1. "I hate getting that treatment."
    2. "The doctor isn't sure if I really have cancer."
    3. "I have a collection of pretty scarves that I am wearing a lot now."
    4. "I don't go anywhere except for my treatments because I look so weird."

74. A hospitalized client asks what is wrong with the person in the next bed. How should the nurse reply?

    1. Ask the client why he wants to know.
    2. Give the client a vague answer.
    3. Tell the client that information is confidential.
    4. Tell the client to ask the head nurse.

75. An adult is being admitted with possible pneumonia. His history indicates he had a tonsillectomy as a child and tuberculosis 10 years ago, which was arrested. Which room assignment is most appropriate?

    1. A room without a roommate
    2. Isolation
    3. A double room with a client who also has pneumonia
    4. A double room with a client who has angina

76. Which activities are appropriate to assign to a certified nursing assistant?

    1. Evaluate vital signs.
    2. Monitor tube feedings.
    3. Assist with activities of daily living.
    4. Discuss discharge insturctions.

77. An adult who recently had an amputation has an above-the-knee prosthesis. Which nursing action will do the most to help the client adjust to the prosthesis?

    1. Adjust the prosthesis for the client.
    2. Offer the client a cane or a walker for ease of movement.
    3. Place an "at risk for fall" sign on the client's door.
    4. Allow the client to manage his own care.

78. The nurse is monitoring a client who is going through barbiturate withdrawal. Which symptom is of most concern to the nurse?

    1. Nausea and vomiting
    2. Anxiety
    3. Hallucinations
    4. Seizures

79. An adult has a substance abuse problem. Which statement, if made by the client, indicates the best understanding of the problem?

1. "I can never use that drug again."

2. "When I am off the drug for two years, I will be cured."

3. "At least I shall be able to go to parties and limit my drugs."

4. "When I feel upset, I can call the support group."

80. The nurse is caring for a woman whose husband beats her regularly. Which is the most important long-term goal for this woman?

    1. Provide a long-term support group.

    2. Help her feel like a survivor.

    3. Point out the ways she behaved.

    4. Be able to blame the abuser.

81. The nurse has delegated the task of taking the temperature of a client with a new tympanic thermometer to a certified nursing assistant. The nursing assistant says, "This looks easy. I am good at figuring things out." What is the nurse's responsibility?

    1. Allow the nursing assistant to proceed.

    2. Assign the task to another nursing assistant.

    3. Ask another nursing assistant to demonstrate this task to the nursing assistant.

    4. Demonstrate the proper use of the thermometer and observe the nursing assistant.

82. While the nurse is preparing medications a code occurs. One of the nursing assistants offers to help by administering the medications. What is the best response by the nurse?

    1. Allow the nursing assistant to give the medications.

    2. Hold the medications until after the code.

    3. Give the medications and then help with the code.

4. Ask the nursing assistant when she was checked off on giving medications.

83. The nurse enters the room of a woman who had a vaginal hysterectomy three days ago and finds her crying. What is the best initial approach for the nurse?

    1. Ask her what seems to be troubling her.

    2. Reassure her that feeling depressed is normal after this type of surgery.

    3. Tell her that the nurse will ask the doctor to order hormones for her.

    4. Leave the room so she can work out her feelings.

84. A client who is scheduled for surgery today says to the nurse, "Do you think I'll survive the surgery?" What is the best initial response for the nurse?

    1. "Don't worry, your surgeon is good."

    2. "Tell me about your concerns."

    3. "I can call your clergyman."

    4. "We do a lot of these surgeries here; everything will be okay."

85. The nurse is assessing a client's emotional state and coping strategies. Evidence of which behavior is of most concern to the nurse?

    1. Anxiety

    2. Dysfunctional family unit

    3. Social isolation

    4. Self-mutilation

86. Following a motor vehicle accident the client does not know where he is or what year it is and has short-term memory impairment. Which nursing action is most appropriate?

    1. Offer several choices to the client.

    2. Give simple directions to the client.

    3. Give the client the details of the care.

    4. Offer written instructions to the client.

87. The nurse is changing a wet to dry dressing. Which action is appropriate?

    1. Pouring a sterile solution directly into a sterile container.
    2. Removing the old dressings with sterile gloves.
    3. Opening the sterile dressings wearing sterile gloves.
    4. Packing the wound wearing sterile gloves.

88. The nurse is providing home care for a client who is visually impaired. What safety precautions are most appropriate for this client?

    1. Remove scatter rugs.
    2. Have hand rails in the bathroom.
    3. Have side rails up whenever the client is in bed.
    4. Have a bell to call for help.

89. An adult client complains of dizziness when getting out of bed in the morning. Which instruction should the nurse give the nursing assistant regarding care of this client?

    1. Have the client wear slippers when getting out of bed.
    2. Have the client sit on the edge of the bed for a few minutes.
    3. Offer the client some juice before getting out of bed.
    4. Tell the client to stay in bed until she is no longer dizzy.

90. An adult had exploratory surgery and post-operatively had an exacerbation of asthma. The client is on a rebreathing mask and seems upset and angry. What is the best nursing approach?

    1. Ask the physician for an order for Ativan.
    2. Spend some time with the client.
    3. Ask the family to have someone stay with the client.
    4. Apply wrist restraints.

91. An adult client became incontinent while hospitalized. The client now drinks very little. The nurse understands that this is

    1. a coping strategy.
    2. a defense mechanism.
    3. a way to not bother the nurse.
    4. regression.

92. The nurse is evaluating the progress of a client who has had a cerebral vascular accident and realizes there has been limited progress. What should the nurse do?

    1. Transfer the client to another caregiver.
    2. Reassess the goals with the client.
    3. Request a longer hospital stay.
    4. Role-play the current plan with the client.

93. The nurse is assessing a client who may be bulimic. What objective finding indicates bulimia?

    1. Low self-esteem
    2. Loss of tooth enamel
    3. Feeling of loss of control
    4. Feeling of social inadequacy

94. When caring for an abused client, what is most important for the nurse to do initially?

    1. Provide a safe place for the victim.
    2. Refer the victim to a long-term support group.
    3. Make an appointment with a counselor.
    4. Make arrangements for the victim to confront the abuser.

95. The nurse is bathing a client who has contact isolation ordered. The nurse wears gloves. What else is needed?

    1. Face mask
    2. Sterile gloves
    3. Isolation cap
    4. Isolation gown

96. The nurse is performing a sterile dressing change. Which action is essential?

   1. Touching the corners of the dressing with clean gloves
   2. Discussing the wound with the client during the dressing change
   3. Irrigating the wound with an antiseptic solution
   4. Wearing sterile gloves during the dressing change

97. The nurse is teaching a client who has short-term memory loss how to use the call light. Which factor is least essential for the nurse to assess when teaching this client?

   1. Visual status
   2. Ambulatory difficulty
   3. Orientation to time, place, and person
   4. Understanding of the English language

98. An adult asks the nurse why she must have her skin shaved prior to surgery. What is the best nursing response? Reducing the hair by shaving

   1. reduces infection by removing hair, which harbors bacteria.
   2. provides a clean area on which to operate.
   3. disinfects the skin.
   4. makes it easier to see the surgical incision.

99. An adult who is undergoing diagnostic tests to diagnose a possible malignancy angrily says to the nurse, "You don't know anything. I want someone competent caring for me." What is the best initial nursing response?

   1. "I am a competent nurse. What would you like?"
   2. "It must be difficult having all those tests. How can I help you?"
   3. "I will get the supervisor who should be able to help you."
   4. "I will care for you, but you may not talk to me in that manner."

100. A client who is admitted for surgery reports drinking eight or nine beers everyday. Two days after surgery the nurse notes the client is shaking and seems disoriented. The nurse's response is based on which understanding of his behavior?

   1. The client has probably consumed alcohol since surgery.
   2. The client may be having a reaction to the narcotics used for pain control.
   3. The client is exhibiting signs of alcohol withdrawal.
   4. The client is most likely in severe pain.

Answers and Rationales for Practice Test Four

Answer	Rationale	NP	CN	SA

#1. **1.** **In Cushing's syndrome there are increased amounts of cortisol, which causes osteoporosis. This is an appropriate nursing diagnosis for someone who has Cushing's syndrome.**   Pl   Ph/9   1

    2. Pain related to cold intolerance would be an appropriate nursing diagnosis for someone who has hypothyroidism. Persons with Cushing's syndrome would be more apt to be warm than cold.

    3. Risk for deficient fluid volume would be an appropriate nursing diagnosis for someone with Addison's disease. The persons with Cushing's syndrome will have high risk for fluid volume excess due to increased amounts of aldosterone, which causes sodium and fluid retention.

    4. Risk for injury related to hypotension would be an appropriate nursing diagnosis for a person who has Addison's disease. A person with Cushing's syndrome will have hypertension.

#2. **3.** **Placenta previa is usually painless, and the client has bright red bleeding from the vagina.**   Dc   Ph/10   3

    1. Sudden knife-like pain in the lower abdomen accompanied by profuse vaginal bleeding is characteristic of abruption of the placenta.

    2. Dark red vaginal discharge can be normal following a pelvic exam at this point in pregnancy.

    4. A tender uterine wall and abdomen with no obvious vaginal bleeding is typical of abruption of the placenta.

#3. **1.** **The normal range for walking is about 7 months to 18 months. Not walking at 13 months is perfectly normal.**   Dc   He/3   4

    2. The normal range for walking is about 7 months to 18 months. Not walking at 13 months is perfectly normal.

    3. This response is inappropriate. The normal range for walking is about 7 months to 18 months. Not walking at 13 months is perfectly normal.

    4. This response is not appropriate and is incorrect information. The normal range for walking is about 7 months to 18 months. Not walking at 13 months is perfectly normal.

#4. 2. **The mother needs positive reinforcement for bringing the baby in,**   Im   He/3   4
but the immunizations will be delayed until the baby is well.

   1.   This is not correct. Immunizations are not given when the child has a
cold.

   3.   This is an inappropriate response. The shots do make the child
irritable, but they are not given when the child has a cold.

   4.   This is poor communication with the parent.

#5. 3. **The protrusion reflex disappears around four months of age.**   Im   He/3   4
Babies are usually ready for solids about this time.

   1.   Two months is too young for solids. The baby still has a strong
protrusion reflex.

   2.   The baby usually takes a quart of formula a day before the age of four
months.

   4.   There may be some truth to this statement, but it offers no guidelines
to the mother.

#6. 2. **Coarctation of the aorta is a narrowing of the descending aorta**   Dc   Ph/10   4
that causes a decrease in blood flow to the lower part of the body.
The classic sign of coarctation of the aorta is that the blood
pressure is higher in the upper extremities than in the lower
extremities.

   1.   Tachypnea (rapid respirations) is common in heart disease but is not
specific to coarctation of the aorta.

   3.   There is no murmur in coarctation of the aorta. A murmur is caused
when blood flows somewhere it doesn't usually go. This is not the
case with coarctation. Coarctation is a narrowing of the aorta.

   4.   Heart rate of 150 per minute is normal for an infant.

#7. 1. **Barbiturates such as phenobarbital frequently cause drowsiness.**   Im   Ph/8   5

   2.   Drowsiness does occur in the post-ictal phase (after a seizure).
However, the question says the child has not had a seizure so this is
not the cause of the drowsiness.

   3.   The drowsiness is probably related to the phenobarbital used to treat
the seizures.

   4.   Some persons do have an aura or a sensory experience that usually
occurs before a seizure. It is not usually drowsiness. The question
says that the child has had no seizures, so this is not likely to be the
cause of his drowsiness.

#8. 3. The blood volume increases by 50 percent by the end of the second trimester.

    1. Oxygen consumption is increased during pregnancy.

    2. The rate of peristalsis is decreased during pregnancy.

    4. Metabolic rate will increase during pregnancy.

#9. 2. Chlamydia, the most common sexually transmitted disease, and gonorrhea are the two major cuases of neonatal eye infections which, if untreated, could lead to blindness.

    1. Chlamydia is transmitted to the baby during the birth process. It is not transmitted through the placenta. Syphilis and HIV are blood-borne and can be transmitted through the placenta.

    3. Chlamydia infection is unrelated to pregnancy-induced hypertension.

    4. Chlamydia is unrelated to congenital (born with) anomalies. If picked up by the baby during the birth process, the baby can develop an eye infection, which could lead to blindness.

#10. 4. High blood sugar levels in the mother probably increased pancreatic production of insulin in the infant, and he may use his stores of sugar quickly. He now has no influx of sugar from the mother and is at risk for hypoglycemia.

    1. The baby of a diabetic woman is not at increased risk of infection.

    2. The baby of a diabetic woman is not at increased risk for hyperglycemia.

    3. The baby of a diabetic woman is not at increased risk for acidosis.

#11. 4. The woman may be turned and may receive oxygen, but the most important first action is to remove the source of the tetanic contraction, which is oxytocin.

    1. The nurse should stop the oxytocin. Slowing it down is not sufficient.

    2. The woman may be turned and may receive oxygen, but the most important first action is to remove the source of the tetanic contraction, which is oxytocin.

    3. The woman may be turned and may receive oxygen, but the most important first action is to remove the source of the tetanic contraction, which is oxytocin.

#12. 1. **The nurse should always listen to a laboring mother. This woman needs to be assessed again.**   Dc   He/3   3

     2. The nurse should always listen to a laboring mother. After she is checked, it may be appropriate to reassure the woman.

     3. A laboring woman does not push unless it is confirmed that she is fully dilated.

     4. The nurse should initially determine if the woman has progressed in labor. There is no data in the question to indicate the woman needs medication to relax.

#13. 1. **Airway takes priority over the other items.**   Im   He/3   4

     2. The nurse will keep the baby warm, but the highest priority is establishing an airway.

     3. The nurse will apply identification bracelets, but the highest priority is establishing an airway.

     4. The LPN/LVN does not legally determine APGAR scores.

#14. 1. **Long pants and long shirts are the best ways to prevent tick bites. Deer ticks transmit Lyme disease, and dog ticks transmit Rocky Mountain spotted fever. Both are serious diseases.**   Pl   He/4   1

     2. Sunscreen is important to prevent exposure to ultraviolet rays. Prolonged exposure to ultraviolet rays predisposes to the development of skin cancer. If the person perspires and the sunscreen is removed, more should be applied.

     3. The most important thing is to replace fluids. The person should bring plenty of water. Salt tablets are not recommended.

     4. Sensitive individuals can get severe poison ivy from the slightest exposure to the oils. If clothing rubs against the plant and the person touches the clothing, an allergic reaction can develop.

#15. 2. **Most cancer chemotherapeutic agents cause nausea as a side effect. Taking it in the evening means there is less nausea during meal times and awake times. It is often better tolerated.**   Im   Ph/8   5

     1. It is important to have a regular time to take medication. However, it does matter when the drug is taken. Most cancer chemotherapeutic agents cause nausea as a side effect. Taking it in the evening means there is less nausea during meal times and awake times. It is often better tolerated.

     3. Drowsiness is not a major side effect of most cancer chemotherapeutic agents. Lack of energy may develop as the bone marrow is depressed and the client has fewer red blood cells. Fatigue due to anemia is not related to the time when the medication is taken.

     4. Activity level does not alter the effectiveness of the cancer chemotherapeutic agents.

#16. 2. **The client has crackles and is beginning to collect fluid in the air spaces. The best thing for the nurse to do is to deep-breathe and cough the client every two hours. This should resolve the problem. The nurse will also record the findings and nursing actions.**   Pl   Ph/9   1

1. The client has crackles and is beginning to collect fluid in the air spaces. The best thing for the nurse to do is to deep-breathe and cough the client every two hours. This should resolve the problem. There is no need to start emergency oxygen. The nurse will record the findings and actions taken.

3. The client has crackles and is beginning to collect fluid in the air spaces. The best thing for the nurse to do is to deep-breathe and cough the client every two hours. This should resolve the problem. The nurse will record the findings and actions. There is no need for an emergency call to the physician and no need for a tracheostomy.

4. The client has crackles and is beginning to collect fluid in the air spaces. The best thing for the nurse to do is to deep-breathe and cough the client every two hours. This should resolve the problem. The nurse will continue to observe the client. This finding does not suggest an immediate risk of cyanosis.

#17. 1. **The nurse should have a tracheostomy set at the bedside along with oxygen and suction. The client is at risk for airway obstruction.**   Pl   Ph/9   1

2. There is no need for a catheterization tray at the bedside for a thyroidectomy client.

3. There is no need for a sterile dressing set at the bedside for a thyroidectomy client.

4. There is no need for a ventilator at the bedside for a thyroidectomy client.

#18. 4. **Iron colors the stools black.**   Ev   Ph/8   4

1. The child's color should improve and the energy level should increase if the child is receiving the iron regularly. This observation may indicate the child is not receiving the medication.

2. Oral administration of iron should not cause brown spots on the skin. IM iron could cause brown spots.

3. Iron should not cause dark-colored urine.

#19. 2. Hydration is important to prevent sickling episodes. Dehydration causes a decrease in oxygen tension, which causes sickling. This response indicates that the parents understand how to reduce the incidence of sickling.   Ev   Ph/9   4

  1. The child can play outdoors. The child should be adequately hydrated, especially when the weather is hot. This response indicates the parents do not understand how to reduce the incidence of crisis.

  3. The child with sickle cell should not receive aspirin. Aspirin is acetyl salycylic acid. Acidosis causes sickling. The child should receive acetaminophen and lots of fluids if he develops a fever. This response indicates the parents do not understand how to reduce the incidence of crisis.

  4. Flying is dangerous for the person who has sickle cell. The oxygen saturation is less at high altitudes. Low oxygen saturation can cause sickling. It would be better for the child to ride in a car than fly in an airplane. This response indicates the parents do not understand how to reduce the incidence of crisis.

#20. 2. When coal tar preparations are used, the client should protect the areas from sunlight for 24 hours.   Im   Ph/8   1

  1. Nausea and vomiting are not frequent side effects of coal tar preparations.

  3. The substance stays on for at least 24 hours. It should not be washed off in 6-8 hours.

  4. Coal tar is black and may make the skin look dark.

#21. 2. When the client is in shock the pulse rate increases, the blood presure decreases, and the pulse pressure decreases.   Dc   Ph/10   1

  1. The BP is higher than the baseline and the pulse pressure is wider. This finding is suggestive of increased intracranial pressure, not shock.

  3. This blood pressure reading is so close to the baseline any change is insignificant.

  4. A pulse rate of 60 in this client would suggest rising intracranial pressure, not shock.

#22. 3. Rather than responding specifically to the complaint that the assignment is unfair, the nurse should determine what the nursing assistant's real concern is and help her to address that.   Im   Sa/1   1

    1. This is a very authoritarian response and does nothing to ease the situation.

    2. This approach will not solve the problem and may be impossible to carry out.

    4. The charge nurse could assign the other nurse to assist as needed. However, discussing the real issues and concerns is much more appropriate.

#23. 3. Tremors are consistent with alcohol withdrawal. The other signs and symptoms are consistent with blood loss and shock.   Dc   Ph/10   1

    1. BP of 90/60 is consistent with blood loss and shock from the GI bleed. It is not symptomatic of alcohol withdrawal.

    2. Dizziness is consistent with blood loss and shock from the GI bleed. It is not symptomatic of alcohol withdrawal.

    4. Pallor is consistent with blood loss and shock from the GI bleed. It is not symptomatic of alcohol withdrawal.

#24. 2. Heavy alcohol intake can damage the liver and cause a prolonged prothrombin time.   Dc   Ph/9   1

    1. Eating or not eating meat is not likely to affect the prothrombin time.

    3. Heparin does not affect prothrombin time. Heparin affects partial thromboplastin time and clotting time.

    4. A recent injury should not cause the prothrombin time to be prolonged.

#25. 3. Walking may help the stone to move down through the urinary tract and be passed in the urine. The client who has kidney stones is often more comfortable ambulating.   Im   Ph/10   1

    1. Walking may help the stone to move down through the urinary tract and be passed in the urine. The client who has kidney stones is often more comfortable ambulating.

    2. Walking may help the stone to move down through the urinary tract and be passed in the urine. The client who has kidney stones is often more comfortable ambulating.

    4. There is no need to limit ambulation to once a day. Walking may help the stone to move down through the urinary tract and be passed in the urine. The client who has kidney stones is often more comfortable ambulating.

#26. 4. **The recommendation is that all women age 50 and over have annual mammograms. Symptoms are a late sign of breast cancer.**   Im   He/4   3

    1. It is normal for breasts to be tender before the period. She is younger than the age recommended for regular mammography. Mammograms are not indicated for this client.

    2. There is no need to do a mammogram for a sports injury. There is a common misconception that a physical injury to the breast causes cancer. This does not appear to be true.

    3. There is no need to do a mammogram for a woman who has been breastfeeding. In fact, breastfeeding is thought to help protect a woman from breast cancer.

#27. 3. **Older persons are particularly at risk for pneumonia. Pneumovax is highly recommended.**   Dc   He/4   1

    1. DPT is diphtheria, pertussis, and tetanus. Pertussis is not given after the age of six. If she hasn't had a tetanus shot in the last 10 years, she may need a booster shot. DPT or pertussis (whooping cough) is not given.

    2. MMR is measles, mumps, rubella. Pneumovax is more important than MMR. Most persons in this age group had these diseases as children. The immunization was not available when they were children.

    4. HIB is hemophilus influenza B which is given to infants to help prevent meningitis caused by h. influenza B. This is not given to adults.

#28. 1. **Preadolescent and early adolescent girls are at the most risk for scoliosis (lateral curvature of the spine). They should be told to wear a bathing suit under their clothing the day of the exam. During the exam they will remove their outer clothing, and the nurse will examine them. They will be asked to bend over and hang their arms down so the nurse can assess whether the shoulders and the hips are even.**   Dc   He/4   4

    2. Scoliosis is a lateral curvature of the spine. A urine test is not the screening approach.

    3. Scoliosis is a lateral curvature of the spine. Hair washing is not related to the assessment process.

    4. Scoliosis is a lateral curvature of the spine. There is no examination of the feet when assessing for scoliosis.

#29. 2.   Induration or a raised area 10 mm or more indicates a positive   Dc   He/4   1
reaction and should be referred for follow-up.

1.   A red area does not indicate a positive response. A tuberculin skin
test should be read with the fingers (feeling a raised area), not the
eyes.

3.   Itching does not indicate a positive response to a tuberculin skin test.
A tuberculin skin test should be read with the fingers (feeling a raised
area), not the eyes.

4.   A rash does not indicate a positive response to a tuberculin skin test.
A tuberculin skin test should be read with the fingers (feeling a raised
area), not the eyes.

#30. 1.   A tuberculin skin test is given intradermally, at a 10-degree angle.   Im   He/4   1

2.   A tuberculin skin test is given intradermally, at a 10-degree angle.

3.   A 60-degree angle is appropriate for a subcutaneous injection. A
tuberculin skin test is given intradermally, at a 10-degree angle.

4.   An intramuscular injection is given at a 90-degree angle. A tuberculin
skin test is given intradermally, at a 10-degree angle.

#31. 4.   Medicines should be in a locked cabinet. Toddlers are good   Ev   He/4   4
climbers. A high shelf is not adequate to prevent curious toddlers
from ingesting medicines. This statement indicates a need for
more instruction.

1.   This statement is correct. Toddlers should be in front facing car seats
in the back seat. This statement indicates the mother understands
child safety.

2.   Toddlers need constant supervision. This statement indicates the
mother understands child safety.

3.   Any household that has toddlers should have syrup of ipecac to
administer in case the child accidentally ingests a poison. This
statement indicates the mother understands child safety.

#32. 2.   Black stools can be an indication of upper GI bleeding. The nurse   Dc   Ph/7   1
should ask the client if he is taking iron. Iron causes stools to be
black.

1.   A bowel movement every other day is normal for many people.

3.   Sometimes straining at stool is normal. The client should be told to
eat more roughage to promote a softer stool.

4.   Three stools a day is normal for many people, especially if they eat a
lot of fruits and vegetables.

#33. 3.   The colostomy should be irrigated at the same time each day. This helps to promote regular function. This answer indicates the client understands the care of his colostomy.

Ev   Ph/7   1

1.   The client should use warm water, not hot water to irrigate the colostomy. Hot water is too irritating. This answer indicates the client does not understand the care of his colostomy.

2.   Alcohol causes pain if applied to irritated skin. This answer indicates the client does not understand the care of his colostomy.

4.   When possible, the irrigation should be performed in the bathroom in an upright position. This is the normal place and position for moving the bowels. This answer indicates the client does not understand the care of his colostomy.

#34. 3.   Pain is what the client says it is. Autonomic symptoms such as changes in vital signs are usually not seen in chronic pain.

Dc   Ph/7   1

1.   Persons with chronic pain often do not exhibit grimaces and other physical signs of pain.

2.   Autonomic symptoms such as changes in vital signs are usually not seen in chronic pain.

4.   Autonomic symptoms such as changes in vital signs are usually not seen in chronic pain.

#35. 3.   This response best meets her needs for rest and activity. Since she has been very ill and on bed rest for several days, the nurse should increase her activity slowly.

Pl   Ph/7   1

1.   This option does not allow the client to rest after the bath before getting her out of bed. She has been very ill with a respiratory condition and has limited oxygenation. Her activities should be spaced.

2.   Having her get out of bed for the first time and bathe herself for the first time is probably too much for this older woman, who has been very ill.

4.   Having her give herself the bed bath and then immediately get up in a chair is probably too much for this older woman, who has been very ill.

#36. 2. **Red drainage in the nasogastric tube immediately following surgery is normal. The nurse should record the amount and color and continue to observe the client.**   Dc   Ph/7   1

    1. The drainage as described is normal. There is no need to report this immediately. It should be recorded and the nurse should continue to observe the client.

    3. The drainage is normal. The nurse should not apply pressure to the operative site.

    4. There is no need to place the client in Trendelenburg's position. Bloody drainage in the nasogastric tube during the first few hours after surgery is normal.

#37. 2. **Prior to administering a tube feeding, it is essential for the nurse to be sure the tube is in the stomach. One of the best ways is to aspirate drainage and check the pH. Stomach contents are acid.**   Im   Ph/7   1

    1. The client should be positioned in a semi-Fowler's position for a tube feeding. Supine position increases the risk of aspiration.

    3. The nurse may routinely check vital signs. However, checking vital signs is not essential before administering a tube feeding.

    4. The nurse might ask the client if she feels full. However, aspirating the contents is essential. When aspirating the contents to check for proper position of the tube, the nurse will also note the amount of feeding returned. This is a better indication of residual than asking the client if she feels full.

#38. 2. **The nurse should instruct the client to splint (hold) the incision when deep-breathing and coughing to prevent pressure on the suture line.**   Im   Ph/9   1

    1. The nurse should instruct the client to take in several deep breaths and then cough while exhaling the last one, then repeat the cycle.

    3. The client needs to take deep breaths when lying in bed. The moving client has less need of deep-breathing exercises than the one who does not move.

    4. Deep-breathing exercises are most needed for those who are confined to bed.

#39. 1. **All of the clients are older. The one who has a broken hip will likely be most immobile and thus most at risk for skin breakdown.**   Pl   Ph/9   1

    2. There is no data to suggest that this client is immobile. Most persons with angina are somewhat mobile.

    3. There is no data to suggest that this client is immobile.

    4. There is no data to suggest that the asthma client is immobile.

#40. 2. **A blood glucose check or Accucheck is performed by puncturing the finger on the side.**   Im   Ph/9   1

    1. The thumb is not the appropriate place to puncture.

    3. The LPN/LVN does not perform venipunctures for a routine blood glucose check.

    4. Blood is not collected in a vial when a routine blood glucose check is performed.

#41. 1. **The client's symptoms suggest a urinary tract infection. The specimen for culture should be obtained before medications are administered. After getting the specimen for culture, the client will want the pyridium, which is a urinary tract anesthetic.**   Pl   Ph/9   1

    2. Gantrisin is a sulfa drug. The nurse should ask the question about allergies before administering the drug. However, the nurse should initially obtain the clean catch urine for culture to confirm the diagnosis and allow identification of the causative organism.

    3. The nurse should initially obtain the clean catch urine for culture to confirm the diagnosis and allow identification of the causative organism. Before administering the Gantrisin the nurse should ask the client if she is allergic to sulfa drugs. Gantrisin is a sulfa drug.

    4. Pyridium is a urinary tract anesthetic that is commonly given to clients who have urinary tract infections. The nurse should obtain the clean catch urine first to confirm the diagnosis and identify the causative organism.

#42. 2. **The parents should check the toes for warmth. Cold toes would indicate the leg was not receiving adequate blood. The cast may be too tight.**   Im   Ph/10   4

    1. A fiberglass cast does not dissolve in water. However, the casted extremity cannot be put in water. Water will get under the cast and cause skin damage because it cannot evaporate under a fiberglass cast. To take a bath the child must either keep his leg out of the tub or wrap both ends of the fiberglass cast in plastic to prevent water from getting under the cast.

    3. A fiberglass cast dries almost instantly. There is no need to keep it uncovered. This would be necessary for a plaster cast.

    4. The casted leg should be kept elevated for the first couple of days to prevent swelling.

#43. 2. **Thrombocytopenia is a condition in which the client has too few**   Im   Ph/10   1
            thrombocytes or platelets. Platelets clot blood. The client is at risk
            for bleeding and should not use dental floss or a firm bristle
            toothbrush.

   1. There is no particular need for the client with thrombocytopenia to
       call the nurse when going to the bathroom.

   3. The client with thrombocytopenia is not infectious and not
       particularly at risk for infection. Thrombocytopenia is a condition in
       which the client has too few thrombocytes or platelets. Platelets clot
       blood.

   4. The client with thrombocytopenia is not at great risk for infection.
       Thrombocytopenia is a condition in which the client has too few
       thrombocytes or platelets. Platelets clot blood.

#44. 3. **The data all suggest the client is hypoglycemic. The appropriate**   Im   Ph/10   1
            intervention for hypoglycemia is to give something that has
            sugar in it. Cola has sugar.

   1. The data all suggest the client is hypoglycemic. Administering insulin
       would make the client worse. The client needs sugar.

   2. The nurse should be able to determine from the client's signs and
       symptoms that she is hypoglycemic. It would be appropriate for the
       nurse to do a blood glucose check. It is not necessary for the nurse to
       call the lab and wait for the results. The nurse should be able to
       determine the client's condition and act immediately.

   4. All the data suggest that the client is hypoglycemic. The client needs
       sugar, not water.

#45. 4. **The baby's eyes should be covered during the time the light is on**   Pl   Ph/10   4
            to prevent damage to the eyes.

   1. There is no need to keep the infant NPO before the treatment. The
       baby needs adequate fluids.

   2. There is no need to keep the mother away from the baby. The
       treatment may be done in the nursery but standard rules would apply.
       Parents can administer phototherapy at home.

   3. The nurse would do routine monitoring of the infant's vital signs, but
       no special monitoring of pulse rate beyond that is needed.

ANSWER	RATIONALE	NP	CN	SA

#46. 3. **The data suggest that the child probably has either a sprained ankle or a broken ankle. The nurse should elevate the foot and apply a cold pack to reduce bleeding and swelling at the site.**

Im   Ph/10 4

1. The foot should be elevated, not put down. Putting the foot down causes more swelling.

2. Cold, not heat, should be applied to a freshly injured ankle. Heat would encourage bleeding and swelling.

4. The data suggest the child has either a sprain or a break. The nurse does not need to risk further injury by asking the child to move the ankle.

#47. 2. **The focus of the question was evaluation of the client's response to oxygen. Oxygen should decrease the client's respiratory rate.**

Ev   Ph/10 1

1. The client may have chest pain with congestive heart failure. However, decrease in chest pain may be due to several factors. It is not the best indicator of the effectiveness of oxygen.

3. A person who has congestive heart failure will also be given furosemide (Lasix). A large urine output indicates the Lasix was effective. Oxygen does not increase urine output.

4. A person who has congestive heart failure will also be given furosemide (Lasix). A decrease in edema indicates the Lasix was effective. Oxygen does not decrease edema.

#48. 4. **Darkening the client's room reduces stimuli, which can cause seizures.**

Pl   Ph/10 1

1. Playing the client's favorite music may be appropriate later. To prevent seizures, the client's room should have as few auditory and visual stimuli as possible.

2. The client should have neurological checks periodically, but stimulating the client would be apt to cause seizures, not prevent them.

3. Keeping a padded tongue at the bedside does not prevent seizures. It was formerly used during a seizure. Now, it is no longer recommended that something be put in the client's mouth during a seizure.

ANSWER   RATIONALE   NP   CN   SA

#49. 1. **Bright red drainage from a nasogastric tube on the day of**   Im   Ph/10 1
surgery is normal. The nurse should chart color and amount.

2. This finding is normal. There is no need to report immediately to the charge nurse.

3. This finding is normal. The suction system does not need to be turned off.

4. This finding is normal. There is no need to apply pressure to the wound. Bloody drainage in the NG tube on the day of surgery does not mean the client is hemorrhaging from the wound.

#50. 2. **A transphenoidal hypophysectomy is the removal of the pituitary**   Im   Ph/9   1
gland. The incision is in the mouth above the gum line and goes
through the sphenoid sinuses into the brain. Drainage in the
mouth could be cerebrospinal fluid. The nurse should test the
secretions for glucose. Cerebrospinal fluid tests positive for
glucose. If cerebrospinal fluid is leaking out, organisms can
enter the brain.

1. A person who has had a transphenoidal hypophysectomy recently should not blow his nose. A transphenoidal hypophysectomy is the removal of the pituitary gland. The incision is in the mouth above the gum line and goes through the sphenoid sinuses into the brain.

3. Having the client rinse his mouth is not the essential nursing action.

4. There is no data to suggest that this client needs an antiemetic.

#51. 2. **The nurse should initially palpate the abdomen. If the client's**   Im   Ph/10 1
ulcer has perforated or ruptured, the client's abdomen will be
rigid and board-like. After palpating the abdomen the nurse
should call the physician or notify the charge nurse.

1. The nurse should call the physician after palpating the client's abdomen.

3. The nurse should call the physician before obtaining a stool for guaiac.

4. The client will be placed in a semi-Fowler's position.

#52. 1. **An elevation in temperature is often the first sign of a transfusion**   As   Ph/8   1
reaction. Temperature should be monitored every 15 minutes
times 2, then in 30 minutes, and then hourly during the rest of
the transfusion.

2. Blood pressure may be monitored, but the most important thing to monitor is the temperature.

3. The nurse may assess respirations, but the most important thing to monitor is the temperature.

4. Pulse may be assessed, but the most important thing to monitor is the temperature.

#53. 2. **O negative is the universal donor and can be given to anyone.**   Im   Ph/8   1

     1. O negative is the universal donor and can be given to anyone.

     3. O negative is the universal donor and can be given to anyone. AB positive is the universal recipient.

     4. O negative is the universal donor and can be given to anyone.

#54. 4. **The client who is vomiting will go into metabolic alkalosis.**   Dc   Ph/10   1

     1. These values indicate respiratory acidosis, which might occur with chronic lung disease.

     2. These values indicate metabolic acidosis, which might occur with diabetes and diarrhea.

     3. These values indicate respiratory alkalosis, which might occur with hyperventilation.

#55. 3. **A walker is the best choice for a client who had foot surgery yesterday, had a recent broken arm, and suffers from arthritis, which also is likely to decrease mobility.**   Pl   Ph/7   1

     1. An elderly person who had surgery on her right foot yesterday is probably not ready for a quad cane. A cane is held on the nonaffected side. A recently broken left arm would make using a cane difficult.

     2. A client who has had foot surgery and a recent broken arm is not a candidate for crutches. The weight-bearing necessary for crutch walking is likely to reinjure her arm. She will be unable to bear weight on her foot.

     4. An elderly person who had foot surgery yesterday is probably not ready for a tripod cane. She will be unable to bear weight on her foot. A cane is held on the nonaffected side. A recently broken left arm would make using a cane difficult.

#56. 4. **The ratio of chest compressions to breaths for one-person rescue is fifteen to two.**   Im   Ph/10   1

     1. The ratio of chest compressions to breaths for one-person rescue is fifteen to two. Five to one is the ratio for two-person rescue.

     2. The ratio of chest compressions to breaths for one-person rescue is fifteen to two.

     3. The ratio of chest compressions to breaths for one-person rescue is fifteen to two.

#57. 2. **Continuous bubbles in the suction control chamber indicate the system is functioning correctly.**   Ev   Ph/9   1

1. There should be bubbles in the water seal chamber. No bubbles in the water seal chamber indicates either that the lung has re-expanded or that there is an obstruction in the tubing. The tube was inserted today. The lung is not likely to have re-expanded.

3. There should not be bubbles in the drainage chamber.

4. The fluid in the water seal chamber should fluctuate slightly with respiration.

#58. 2. **Portable wound suction ahould always be maintained below the level of the wound. Otherwise it will not drain.**   Im   Ph/9   1

1. The drainage device should not be removed until the physician removes it.

3. There is no need to completely empty the collection device before ambulating. If it is full, it could be emptied.

4. The suction apparatus should not be disconnected before ambulating. The physician will remove the device.

#59. 3. **The client who has had a hip replacement should keep the hip extended and abducted. A pillow between the legs will keep the hip abducted and prevent adduction.**   Im   Ph/7   1

1. The client should have his position changed frequently (every two hours).

2. The client who has had a total hip replacement should be maintained in extension.

4. The client who has had a total hip replacement should be maintained in abduction.

#60. 3. **Many older persons nap during the day and then have difficulty sleeping during the night. The client should be encouraged to stay awake during the day to see if this will improve nighttime sleeping.**   Im   Ph/7   1

1. The nurse should initially try nonpharmacologic methods to help the client sleep. If these are not successful the nurse may ask the physician for an order for sleeping medication.

2. Exercises tend to increase metabolism and keep people awake. Exercises should not be done just before bedtime.

4. Coffee and other caffeine-containing beverages should not be consumed during the evening as they are stimulants and keep people awake. Many older persons can no longer drink caffeine-containing drinks after noon because it keeps them awake.

#61. 4. The chair should be put on the unaffected side when transferring a hemiplegic to a chair. The daughter's technique is not correct and she needs more instruction.

Ev   Ph/7   1

1. It is appropriate to exercise the client's arms and legs every day. This does not indicate a need for further instruction.

2. It is appropriate for the daughter to get her mother out of bed several times a day. This does not indicate a need for further instruction.

3. It is appropriate to give a shower every other day to an 80-year-old woman. Most older clients do not need a daily shower. This action does not indicate a need for further instruction.

#62. 1. Deep-breathing and coughing expands alveoli and helps the client to move secretions so she will not develop pneumonia.

Im   Ph/7   1

2. Leg and foot exercises help to prevent deep-vein thrombophlebitis which usually causes blood clots in the lungs. Deep-breathing and coughing expands alveoli and helps the client to move secretions so she will not develop pneumonia.

3. There may be some truth to this statement. However, the major reason deep-breathing and coughing is encouraged is to expand alveoli and prevent the accumulation of secretions in the lungs.

4. There may be some truth to this statement. However, the major reason deep-breathing and coughing is encouraged is to expand alveoli and prevent the accumulation of secretions in the lungs.

#63. 3. Compazine is an antiemetic and is given for nausea and vomiting. Because the client has nausea but is not vomiting, the oral route is indicated. Imodium is for diarrhea. The client has had an episode of diarrhea, so the Imodium should be given.

Im   Ph/8   5

1. The client has nausea but is not vomiting. The prochlorperazine can be given by mouth. The client also has diarrhea and so should be given loperamide.

2. Loperamide is appropriate. However, the client also has nausea and should receive prochlorperazine as well.

4. The client is not vomiting and so can probably take the prochlorperazine by mouth. The client also has diarrhea and should receive loperamide as ordered.

#64. 1. Ice cream is a milk product and is not a clear liquid.

Im   Ph/7   6

2. Beef broth is a clear liquid.

3. Apple juice is a clear liquid.

4. Iced tea is a clear liquid.

#65. 1. **When an infant's apical heart rate is below 100, the nurse should**   Dc   Ph/8   4
        withhold the medication and notify the charge nurse or the
        physician.

2. An infant who needs digoxin may well have little energy and appear
    lethargic. Lethargy is not necessarily a side effect of digoxin.

3. Circumoral cyanosis is common in infants who have cardiac disease.
    Digoxin is a heart drug. Circumoral cyanosis is not a side effect of
    digoxin.

4. A respiratory rate of 38 is normal for a six-month-old infant.

#66. 1. **The client should not change the bag each time it gets full. The**   Ev   Ph/7   1
        client should empty the bag when it is half full. This comment
        indicates incorrect behavior and a need for more instruction.

2. The toilet is the ideal place for irrigating a colostomy. This behavior
    indicates the client understands the procedure.

3. The irrigating solution container should be placed at shoulder height.
    This behavior indicates the client understands the procedure.

4. Chlorophyll tablets are used to prevent odors in the colostomy bag.
    This behavior indicates the client understands how to care for the
    colostomy.

#67. 3. **There is no need to rinse the dentures with hydrogen peroxide.**   Im   Ph/7   1
        Dentures should be rinsed with water.

1. A washcloth should be placed in the bottom of the sink to prevent
    breakage of dentures if they should drop.

2. Dentures can be brushed with toothpaste.

4. Dentures should be removed from the mouth for cleaning.

#68. 2. **A nursing assistant should be able to handle a client who has**   Pl   Sa/1   1
        Alzheimer's and Parkinson's and is ambulatory with assistance.

1. The new nursing assistant should probably be able to care for a client
    who has dementia. However, this client also has advancing
    congestive heart failure. A new nursing assistant is not likely to have
    the skills needed to monitor a client who has advancing CHF.

3. The client is a new client who has had a total hip replacement. The
    client needs special positioning. A new nursing assistant is not likely
    to be skilled in caring for this client.

4. A new nursing assistant is not likely to be skilled in caring for a client
    who has a tracheostomy and a gastrostomy.

#69. 2. **The nurse should discuss the client's advance directives with the daughter. Advance directives are the client's wishes and should be followed.**   Im   Sa/1   1

    1.   The nurse does not have the authority to change the order. The client's wishes are not to be resuscitated, and the physician has written the order.

    3.   The purpose of an advance directive is to be sure the client's wishes are followed even when the client is no longer able to make decisions. The nurse cannot simply have the daughter sign away her mother's wishes.

    4.   The client made advance directives so she would not have to make decisions at this time. There is no need to bother her with this again. If this is to be discussed with the client at this time, it should be the daughter who does it.

#70. 4. **The primary purpose of Universal Precautions is to reduce the spread of disease by preventing the mode of transmission of the organism.**   Pl   Sa/2   1

    1.   Reverse or protective precautions are used to protect the client who has a weak immune system.

    2.   Diseases other than AIDS are prevented by the use of Universal Precautions.

    3.   Nosocomial infections are hospital-acquired infections. Universal Precautions will help to prevent nosocomial infections; however, this is not the primary purpose.

#71. 2. **The nurse should initially remove the client from the room. Remember RACE (Rescue, Alarm, Contain, Evacuate).**   Im   Sa/2   1

    1.   The nurse should initially rescue the client and sound the alarm.

    3.   The nurse should not close the door to the room until removing everyone from the room.

    4.   The nurse should initially remove the client from the room. Remember RACE (Rescue, Alarm, Contain, Evacuate.)

#72. 1. **The most common defense mechanism in substance abusers is denial. Denial is also the most common initial response to a bad diagnosis.**   Dc   Ps/6   2

    2.   Anger response is not usually the initial response to a diagnosis of a serious illness.

    3.   Most persons who are confronted with being an alcoholic are not initially going to ask how to get help.

    4.   The person who is addicted to alcohol and is confronted with the effects of this addiction is not likely to initially ask for help.

#73. 3. **Chemotherapy often causes allopecia (loss of hair). Wearing scarves indicates the client has accepted the side effects of chemotherapy.**   Ev   Ps/5   2

   1. This statement does not indicate acceptance of the diagnosis and treatment.

   2. This statement indicates the client has not accepted her diagnosis.

   4. This statement idnciates the client has not accepted her diagnosis.

#74. 3. **The nurse should tell the client in a nice way that information about other clients is confidential.**   Im   Sa/1   1

   1. The nurse should tell the client in a nice way that information about other clients is confidential.

   2. The nurse should tell the client in a nice way that information about other clients is confidential.

   4. The nurse should tell the client in a nice way that information about other clients is confidential.

#75. 2. **A client who has a history of tuberculosis should be isolated when admitted with a respiratory infection. Even after the disease is arrested, the tuberculosis organism is apt to remain walled off in the person's lungs and may activate when the person is under extreme stress or has a respiratory infection. The person should be isolated until sputum cultures prove that tuberculosis has not recurred.**   Pl   Sa/1   1

   1. A private room does not protect staff from tuberculosis. A client who has a history of tuberculosis should be isolated when admitted with a respiratory infection. Even after the disease is arrested, the tuberculosis organism is apt to remain walled off in the person's lungs and may activate when the person is under extreme stress or has a respiratory infection. The person should be isolated until sputum cultures prove that tuberculosis has not recurred.

   3. A client who has a history of tuberculosis should be isolated when admitted with a respiratory infection. Even after the disease is arrested, the tuberculosis organism is apt to remain walled off in the person's lungs and may activate when the person is under extreme stress or has a respiratory infection. The person should be isolated until sputum cultures prove that tuberculosis has not recurred.

   4. A client who has a history of tuberculosis should be isolated when admitted with a respiratory infection. Even after the disease is arrested, the tuberculosis organism is apt to remain walled off in the person's lungs and may activate when the person is under extreme stress or has a respiratory infection. The person should be isolated until sputum cultures prove that tuberculosis has not recurred.

#76. 3. **Assisting with ADLs is an appropriate activity for the nursing assistant.** Pl   Sa/2   1

    1. A nursing assistant may take the vital signs, but the nurse is responsible for evaluating them.

    2. Monitoring tube feedings is the responsibility of the nurse.

    4. The discussion of discharge instructions is the responsibility of the nurse.

#77. 4. **The nurse should respect the client's dignity and self-esteem. Allowing the client to manage his own care as much as possible will promote self-esteem.** Pl   Ps/5   1

    1. The nurse should encourage the client to adjust the prosthesis as this is a task he must learn to do by himself.

    2. There is no data to suggest the client needs a cane or a walker.

    3. There is no data to suggest the client is at risk for falls.

#78. 4. **Seizures can be life-threatening and are the most dangerous of the symptoms.** Dc   Ps/6   1

    1. Nausea and vomiting are unpleasant but are not life-threatening symptoms.

    2. Anxiety is unpleasant but is not life-threatening.

    3. Hallucinations can be frightening but are not life-threatening.

#79. 1. **Persons who are addicted to a substance should never use that substance again.** Ev   Ps/6   2

    2. Persons who are addicted to drugs are not cured. Once they are no longer using the substance they must avoid the substance. If they start to use the substance again, the inability to control the use of the substance returns. This response indicates either a lack of knowledge or denial by the client.

    3. Persons who are addicted to drugs are not cured. Once they are no longer using the substance they must avoid the substance. If they start to use the substance again, the inability to control the use of the substance returns. This response indicates the client lacks understanding of the problem.

    4. The client should be participating in the support group on a regular basis, not just when upset.

#80. 2. **The most important long-term goal is for the victim to feel as though she has survived the ordeal and can rebuild her self-esteem.**   Pl   Ps/6   2

    1. A long-term support group is helpful but is not the most important long-term goal for this client.

    3. Pointing out her behavior is not helpful to the victim. She needs to rebuild her life.

    4. Blaming the abuser serves no useful purpose. The victim needs to rebuild her life.

#81. 4. **The nurse is responsible for assigning and supervising the tasks assigned to the nursing assistant.**   Im   Sa/1   1

    1. Personnel should not be allowed to use equipment if they have not been instructed in how to use it.

    2. The problem is the nursing assistant does not know how to use the new thermometer. The nurse should instruct the staff member on how to use the equipment. There is no data to suggest the need for the temperature is so immediate that another person must be assigned to the task.

    3. Nursing assistants are not responsible for teaching other nursing assistants. Teaching the nursing assistant is the nurse's responsibility.

#82. 2. **The code takes priority. The need is immediate. Most medications can safely be administered slightly late.**   Pl   Sa/1   1

    1. The nursing assistant is not qualified or licensed to give medications. Medications should only be administered by the person who prepared them.

    3. The code takes priority over administering medications.

    4. Giving medicatons is not a function of the nursing assistant. Because this is not a task that the nursing assistant can do, it is not possible for the nursing assistant to have been checked off on this procedure.

#83. 1. **The nurse should initially assess the client.**   Im   Ps/5   1

    2. This response minimizes the client's feelings and does not help the nurse to determine what the client's problem is.

    3. The best initial response is for the nurse to assess the client and allow her to express her feelings.

    4. Avoiding the client is not the best initial response. The nurse should initially determine the nature of the client's concerns.

#84. 2. This open-ended comment will allow the client to express thoughts and fears. — Im / Ps/5 / 2

  1. This stereotypical response minimizes the fears of the client.

  3. Calling the clergyman is not the best initial response. The nurse should explore the client's concerns and then call the clergyman if appropriate for this client.

  4. False reassurance is not helpful to the client.

#85. 4. Self-mutilation is a cry for help and needs to be addressed immediately because it shows ineffective coping strategies. — Dc / Ps/5 / 2

  1. Anxiety is not as serious a concern as self-mutilation.

  2. A dysfunctional family unit is of concern but not as serious a concern as self-mutilation.

  3. Social isolation is a cause of concern but not as serious a concern as self-mutilation.

#86. 2. The client may be able to process simple instructions. Too much information is likely to confuse the client further. — Pl / Ps/5 / 1

  1. Offering several choices is likely to further confuse the client.

  3. The client has short-term memory loss. Giving details of care is likely to cause further confusion.

  4. The client may not be able to interpret the written word.

#87. 4. The wound is considered the center of the sterile field. The nurse must wear sterile gloves whenever in contact with the area. — Im / Sa/2 / 1

  1. Pouring sterile solution directly into a sterile container is not appropriate. The nurse should pour some solution out of the container first to eliminate bacteria on the lip of the container.

  2. There is no need to wear sterile gloves when removing a dressing. The nurse should wear clean gloves to protect the nurse.

  3. Wearing sterile gloves to open sterile dressings contaminates the sterile gloves when the unopened packages are touched.

#88. 1. A visually impaired client may have difficulty seeing the rugs and fall. — Pl / Sa/2 / 1

  2. Handrails are nice to have but are not particularly indicated because the client is visually impaired.

  3. There is no indication the client is at risk for a fall from the bed.

  4. Having a bell is not especially helpful for the visually impaired. They may have difficulty locating the bell.

ANSWER	RATIONALE	NP	CN	SA

#89. 2. **Sitting on the edge of the bed for a few minutes gives time for the body to adapt to an upright position. This decreases dizziness and reduces the chance the client will fall.**   Pl   Sa/2   1

1. Wearing slippers when getting out of bed will not help the dizziness. Wearing slippers may be appropriate but is not related to the client's complaint of dizziness when getting up.

3. The client complained of dizziness when getting out of bed in the morning. The most likely problem is orthostatic hypotension. Drinking juice will not help this problem. Drinking juice might be appropriate if the client had low blood sugar.

4. The client complained of dizziness when getting out of bed in the morning. The data does not indicate the client is dizzy before getting up. Staying in bed is not likely to solve the problem and will create additional problems.

#90. 2. **Spending time with the client will give the nurse the opportunity to listen to concerns and find the source of the client's anger.**   Im   Ps/5   1

1. Chemically restraining the client will not help to identify the problem. Use of chemical restraints is not the first choice.

3. Having someone stay with the client might be helpful, but it does not help the nurse find out what is bothering the client.

4. Wrist restraints should only be applied when the client is in danger of hurting himself or others. There is no data to suggest that wrist restraints are necessary. Applying restraints is likely to make the client more upset and angry.

#91. 1. **This is a coping strategy on the part of the client.**   Dc   Ps/5   2

2. The behavior described is a coping strategy, not a defense mechanism.

3. The behavior described is a coping strategy. There is no data to suggest what the client is thinking when adopting this coping strategy.

4. The behavior described is a conscious choice and does not indicate regression-adopting behaviors more appropriate for an earlier age.

#92. **2.** **The nurse should work with the client to set goals. Sometimes the goals have to be changed or adapted to the progress the client is making.**   Ev   Sa/1   1

　　1. Transferring the client to another caregiver does not solve the problem. There is no data to suggest that the nurse is not giving adequate care.

　　3. A longer stay may not be the solution to the problem. The nurse should involve the client in the care plan.

　　4. Role-playing the current care plan is not likely to be an effective solution to the problem.

#93. **2.** **Loss of tooth enamel is an objective sign of bulimia.**   Dc   Ps/6   1

　　1. Low self-esteem is a subjective symptom often associated with bulimia.

　　3. Feeling loss of control is a subjective symptom often associated with bulimia.

　　4. Feeling social inadequacy is a subjective symptom often associated with bulimia.

#94. **1.** **The nurse should first provide for the client's safety.**   Pl   Ps/6   2

　　2. Referral to a long-term support group is appropriate but is not the initial priority. Safety is the initial priority.

　　3. Making an appointment with a counselor is appropriate but is not the initial priority. Safety is the first priority.

　　4. Confronting the abuser is dangerous and not an appropriate action.

#95. **4.** **An isolation gown is needed because the nurse is in direct contact with the client.**   Im   Sa/2   1

　　1. A face mask is indicated for respiratory conditions.

　　2. Sterile gloves are not needed for contact isolation. Sterile gloves are used when dealing with open wounds to protect the client from the nurse.

　　3. An isolation cap is not needed for contact isolation.

#96. **4.** **Sterile gloves must be worn during the dressing change.**   Im   Sa/2   1

　　1. Touching the corners of the dressing with clean gloves is a violation of sterile technique and introduces organisms. Sterile gloves should be worn when touching the dressing.

　　2. Talking over a sterile field is not appropriate. Bacteria may enter the wound.

　　3. Irrigating the wound might be done if ordered by the physician. There is no data in this question to indicate such an order.

#97. 2. The nurse is teaching the client how to use the call light. Problems with ambulation are not relevant.   Dc   Sa/2   1

  1. The nurse should assess the client's ability to see the call light.

  3. The nurse should assess the client's orientation status as this will help determine the client's ability to learn.

  4. The client should be able to understand the instructions.

#98. 1. Hair habors bacteria, which can cause infections.   Im   Sa/2   1

  2. There is some truth to this answer. However, the best response is the primary reason for removing hair, which is the removal of a source of bacteria.

  3. Removing hair does not disinfect the skin.

  4. There is some truth to this answer. However, this in not the best answer because it is not the major reason for removing hair.

#99. 2. The nurse should initially respond with empathy and recognition of the client's feelings. The client's anger is probably stemming from the possible diagnosis and the tests, not the nurse's actions. An empathetic response will help to establish rapport with the client and is appropriate initially.   Im   Ps/5   2

  1. The nurse should not initially respond with a defensive reaction. This is likely to escalate the situation. The nurse should recognize that the client's anger is most likely the result of the possible diagnosis and the tests, not the nurse's behavior.

  3. Getting the supervisor is not the best initial response. The nurse should recognize that the client's anger is most likely a result of the possible diagnosis and the tests, not the nurse's behavior.

  4. Trying to change the client's behavior is not the best initial response. The nurse should recognize that this client's anger is most likely related to the possible diagnosis and the tests, not the nurse's behavior. The client's behavior is not likely to be a deliberate attempt to put the nurse down.

#100. 3. **Tremors (shaking) and disorientation are suggestive of alcohol withdrawal. Consuming eight or nine beers daily is evidence the client is an alcoholic. Suddenly stopping alcohol intake will cause withdrawal symptoms.**

1. If the client had consumed alcohol since surgery he would not be having symptoms of withdrawal. Shaking and disorientation are symptoms of withdrawal.

2. The symptoms of shaking and disorientation are suggestive of withdrawal, not a reaction to narcotic analgesics.

3. The symptoms of shaking and disorientation are consistent with withdrawal. It may be possible that shaking and disorientation could be due to pain. However, given the history of heavy alcohol abuse, the nurse should consider this option.

Practice Test Five

1. An infant had a repair of a myelomeningocele two days ago. Which assessment is most important to detect a problem commonly seen following myelomeningocele repair?

   1. Bowel sounds

   2. Neuro checks

   3. Blood pressure in all four extremities

   4. Head circumference

2. The mother of a two-year-old tells the nurse she is embarrassed when her child plays with other children because he does not share his toys or even interact with the other children. The nurse's response to the mother is based on the knowledge that a two-year-old usually engages in which type of play?

   1. Solitary

   2. Parallel

   3. Cooperative

   4. Collaborative

3. The parents of a child with Tetralogy of Fallot ask the nurse why it is called a cyanotic heart defect. The nurse responds that it is called a cyanotic heart defect because

   1. It has four separate defects.

   2. It involves left-to-right shunting.

   3. It involves right-to-left shunting.

   4. Blood flow to the lungs is poor.

4. A mother brings her one-month-old son to the clinic for a well-baby visit. The child has a moderately severe hypospadias that was seen by a urologist in the newborn nursery. The mother is upset that the doctors would not circumcise her son before he was discharged. What information should the nurse include when responding to the mother?

   1. The foreskin should not be removed, as it will be used in the repair of the hypospadias.

   2. The child's condition did not allow for elective surgery. It will be done at a later date when he is stronger.

   3. Circumcision is a surgical procedure. Because he will have surgery in the near future, it will be done at the same time to avoid two surgeries close together.

   4. The procedure was not done because circumcision is medically unnecessary, not because he has a hypospadias.

5. An eight-year-old is admitted to the hospital with pneumonia. The child has had frequent respiratory infections. A chloride sweat test is ordered. The nurse knows the reason for this test is to rule out which condition?

   1. Pernicious anemia

   2. Diabetes insipidus

   3. Cystic fibrosis

   4. Glomerulonephritis

6. Written instructions to pregnant women include instructions to perform Kegel's exercises. One of the women asks the nurse why these exercises are important. The nurse should reply that the purpose of these exercises is to

   1. Increase circulation to the uterus

   2. Strengthen the muscles of the pelvic floor

   3. Prepare the breasts for nursing

   4. Condition the pregnant woman for the "work" of childbirth

7. A 26-year-old woman with a history of heart disease is admitted in labor. She has been on bed rest for four months to prevent dyspnea. During labor this client is likely to receive which of the following?

1. Extra intravenous fluid to expand her blood volume
2. General anesthesia
3. Instruction to push by holding her breath and bearing down
4. Epidural anesthesia

8. All of the following women are seen in the physician's office. Which is at greatest risk for pre-term labor?

   1. A primigravida who has gained 30 pounds during her pregnancy
   2. A 35-year-old carrying a small baby
   3. A 21-year-old pregnant with twins
   4. A 40-year-old who has four other children

9. A new mother asks the nurse when the baby's umbilical cord will fall off. The nurse replies that it usually takes how many days to detach?

   1. 1–2 days
   2. 3–5 days
   3. 7–10 days
   4. 15–20 days

10. A new mother is two days postpartum, is breastfeeding her infant, and now is preparing for discharge. She states that for contraception she is going to use her diaphragm, which she still has. The nurse's response should be based on which information?

    1. Diaphragms need to be refitted after the birth of a baby.
    2. As long as the diaphragm is in good shape, the client can continue to use it.
    3. Diaphragms are not good contraceptives for postpartal women.
    4. Since the client is breastfeeding, she will not need her diaphragm for four to six months.

11. A laboring woman has been pushing for one hour and is not making progress. The nurse knows that which of the following could hinder the descent of the fetus in the second stage of labor?

    1. A full bladder
    2. Paracervical block given during the first stage of labor
    3. Mother placed in a side-lying position
    4. Fetus in LOA (left occiput anterior) position

12. The nurse is providing home care to a man who had a transphenoidal hypophysectomy. Which behavior by the client indicates a need for more teaching?

    1. He bends over to tie his shoes.
    2. He tells the nurse he takes a lot of pills every day.
    3. He ambulates daily.
    4. He tells the nurse he has ordered a medical identification bracelet.

13. An adult has been diagnosed with Bell's palsy and asks what causes it. The nurse knows that which of the following is correct?

    1. Bell's palsy is caused by the chickenpox virus.
    2. The cause is unknown.
    3. Bell's palsy usually follows a cold or influenza.
    4. Trauma to the area brings on the symptoms.

14. Magnetic resonance imaging has been ordered for a client. Which factor should the nurse report to the physician?

    1. The client states she had an allergic reaction to iodine.
    2. The client has a pacemaker.
    3. The client wears a hearing aid.
    4. The client takes digoxin.

15. A woman is admitted with Hodgkin's disease. Which does the nurse expect the client to report?

    1. Swollen lymph nodes
    2. A painful rash
    3. Stomach pain
    4. Joint pain

16. A client who has congestive heart failure is being admitted. How should the nurse position this client?

    1. Supine
    2. Sim's
    3. Semi-Fowler's
    4. Side-lying

17. Which assessment is most essential before administering digoxin to an adult?

    1. Ask the client if he has chest pain.
    2. Take an apical pulse.
    3. Take the client's blood pressure.
    4. Ask the client if he is short of breath.

18. The LPN/LVN is caring for an adult who has pneumonia. The nurse should instruct the nursing assistant to report which information immediately?

    1. Restlessness
    2. Pink-colored skin
    3. Nonproductive cough
    4. Dry mouth

19. A low-sodium, high-potassium diet is ordered for a client. Which food selection made by the client indicates understanding of the prescribed diet?

    1. Orange juice, baked chicken, and a cucumber and tomato salad
    2. Milk, roast beef, and spinach salad
    3. Iced tea, fish sandwich, and mixed vegetables

4. Cola, fried shrimp, and coleslaw

20. The nurse is teaching unlicensed personnel about preventing the spread of disease in the health care environment. The nurse knows the personnel understand when they state that which is the most important way to prevent the spread of disease?

    1. Isolating infected clients
    2. Consistently washing hands
    3. Wearing a gown when there is a client with a questionable disease
    4. Wearing gloves whenever giving care

21. The LPN/LVN is to perform a sterile procedure. Which action will maintain a sterile field?

    1. Keeping the sterile field within the line of vision
    2. Opening sterile packages with sterile gloves
    3. Talking to others over the sterile field
    4. Handing the physician medicine over the sterile field

22. A 56-year-old man is visiting the doctor for the first time in seven years for treatment for an infected finger. The office nurse wants him to make an appointment for a physical. The nurse knows he does not understand the importance of a physical when he makes which statement?

    1. "I know my blood sugar and weight should be monitored."
    2. "I am healthy. If I wasn't, I'd have some problems."
    3. "I don't smoke and I exercise daily."
    4. "I understand checking my blood pressure is important."

23. The nurse is preparing a client for a KUB (kidney-ureter-bladder x-ray). What is included in the preparation?

1. Keeping the client NPO
2. Explaining the procedure
3. Catheterizing the client
4. Administering an enema

24. The nurse is caring for a client who has a cervical radioactive implant. Which action is not appropriate for the nurse when caring for this client?

   1. Post a radioactive symbol on the client's chart and the door to the room.
   2. Put on gloves to remove any radioactive implant that may have come out.
   3. Wash hands with soap and water after caring for the client.
   4. Limit the amount of time with the client.

25. The nurse is preparing a client environment that will reduce the chance of falls. Which action is appropriate?

   1. Keep the side rail down on the side the client gets out of bed.
   2. Keep the lights down since glare bothers some clients.
   3. Call housekeeping to clean up the spilled water.
   4. Make sure that a path is cleared to assist the client when walking.

26. A nurse's aide who had a tuberculosis test planted two days ago has a reddened area 15-mm in diameter. The aide asks the nurse what this means. The nurse understands that the test result is

   1. positive, indicating the aide has been exposed to tuberculosis.
   2. positive, indicating the aide has active tuberculosis.
   3. a false negative and must be repeated.
   4. negative; redness without induration is of no significance.

27. A woman who has emphysema is on continuous oxygen therapy. She appears anxious and short of breath. Her husband increases the oxygen flow to 6 liters/min. The nurse knows this action is most likely to

   1. make breathing easier.
   2. decrease her blood oxygen levels.
   3. have no impact on blood oxygen levels.
   4. cause her to stop breathing.

28. An adult who is waiting for a cardiac catheterization is joking with the staff. The nurse understands that this behavior is most likely

   1. a coping mechanism for the client.
   2. an inappropriate behavior for a serious procedure.
   3. a defense mechanism of denial.
   4. a defense mechanism of rationalization.

29. An adult had an open cholecystectomy and has an open wound. The client refuses to look at the area during the dressing change. What is the most likely reason for this behavior?

   1. Denial of surgery
   2. Change in body image
   3. The client fears becoming nauseated at the sight of the wound
   4. The client does not like the sight of blood

30. The nurse is supervising an unlicensed person who is giving oral care to an unconscious client. Which observation indicates that the unlicensed person needs further instruction?

   The client
   1. is in a lateral position with the head turned to the side during oral care.
   2. is positioned in high-Fowler's position.
   3. has a towel placed under the chin.
   4. remains in the lateral position for 30 minutes after oral care.

31. Which activity should not be assigned to an unlicensed person?

    1. Record all oral intake.
    2. Measure all output.
    3. Record output on appropriate graphs.
    4. Complete the 24-hour I & O record.

32. The nurse observes a client using a walker. Which observation indicates the client needs more instruction?

    1. The client uses the walker to pull herself out of a chair.
    2. The client moves the walker forward, then takes a step.
    3. The client complains the walker is not waist-high.
    4. The client sometimes does not use the walker.

33. A hearing-impaired client is becoming withdrawn and depressed. He reports that even with a hearing aid he is having increased difficulty hearing. Which suggestion is least likely to be helpful?

    1. Get a hearing guide dog.
    2. Join a social club.
    3. Get a telephone TDD.
    4. Get a closed-caption TV.

34. An adult is taking phenazopyridine hydrochloride (Pyridium) 200 mg PO TID after meals. Which comment by the client indicates a lack of understanding about the medication?

    1. "If I take my medications after meals I avoid upsetting my stomach."
    2. "I am concerned that my urine is bright orange."
    3. "I do not have as great an urge to urinate since I have been on Pyridium."
    4. "I have to let my doctor know if my skin or eyes turn yellow."

35. An adult who is hospitalized with congestive heart failure is receiving an intravenous infusion. The nurse is checking the IV. Which of the following is of greatest concern to the nurse?

    1. The insertion site
    2. The volume infused
    3. The frequency with which the tubing is changed
    4. The presence of a flashback

36. The nurse is working to prevent falls in a restraint-free environment. Which of the following is inappropriate for the nurse to delegate to assistive personnel?

    1. Making sure the bed is in low position
    2. Making sure the bedside table is within reach of the client
    3. Assessing the safety needs of the client
    4. Monitoring client behavior for potential falls

37. Prior to administering a feeding, the nurse checks for placement of a feeding tube. What is the best way to do this?

    1. Check for residual.
    2. Measure the pH of aspirated gastrointestinal fluid.
    3. Inject 10–20 ml of air while auscultating over the epigastric area.
    4. Ask the client to talk or hum.

38. The nurse has assigned a nursing assistant to give the client a bath. Which observation reported by the nursing assistant requires immediate attention by the nurse?

    1. A red area on the back that disappears after it is massaged.
    2. A red area on the hip that does not go away after the area is massaged.
    3. The client's insistence on doing most of the bath.

4. The indwelling urethral catheter is draining clear, amber urine.

39. The nurse is evaluating how a client who has a halo brace is reacting to this change in his body image. Which statement by the client indicates a need for additional support in adjusting to the brace?

   1. "I shall avoid going out in public since I may bump into people."
   2. "I don't mind that people look at me."
   3. "I told my grandchildren that this looks like a space helmet."
   4. "I like to sleep in the reclining chair that we have."

40. A throat culture is ordered for an adult who has a sore throat. The nurse asks the client if he has taken any medications to treat himself. Which medication, if reported by the client, would be of greatest concern to the nurse?

   1. Aspirin
   2. A throat lozenge
   3. Acetaminophen
   4. An antibiotic

41. The nurse is preparing to give an adult a subcutaneous injection of heparin. What should the nurse check prior to giving the medication?

   1. International Normalized Ratio (INR)
   2. Bleeding time
   3. Prothrombin time
   4. Partial thromboplastin time

42. A young woman has routine blood work done at her prenatal appointment. The results indicate she has a hemoglobin of 10 gm/dl. The nurse explains to her that this result is

   1. high.
   2. insignificant.
   3. low.
   4. normal.

43. The nurse is caring for a client who has congestive heart failure. Which finding indicates her condition is getting worse?

   1. An increase in urine output
   2. A decrease in blood pressure
   3. A decrease in heart rate
   4. Warm, moist skin

44. A seventy-two-year-old woman is being treated for pneumonia. Physician's orders include an antibiotic, oxygen PRN for O2 saturation less than 90, pulse oximetry every 4 hours. The nurse obtains a pulse oximetry reading of 82% on room air. What is the best action for the nurse to take?

   1. Report the finding to the physician.
   2. Report the finding to the registered nurse to get instructions.
   3. Start supplemental oxygen.
   4. Start oxygen and repeat the pulse oximetry in 20 minutes.

45. A fourteen-year-old is going home with a permanent tracheostomy. Which comment by the child's parent indicates to the nurse that the parent needs more instruction?

   1. "I need to ask the doctor how many times a day I can suction my child."
   2. "I will suction if my child cannot effectively cough up sputum."
   3. "I know my child will not need the same amount of suctioning every day."
   4. "I know I should only suction my child if it is really necessary."

46. The nurse is working on a plan to assist an abused client back into the work situation. Which will most likely be most helpful in decreasing the trauma for the client?

    1. Support from significant others
    2. Support from a counselor
    3. Support from friends
    4. Support from coworkers

47. A ten-year-old child is admitted to the hospital with injuries. Which finding most suggests that additional assessment for child abuse is indicated?

    1. The child asks to have friends visit.
    2. The child asks to have a teacher bring in homework.
    3. The child's parents state that they need to spend some time with the child's siblings.
    4. The child's parents will not leave the child alone while in the hospital.

48. The nurse is to move a client up in bed without any help. Where should the nurse place the client's pillow?

    1. At the bottom of the bed
    2. On the bedside stand
    3. At the head of the bed
    4. Under the client's head

49. The nurse's neighbor complains to the nurse that he feels tired all the time. Which comment suggests to the nurse that the man may have a serious sleep disorder?

    1. "My wife complains because I snore off and on all night."
    2. "I like to nap in the afternoon."
    3. "I wake up early every morning."
    4. "My muscles seem to jerk as I fall asleep."

50. A mentally retarded, nonverbal, ambulatory client is found sitting on the floor unable to get up. The LPN/LVN notes the client appears to be in great pain and his right leg is out of alignment. What is the most important action for the nurse to take as the client is readied for ambulance transport?

    1. Give the client pain medication.
    2. Immobilize the leg.
    3. Gather any medical records that need to accompany the client.
    4. Complete the incident report and other documentation.

51. The nurse enters an adult's room to premedicate for surgery. The client says, "You know, nurse, that form I signed said something about a nephrectomy. What does that mean?" How should the nurse respond initially?

    1. "What did your surgeon explain to you about your operation?"
    2. "Don't worry about the technical terms. We'll take good care of you."
    3. "I think you're just nervous about the surgery. This injection will make you feel calmer."
    4. "It is a kidney operation."

52. An insulin-dependent diabetic is admitted with a blood sugar of 415 mg/dL. His wife states, "He always follows his diabetic diet religiously and administers his insulin using a sliding scale twice a day." Upon reviewing his chart, the nurse notes that the client has been hospitalized four times during the past three months for a medical diagnosis of hyperglycemia secondary to noncompliance with medical regimen. When questioned, he says, "It's a little too complicated to keep track of when I need to eat, and when I need to check my blood and take my medicine."

    Which nursing diagnosis is most appropriate?

    1. Impaired adjustment
    2. Impaired home maintenance

3. Ineffective therapeutic regimen management

4. Noncompliance

53. The nurse who is the primary caregiver for an adult client receives a telephone report from the Microbiology Department that the client's blood culture is positive for gram negative rods. The client is not on antibiotics. What should the nurse do first?

1. Document the result in the appropriate area of the chart.

2. Inform the client that we now know what is causing his illness.

3. Place a call to the physician and document the results of the lab work and the notification of the physician in the nurse's notes.

4. Place the laboratory report on the client's chart as soon as possible.

54. While giving a report at 3:15 in the afternoon, the nurse realizes that she/he forgot to chart the client's physical therapy, which occurred at 10:30 A.M. Which is the appropriate action for the nurse to take?

1. Ask the incoming nurse to record it.

2. Date and time and entry for 3:15 P.M. "Late entry (date: 10:30 A.M.)" before making the addition.

3. Do not add the information to the chart. Complete an incident report for the omitted charting and forward it to the risk management department.

4. Because it is already charted by the physical therapists in their progress notes, the nurse does not need to "double chart" the same information. The nurse does not have to do anything.

55. The nurse notes a client has received a medication by mistake. What should the nurse do?

1. Notify the physician, complete an incident report and make a separate note, in the nursing documentation, of the error, the client's response, and any treatment received by the client due to the medication error.

2. Complete an incident report and reference it in the nurse's notes.

3. Make a note of the error and any treatment the client receives because of the error in the nurse's notes.

4. Report the error to the nursing supervisor and the client's physician and document any treatment prescribed in the nurse's notes.

56. A newly diagnosed diabetic has worked as a manual laborer all his life. He requires teaching so that he can manage his diabetes after discharge. The nurse has given him booklets designed for clients who need an introduction to diabetes. When the nurse evaluates his learning from the booklets, he says he doesn't have his glasses and couldn't read the booklets. When the nurse offers large-print material, he says his wife usually takes care of things at home, and that you should work with her because she prepares all the meals and keeps track of the medicines for both of them. Which understanding of the client's behavior is most likely correct?

1. He is in denial about his diagnosis.

2. He is not willing to take responsibility for his own learning.

3. He cannot read.

4. He is too anxious about his new diagnosis to be able to process any new information at this time.

57. The nurse is caring for a preschooler who needs stitches resulting from an injury received during play in the yard. What would be the most appropriate way to prepare the child for the treatment he will receive?

1. Tell the child the nurse and the doctor will "make things all better."
2. Use dolls and explain through play and simulation what will be done.
3. Explain to the child slowly and precisely the steps that will be taken in his treatment.
4. Tell the child that he will have minimal scarring and that any marks will diminish over time.

58. A 76-year-old man living at the long-term care facility has lost 10 pounds in the last two months. He states that although he has had dentures for two years, they have not felt comfortable for the past three or four months so he rarely uses them at mealtime. The nurse's first priority would be to ask the client's physician to do which of the following?

1. Order a mechanical soft or edentulous diet for the client.
2. Order a dental consult to correct the client's problem.
3. Order a dietary consult to assist the client in making educated food choices.
4. Talk to the client regarding the proper use of dentures.

59. A client who has hypokalemia asks the nurse for dietary advice on what foods would help this problem. What should the nurse tell the client?

1. Eggs and cheese
2. Fruits, especially oranges, bananas, and prunes
3. Green leafy vegetables
4. Breads and cereals

60. The client complains of frequent insomnia affecting her ability to rest well. Which of the following factors or lifestyle choices in her assessment history most likely contribute to her inability to sleep?

1. Having a slight snack at bedtime
2. Heart disease prevention of one baby aspirin each day
3. Reading in bed prior to going to sleep
4. Smoking packs of filtered cigarettes each day

61. The client is unable to adequately bathe himself because he has dressings on his hands that cannot get wet. What is the most appropriate nursing diagnosis for this assessment finding?

1. Risk for infection
2. Deficient knowledge
3. Pain related to specific illness or disease process
4. Self-care deficit (bathing/hygiene)

62. The nurse has delegated care of a client who is very hard of hearing to an unlicensed person. Which of the following would be the least helpful information to give to the unlicensed person to better facilitate communications with the client?

1. Reduce background noise.
2. Adjust the hearing aid.
3. Anticipate what the client may say and finish the statement for the client.
4. Face the client when speaking to the client.

63. The nurse is assessing a 16-year-old mother for potential child abuse. Which factor is most important when assessing potential for child abuse?

1. Age of the mother
2. Marital status
3. Socioeconomic status
4. Abuse as a child

64. An adult is receiving intermittent tube feedings. When the nurse aspirates and measures the gastric contents, the client's wife asks the nurse what she is doing. What information is most important to include in the response? The procedure is done to

1. test that the tube is working.
2. check the placement of the tube.
3. check for gastric emptying.
4. clear the line.

65. Before giving furosemide (Lasix) to an adult, the nurse checks the laboratory report for the last serum potassium level. Which finding would be of concern to the nurse?

1. 3.2 mEq/L
2. 3.7 mEq/L
3. 4.1 mEq/L
4. 4.9 mEq/L

66. A six-year-old was just diagnosed with pediculosis capitis. Which comment by the mother of the child indicates to the nurse in the physician's office that she does not understand how this condition is spread?

1. "I need to wash all his bedsheets in hot water."
2. "I will call the school nurse and tell her."
3. "I think he got this at our neighbor's house; it's very dirty."
4. "I will tell my son not to wear other children's hats."

67. An 85-year-old woman is hospitalized with a fractured hip. She complains to the LPN/LVN that she feels something is wrong and her chest hurts. The nurse notes the client has tachypnea. What should the nurse do immediately?

1. Administer oxygen.
2. Take vital signs.
3. Elevate the head of the bed.
4. Give aspirin.

68. Joan is at lunch in the hospital cafeteria with a nurse coworker. Joan is very allergic to nuts and always carries her anaphylactic kit with her. Joan tells her coworker that there must have been nuts in something she ate as she is having increasing difficulty breathing. What should the nurse do immediately?

1. Take her to the hospital emergency room.
2. Administer the medication in her friend's anaphylactic kit.
3. Call the floor for help.
4. Monitor the symptoms.

69. A client who had bowel surgery is to be NPO for several days. The nurse anticipates that the client will have an order for

1. diet therapy.
2. enteral nutrition.
3. parenteral nutrition.
4. nasogastric tube feedings.

70. A client who has mycoplasma pneumonia needs to go to the radiology department for a chest x-ray. What should the client wear?

1. A face shield
2. A surgical mask
3. An N 95 respirator
4. Gloves and a gown

71. A new client is admitted with a major abscess on her thigh caused by scratching mosquito bites with dirty hands after digging in her garden. She is on isolation precautions in a private room after surgical debridement. The physician changes her dressings daily. What should the nurse wear when providing care for this client?

1. An N 95 respirator and gloves
2. Eye protection and a face mask
3. Gloves and gown
4. A gown only

72. The nurse is assisting in the attempt to control bleeding from an artery. What personal protection equipment should be worn?

    1. Gloves only
    2. Gown, gloves, mask, and goggles
    3. Mask and gown
    4. None because time should not be wasted

73. A 63-year-old woman is taking digitalis, baby aspirin, K-Dur, and Lasix daily. She complains of multiple symptoms, which include muscle cramps and facial tics. Physical exam reveals positive Chvostek's and Trousseau's signs, hypotension, and confusion. The nurse suspects she has hypomagnesemia. What else should the nurse expect?

    1. Laboratory tests to reveal high serum calcium and potassium levels.
    2. Laboratory tests to reveal low serum calcium and potassium levels.
    3. Altered acid-base balance, which requires administration of $NaHCO_3$ intravenously in addition to treatment for hypomagnesemia.
    4. To monitor cardiac function since hypomagnesemia often causes bradycardia episodes and altered ECG waves.

74. An adult has experienced significant vomiting and diarrhea for the past 24 hours. Her chloride level is 90 mEq/L. What would the nurse expect to find when interpreting her sodium level?

    1. It would be high.
    2. It is impossible to predict the sodium level with this information.
    3. It would be low.
    4. It would be normal.

75. A post-operative client has an NG tube following bowel surgery. The orders read, "acetaminophen 650 PRN for fever above 101°F." The client has a temperature of 101.4°F. What is the most appropriate nursing action?

    1. Administer the acetaminophen by rectal suppository.
    2. Administer the acetaminophen by elixir through the NG tube and turn suction off for 30 minutes.
    3. Administer the acetaminophen by crushing two tablets, giving it through the NG tube, and turning suction off for 30 minutes.
    4. Call the physician and question the order.

76. The nurse is preparing a client with a severe case of inflamed hemorrhoids for a rectal examination by the physician. What is the best position to place her on the examination table?

    1. Dorsal recumbent
    2. Knee-chest
    3. Sim's
    4. Lithotomy

77. The nurse notes that the client has a pulse deficit. What is the most appropriate action for the nurse?

    1. Document this as a normal finding.
    2. Instruct the client to report to the clinic for a weekly re-evaluation.
    3. Report this finding immediately to the client's physician.
    4. Teach the client how to monitor pulse at home.

78. A post-operative client has pain medication ordered PRN for discomfort. During the first assessment, the nurse notes that the client has not received pain medication all day. His vital signs are within normal limits, but he is sweating profusely. He smiles at you while speaking and states that he is not hot but is still experiencing some pain and has been since early this morning. What is the most appropriate nursing action?

1. Administer the largest dose of pain medication allowed because he has been without it all day and then allow him to rest undisturbed.

2. Administer the minimum dose of medication and reassess his level of pain 30 minutes after administration.

3. Hold the pain medication because his vital signs are within normal limits, and he is smiling and showing no evidence of being in pain.

4. Encourage the client to continue to do without pain medication so he won't become addicted to the opioid.

79. A woman is scheduled for a biopsy and possible mastectomy in the morning. She is crying and says, "I am so upset because I watched my mother die from ovarian cancer." What is the most appropriate nursing diagnosis?

   1. Fear
   2. Anxiety
   3. Ineffective family coping
   4. Spiritual distress

80. Which diagnosis for the client with tuberculosis would have the greatest impact on public health?

   1. Ineffective breathing pattern
   2. Deficient knowledge
   3. Fatigue
   4. Ineffective therapeutic regimen management

81. A client comes to the emergency room with complaints of "numbness, tingling, and coldness" of her left leg. She is able to walk. You note that the skin appears pale and is cool to the touch. What should the nurse do first?

   1. Ask if she had had a similar condition in her arms or the other leg.
   2. Notify the physician immediately.

3. Obtain a detailed nursing health history.

4. Palpate and record the femoral, popliteal, posterior tibial, and dorsalis pedis pulses in the affected leg.

82. The nurse has taken vital signs of a 95-year-old client: oral temperature 98.6°F; pulse 84 with a regular irregularity; respirations 18 and blood pressure 140/86. Which nursing assessment(s) should be done first to obtain more data?

   1. Apical pulse for one minute
   2. Carotid pulse and temperature
   3. Full respiratory system assessment
   4. Positional blood pressure readings

83. An adult has returned to the nursing care unit following abdominal surgery. She has an order for meperidine IM prn for severe pain or acetaminophen #3 PO prn for mild to moderate pain. You ask the client if she is experiencing pain now and she states, "Yes, I am." What is the most appropriate initial action for the nurse?

   1. Administer the meperidine since she is less than 24 hours post-op.

   2. Administer the acetaminophen #3 because meperidine can be given if the acetaminophen doesn't relieve the pain.

   3. Assess the client further as to the location and degree of pain using a pain scale.

   4. Reposition the client and help her perform some relaxation exercises to reduce her reliance on opioids.

84. The nurse is admitting an adult woman to the ambulatory surgery unit at 6:30 A.M. The assessment reveals that her blood pressure is elevated, her pulse and respirations are rapid, she is diaphoretic, and she has dilated pupils. The nurse attempts to reinforce her pre-operative teaching for today's surgery, but the woman cannot restate anything about her previous instructions. She is wringing her hands and seems to be on the verge of tears. What is the most appropriate initial nursing action?

1. Administer her prescribed pre-operative medication now.
2. Ask her, "How are you feeling right now?"
3. Repeat all her pre-operative instructions slowly.
4. Notify her surgeon of the client's emotional status.

85. The client states, "My discharge plan leaves me with a lot to do. I don't think I can do it. I'm never good at doing things." The nurse knows the client lacks

1. maturation.
2. organization.
3. a readiness to learn.
4. self-efficacy.

86. The nurse is caring for an older client who insists on having a "hot toddy" laced with liquor at bedtime to help her sleep. How should the nurse respond in order to give culturally sensitive and appropriate care?

1. "Is that something you learned from a relative or a friend?"
2. "No one your age should be drinking at bedtime."
3. "That is an old wive's tale. The doctor can prescribe a sleep aid if you need one."
4. "We don't allow alcohol in the hospital."

87. A 55-year-old woman is recovering from a bowel resection. She is receiving epidural

analgesia. She lived by herself right up until admission and has no cognitive defects. All of the following interventions will reduce the risk of client falls. Which would be most appropriate for this client?

1. Apply a vest restraint around her so she cannot get out of bed.
2. Make sure someone is always present in her room to prevent her from getting out of bed.
3. Keep the bed in low position and the call bell within her reach.
4. Rearrange the room assignments so that she is in a room directly across from the nurse's station.

88. A nurse prepared the 9:00 A.M. medications for his clients and then was called off the unit briefly before he was able to administer them. Who may administer the medications to the clients now?

1. Any licensed nurse assigned to the unit and familiar with the clients
2. A pharmacy technician certified to administer medications
3. The nurse who prepared them
4. The nurse manager of the unit

89. In the past twelve-month period, a man has been arrested twice for driving while intoxicated. He is able to perform his activities of daily living without the use of alcohol and restricts his drinking to weekends. This client meets the criteria for which of the following?

1. Alcohol withdrawal syndrome
2. Bad judgment syndrome
3. Substance abuse
4. Substance dependence

90. A client with a knee injury is scheduled for a MRI examination. The nurse explains the test to the client. Which finding in the client

would make the client ineligible for this type of exam?

1. Presence of a metal plate in the leg from an old fracture

2. Presence of a ceramic artificial hip

3. A history of asthma attacks

4. Allergy to injected dye

91. Which of these clients is at greatest risk for the complications associated with osteoporosis?

    1. A 65-year-old Asian-American man who is sedentary, has a low calcium intake, and takes corticosteroids for chronic obstructive pulmonary disease

    2. A 22-year-old woman with anorexia nervosa who is not having menstrual periods

    3. A 73-year-old postmenopausal woman who has limited mobility due to rheumatoid arthritis, for which she takes corticosteroids, and who drinks a bottle of wine by herself each evening

    4. A 70-year-old woman who takes estrogen therapy, was very athletic in her youth playing tennis and golf, and takes anticonvulsant therapy as a result of a head injury suffered in an auto accident three years ago

92. An adult admitted for surgery also is diagnosed with obsessive-compulsive disorder. The client spends most of her time in the bathroom washing her hands. The client is scheduled for surgery at 8 A.M. and is to be premedicated at 7 A.M. Which nursing action will be most appropriate?

    1. Inform the client at 6:30 A.M. that she will soon be medicated and have to stay in bed after that.

    2. When medicating the client, explain to her that she will not be able to get up after receiving the medication.

    3. After medicating the client, place a wash basin and wash cloth at the bedside for her use.

    4. After medicating the client, assist her in washing her hands at the bedside.

93. A 43-year-old woman with lupus erythematosus expresses frustration about the unpredictable course of her illness and the change in her physical appearance. Which nursing intervention would be most appropriate?

    1. Explore with her the affect the lupus has on her occupation, leisure activities, and personal relationships.

    2. Explain to her that things could be worse, and that she could have a more serious illness, such as terminal cancer, to help her put her situation into perspective.

    3. Help the client reduce conflicts in her personal life.

    4. Teach her what can be expected as the disease progresses.

94. A child's burn is debrided each day with hydrotherapy to remove the eschar. The child's parents ask why this immersion is necessary. What is the most appropriate response for the nurse to make?

    1. "By removing the scab or crusting daily in the special bath, we help prevent infection and then the healthy tissue may be covered by skin grafts."

    2. "By submersion in a whirlpool bath, we can better exercise her limbs to prevent contractures."

    3. "This is a cleansing bath given so that fresh dressings may be applied to the burn areas."

    4. "We decrease her chance of infection by immersion in antibiotic solutions with each debriding bath."

95. The nurse is caring for a client who was admitted for treatment of schizoaffective disorder with visual hallucinations. He tells the nurse that he sees extraterrestrials that are coming to get him. What is the best nursing response?

1. "You know that extraterrestrials are make-believe."
2. Call his physician and report this visual hallucination.
3. Ignore his comment and change the subject.
4. "You think someone is coming after you?"

96. An adult is almost ready for discharge. She has a complicated care regimen to follow. When conducting client teaching, the nurse notes that the client cannot recall basic information that was discussed the day before. The client also appears distracted. When asked if she is feeling comfortable about leaving the hospital, she states, "There's just too much to learn. I know I'm going to get home and mess something up." The nurse realizes that the client may be experiencing

1. mild anxiety.
2. moderate anxiety.
3. severe anxiety.
4. panic anxiety.

97. The family of an 88-year-old woman who was admitted with severe dehydration says to the nurse, "Why don't you just tie down her arms so she won't try to get out her IV?" What is the best response for the nurse to make?

1. Ask the physician for an order to restrain the woman.
2. Explain to the family that restraints are not allowed in the hospital unless the doctor orders them.
3. Assess the client's mental status and safety needs.
4. Tell the family that they can restrain the client, but the nurse cannot.

98. An adult client is to have a portable chest x-ray in his room. The client's wife and pregnant daughter are visiting. Which action is essential for the nurse?

1. Ask the pregnant daughter to leave the room and have the wife assist in holding the client.
2. Have the client wear a lead apron over his chest and abdomen.
3. Close the door to the room securely during the x-ray.
4. Ask the wife and daughter to leave the room.

99. The LPN/LVN is providing home care to an elderly widow who has senile dementia. The woman tells the nurse that her daughter hits her and tells her to shut up. The nurse notes one ecchymotic area on the client's right forearm. The daughter seems attentive to the woman when the nurse is present. What action should the nurse take?

1. Immediately call the police.
2. Ask the daughter why she abuses her mother.
3. Ask the physician to order long bone x-rays.
4. Report the woman's remarks and the nurse's findings to the nursing supervisor.

100. A nurse from the float pool is giving medications on a pediatric unit and is to give medications to a two-year-old in room 534, bed B. The child in that room does not have an identification band. What is the best action for the nurse to take?

1. Ask the child what his name is?
2. Give the medication to the child in room 534, bed B.
3. Refuse to give the medication.
4. Ask the adults beside the bed the name of the child in that bed.

Answer	Rationale	NP	CN	SA

#1. **4.** **Infants who have had a myelomeningocele repair frequently develop hydrocephalus following the surgery. Increased head circumference is an indication of hydrocephalus.**   Dc   Ph/9   4

1. Assessment of bowel sounds is a routine post-operative nursing measure, but it is not related to a common problem seen in these infants.

2. Neuro checks are not a routine post-operative nursing care measure.

3. Blood pressure in all four extremities would be done for infants suspected of having cardiac disease, not surgical repair of myelomeningocele.

#2. **2.** **A two-year-old usually engages in parallel play. They like to be around others and play the same thing, but do not interact and do not share.**   Im   He/3   4

1. Solitary play is characteristic of an infant.

3. Cooperative play is characteristic of a preschool child.

4. Collaborative play is characteristic of preschool and school-age children.

#3. **3.** **The right side of the heart carries unoxygenated blood. When it passes through defects to the left side of the heart, poorly oxygenated blood is mixed with well-oxygenated blood and gives the cyanotic appearance.**   Im   Ph/10   1

1. Tetralogy of Fallot does have four separate defects: pulmonic valve stenosis, right ventricular hypertrophy, ventricular septal defect, and overriding aorta. However, this does not answer the question, which was why it is called a cyanotic heart defect.

2. Left-to-right shunting takes blood that is in the left side of the heart and has been oxygenated to the right side of the heart and through the lungs again. There is no unoxygenated blood in the systemic circulation and no cause for cyanosis.

4. This is true in Tetralogy of Fallot because of the pulmonic valve stenosis. However, this response does not answer the question. This is not the reason it is called a cyanotic heart defect.

		NP	**CN**	**SA**

ANSWER   RATIONALE

#4. 1. The extra tissue in the foreskin is used to help repair the hypospadias.   Im   Ph/9   4

   2. This statement is not true. Hypospadias does not put the child in a weakened condition. The foreskin is not removed because it is used in the repair of the hypospadias.

   3. This statement is not true. The foreskin is not removed because it is used in the repair of the hypospadias.

   4. It is true that circumcision is not medically necessary. However, this is not the reason that the child was not circumcised. The foreskin is not removed because it is used in the repair of the hypospadias.

#5. 3. The sweat test is a diagnostic for cystic fibrosis. In cystic fibrosis there is a salty taste to the sweat and a high concentration of NaCl. Children with cystic fibrosis usually have frequent respiratory infections as well as malabsorption of nutrients and failure to thrive.   Dc   Ph/9   4

   1. Pernicious anemia is unrelated to the history of respiratory infections and a sweat test.

   2. Diabetes insipidus is unrelated to the history of respiratory infections and a sweat test.

   4. Glomerulonephritis is unrelated to the history of respiratory infections and a sweat test.

#6. 2. Kegel's exercises are the tightening and relaxing of the pubococcygeus muscle, which improves the strength of the pelvic floor. It may help prevent cystocele and rectocele.   Im   He/3   3

   1. Kegel's exercises are unrelated to the uterus. They are the tightening and relaxing of the pubococcygeus muscle, which improves the strength of the pelvic floor.

   3. Kegel's exercises are unrelated to the breasts. They are the tightening and relaxing of the pubococcygeus muscle, which improves the strength of the pelvic floor.

   4. Kegel's exercises are the tightening and relaxing of the pubococcygeus muscle, which improves the strength of the pelvic floor. They are not general conditioning for the work of childbirth.

#7. 4. Epidural anesthesia decreases blood flow back to the heart from the lower extremities, decreasing the risk of congestive heart failure.   Pl   Ph/9   3

   1. Giving extra intravenous fluid would increase the blood volume to her heart and increase her risk of congestive heart failure.

   2. General anesthesia increases the risk of maternal death.

   3. Holding her breath and bearing down increases blood volume to the heart and increases risk of congestive heart failure.

#8. 3. **Although there are many unknowns in pre-term labor, a uterus that is overly enlarged by carrying more than one baby is a risk.**   Dc   He/3   3

    1. A 30-pound weight gain is normal.

    2. A small baby is not a risk factor for premature labor; neither is age.

    4. Age and multiparity are not significant risk factors for premature labor.

#9. 3. **The average length of time for the cord to detach is 7–10 days. Longer or shorter can be normal as long as the cord is free from signs of infection or bleeding.**   Im   He/3   4

    1. The average length of time for the cord to detach is 7–10 days. Longer or shorter can be normal as long as the cord is free from signs of infection or bleeding.

    2. The average length of time for the cord to detach is 7–10 days. Longer or shorter can be normal as long as the cord is free from signs of infection or bleeding.

    4. The average length of time for the cord to detach is 7–10 days. Longer or shorter can be normal as long as the cord is free from signs of infection or bleeding.

#10. 1. **Diaphragms must be refitted after the birth of a baby, an abortion, or weight loss or gain of 15 pounds or more.**   Im   He/3   3

    2. Before continuing to use the diaphragm the woman must be resized. If the fit is okay, the previous diaphragm may be used.

    3. Diaphragms are a very acceptable choice for postpartum contraception.

    4. Breastfeeding should not be relied on for birth control.

#11. 1. **A full bladder may prevent descent of the fetus. The mother should be checked.**   Dc   He/3   3

    2. A paracervical block given in the first stage of labor anesthesia will not have an effect in second stage.

    3. Often the side-lying position is helpful when the baby is not descending.

    4. LOA (left occiput anterior) position is a normal position.

#12. **1.** **Bending over to tie his shoes could raise intracranial pressure. A transphenoidal hypophysectomy is the removal of the pituitary gland. The incision is in the mouth above the gum line and goes through the sphenoid sinuses into the brain. This client has had a brain surgery and is at risk for increased intracranial surgery. This behavior indicates the client does not understand the teaching.**   Ev   Ph/9   1

   2. The person who has had the pituitary gland (master gland) removed will be taking a lot of medicines. This comment indicates the client is taking the medications.

   3. There is no reason the client should not ambulate following a transphenoidal hypophysectomy. Ambulation will help to prevent immobility post-operative complications. This behavior indicates understanding of post-operative care.

   4. The client who has had the pituitary (master) gland removed must have a medical identification bracelet. If the client was in an accident and unable to tell anyone about his medications, he might die. The medications are essential for life. This behavior indicates an understanding of his care.

#13. **2.** **The cause of Bell's palsy is unknown.**   Dc   Ph/10   1

   1. Shingles is caused by the chickenpox virus.

   3. Guillain-Barré syndrome usually follows a cold or influenza.

   4. The cause of Bell's palsy is unknown. It does not appear to be related to trauma.

#14. **2.** **A pacemaker is a contraindication for magnetic resonance imaging.**   Dc   Ph/9   1

   1. Iodine is not used during magnetic resonance imaging.

   3. A hearing aid is not a contraindication for magnetic resonance imaging. A hearing aid can be removed during the procedure if needed.

   4. Digoxin is not a contraindication for magnetic resonance imaging.

#15. **1.** **Hodgkin's disease is cancer of the lymphatic system. The client will have one or more swollen lymph nodes.**   Dc   Ph/10   1

   2. A painful rash is not associated with Hodgkin's disease. The client may have severe itching, but it is not associated with a rash.

   3. Stomach pain is not characteristic of Hodgkin's disease.

   4 Joint pain is not characteristic of Hodgkin's disease.

#16. 3. **Semi-Fowler's position is indicated to make breathing easier for the client.**   Im   Ph/7   1

    1. Supine position is not appropriate. The client who is in congestive heart failure has shortness of breath and needs to be positioned in semi-Fowler's position.

    2. Sim's position is not appropriate. The client who is in congestive heart failure has shortness of breath and needs to be positioned in semi-Fowler's position.

    4. Side lying is not appropriate. The client who is in congestive heart failure has shortness of breath and needs to be positioned in semi-Fowler's position.

#17. 2. **The nurse should take an apical pulse before administering digoxin.**   Im   Ph/8   1

    1. Asking the client if he has chest pain is not the most important information for the nurse to obtain from the client before administering digoxin.

    3. Taking the client's blood pressure is not the most importation information for the nurse to obtain from the client before administering digoxin.

    4. Asking the client if he is short of breath is not the most important information for the nurse to obtain from the client before administering digoxin. This information is nice to know but not most essential.

#18. 1. **Restlessness is a sign of hypoxia, which must be further assessed in a person who has pneumonia.**   Pl   Sa/1   1

    2. Pink-colored skin is a normal finding.

    3. A nonproductive cough may occur with pneumonia and should be assessed, but it is not critical and not as significant as restlessness.

    4. Dry mouth is commonly seen in clients with pneumonia because most persons with pneumonia are mouth breathers.

#19. 1. **Orange juice and tomatoes are high in potassium. Baked chicken is low in sodium.**   Ev   Ph/7   6

    2. Milk, roast beef, and spinach are all high in sodium.

    3. A fish sandwich is high in sodium.

    4. Shrimp is high in sodium.

#20. 2. According to the Center for Disease Control, the most effective way to control the spread of disease is consistent hand washing.   Ev   Sa/2   1

1. Isolating infected clients will help. However, most clients are admitted before testing and may not be isolated until after tests have been done and they have been receiving care for some time. The most effective way to control the spread of disease is consistent hand washing.

3. Consistent hand washing is more effective in preventing the spread of disease than occasionally wearing a gown.

4. It is not necessary to wear gloves for *all* care. Consistent hand washing is the most effective way to prevent the spread of disease.

#21. 1. The nurse should keep items above waist level and never turn with the back to a sterile field. The sterile field should always be in the line of vision.   Im   Sa/2   1

2. The outside of a sterile package is contaminated. It may not be opened with sterile gloves because that will contaminate the sterile gloves.

3. Talking over a sterile field may contaminate the field by droplets.

4. Reaching over a sterile field will contaminate the field. The nurse should reach around the field to give another person medicine.

#22. 2. This statement indicates a lack of understanding about health promotion behaviors. Potential health problems can be detected before obvious symptoms are present. Annual physicals are recommended for persons over 50 years old whether or not they are experiencing any problems.   Ev   He/4   1

1. This response indicates understanding of some health promotion activities. The question asked for a response indicating lack of understanding.

3. This response indicates understanding of some health promotion activities. The question asked for a response indicating lack of understanding.

4. This response indicates understanding of some health promotion activities. The question asked for a response indicating lack of understanding.

#23. 2. The nurse should explain the procedure to the client. There is no special preparation for this procedure.   Pl   Ph/9   1

1. There is no need to keep the client NPO before a KUB.

3. There is no need to catheterize the client before a KUB.

4. There is no need to give an enema before a KUB.

#24. 2. **Dislodged radioactive implants would never be picked up with the hands, even with gloves on. Gloves give no protection against radiation. Any dislodged material should be picked up with long-handled forceps and placed in a lead-lined container.**   Im   Ph/10   1

    1. All people caring for the client should be aware of the radiological danger. It is appropriate to label the chart and the door to the room.

    3. Washing hands with soap and water is appropriate after caring for any client. This is good care, but not specifically related to the radiation implant.

    4. Caregivers, including nurses, should spend as little time as possible with the client while the implant is in place. Radiation is cumulative. Limiting time with and increasing distance from the client will reduce nurse exposure to radiation.

#25. 4. **Removing all unnecessary items in the room or hall will reduce the possibility of the client tripping and falling.**   Pl   Sa/2   1

    1. The client can use the side rail to assist himself or herself in getting into and out of bed.

    2. Decreased lighting increases the chance for the client to fall.

    3. All staff members need to take responsibility to clean up wet areas on the floor to prevent falls.

#26. 4. **Redness without induration is generally considered to be of no significance when reading the result of a tuberculin skin test.**   Dc   He/4   1

    1. The correct procedure is to measure the area of induration, not redness. Lack of induration is a negative test.

    2. The correct procedure is to measure the area of induration, not redness. Lack of induration is a negative test. This answer is further incorrect in that a positive test does not mean a person has active tuberculosis.

    3. Redness does not indicate the test is falsely negative.

#27. 4. **Persons who have chronic obstructive pulmonary disease associated with carbon dioxide retention may become insensitive to carbon dioxide levels to stimulate breathing. Instead, they depend on a low oxygen level to stimulate breathing. Excessive oxygen therapy increases the oxygen level above the set point and decreases the drive to breathe.**   Im   Ph/10   1

　　1. In persons with emphysema, low-flow oxygen may be beneficial. High-flow oxygen increases the blood level of oxygen and may stop the stimulus to breathe, which is a low oxygen level in persons who have emphysema. The client will no longer breathe and will die if this continues very long.

　　2. Increased delivery of oxygen will not lower blood oxygen levels. It will raise the oxygen above the level to stimulate breathing.

　　3. High concentrations of oxygen may increase blood levels.

#28. 1. **Humor and joking are often ways to handle stress. This should be considered a coping mechanism.**   Dc   Ps/5   2

　　2. Humor is an appropriate way of coping.

　　3. There is no information to suggest that the client is denying the seriousness of the procedure.

　　4. The behavior described is not rationalization.

#29. 2. **A surgical wound changes the way the body looks. Some clients are unable to accept the change in body image.**   Dc   Ps/5   2

　　1. There is no evidence the client is denying the surgical procedure. The client would say, "The doctor didn't really do an operation."

　　3. There is no indication that the client fears becoming nauseated. This is an assumption on the part of the nurse.

　　4. There is no indication that the client does not like the sight of blood or that there is bleeding at the wound site.

#30. 2. **The unconscious client will not be able to maintain a high-Fowler's position and will fall to the side. The unconscious client should not be placed in this position. This action indicates a need for further instruction.**   Ev   Sa/1   1

　　1. The unconscious client should be placed in a lateral position with the head turned to the side. This indicates that the unlicensed person is performing the procedure correctly.

　　3. Placing a towel under the chin is appropriate during mouth care. It keeps the area clean and dry.

　　4. Keeping the client in the lateral position for 30 minutes after oral care prevents pooling of secretions and aspiration of fluids. This action is appropriate and indicates the person understands how to perform the procedure.

#31. 4. **Completing the 24-hour intake and output record requires analysis and assessment. It must be done by the nurse and should not be assigned to unlicensed personnel.**   Pl   Sa/1   1

    1. Measuring all oral intake is an activity that may be delegated.

    2. Recording all output is an activity that may be delegated.

    3. Unlicensed personnel may enter data on graphs.

#32. 1. **Walkers are not fixed. Pulling on a walker to get out of a chair is a safety problem. The correct method is to push out of the fixed chair and once standing take hold of the walker.**   Ev   Ph/7   1

    2. Moving the walker forward, then taking a step is the correct method for walking with a walker.

    3. The walker should not be waist high. This does not indicate a need for further instruction.

    4. Many clients may not need to use the walker all of the time. This will vary with the reason the client needs a walker and the progress the client is making.

#33. 2. **Joining a social club without addressing the underlying hearing problem may increase his withdrawal and depression.**   Pl   Ph/7   2

    1. Getting a hearing guide dog is one possible solution to a severe hearing deficit. This suggestion may be very helpful.

    3. A telephone TDD is likely to be very helpful for a hearing-impaired client.

    4. A closed-caption TV will make it possible for the severely hearing impaired to watch television. This suggestion will be helpful to the client.

#34. 2. **Pyridium turns urine a red-orange color. This is normal and nothing to be concerned about. This statement indicates the client does not understand about the medication.**   Ev   Ph/8   5

    1. Pyridium should be taken after meals to avoid stomach upset.

    3. Pyridium is a urinary tract anesthetic and antispasmodic. The reason for giving Pyridium is to reduce the bladder pain and spasms that cause the urgency and frequency.

    4. Liver damage is a possible side effect of the drug. The client should inform the health care provider if there is evidence of jaundice.

#35. 2. **Persons who have congestive heart failure are more prone to fluid overload. The volume of fluid infused should be carefully monitored to ensure the client does not receive a volume of fluid greater than intended.**

Dc   Ph/8   1

    1.   The nurse should always check the insertion site, but this is not the focus of particular concern in the client who has congestive heart failure.

    3.   The tubing should be changed at regular intervals according to agency policy. This is not the greatest area of concern in a client who has congestive heart failure.

    4.   The nurse should be aware of a flashback and should report this to the nurse in charge. However, this is not the greatest area of concern for the nurse when the client has congestive heart failure.

#36. 3. **Assessment of safety needs of the client is the role of the nurse and cannot be delegated to assistive personnel.**

Pl   Sa/1   1

    1.   The bed should be in the low position to prevent falling injuries. This can be delegated to assistive personnel.

    2.   Falls occur when clients reach for items on the bedside table that are out of reach. Ensuring that the bedside table is within reach can be delegated to assistive personnel.

    4.   Monitoring behavior may be delegated to assistive personnel. Assessment of the behavior and problem solving are the role of the nurse.

#37. 2. **Although all of these methods are used to check placement, the best method is checking pH. If it is acid, it came from the stomach. The pH should be less than five.**

Im   Ph/7   1

    1.   Checking the residual does not indicate where the fluid came from.

    3.   Injecting air and listening for the "swoosh" does not indicate exact placement in the gastrointestinal tract.

    4.   Asking the client to talk or hum is done to determine that there is nothing in the larynx. However, a small-bore feeding tube may not interfere with the client's ability to talk even if it is in the trachea.

#38. 2. A red area that does not disappear following massage indicates the skin will break down and needs immediate attention.   Pl   Sa/1   1

  1. A red area that disappears with massage is a pressure area that should not break down if the client is turned frequently.

  3. Most clients should be encouraged to perform as much self-care as possible. This information is nice to know but does not require immediate action.

  4. Clear, amber urine draining from an indwelling urinary catheter is normal. This is nice to know but does not require immediate attention from the nurse.

#39. 1. There is no safety reason to avoid going out in public. This statement most likely indicates the client has not adjusted to the halo brace.   Ev   Ps/5   2

  2. Stating that he does not mind if people look at him indicates acceptance of the device.

  3. Telling his grandchildren that the halo brace looks like a space helmet indicates the use of humor in handling the change in image. This is appropriate.

  4. Finding a comfortable way to sleep indicates the client is problem-solving some of the challenges that occur with this brace. This is appropriate.

#40. 4. A throat culture is done to identify any microorganisms that may be present. Antibiotic use inhibits the growth of microorganisms. The throat culture will not be accurate. Cultures should be taken before any antibiotics are given.   Dc   Ph/9   4

  1. Aspirin does not interfere with a throat culture.

  2. Throat lozenges do not interfere with a throat culture.

  3. Acetaminophen does not interfere with a throat culture.

#41. 4. Partial thromboplastin time (PTT) is the test done to monitor effectiveness of heparin therapy.   Dc   Ph/8   5

  1. INR is a way of reporting prothrombin time, which is used to monitor the effectiveness of coumadin therapy.

  2. Bleeding time is not used to monitor the effectiveness of heparin therapy.

  3. Prothrombin time is used to measure the effectiveness of coumadin therapy.

#42. 3.   **A hemoglobin result of 10 gm/dl is below the normal hemoglobin,**   Dc   Ph/9   1
which is 12–16 gm/dl for females and 12–18 gm/dl for males.

    1.   The normal hemoglobin for females is 12–16 gm/dl. A result of 10 gm/dl is low, not high.

    2.   A hemoglobin result of 10 gm/dl is below the normal hemoglobin, which is 12–16 gm/dl for females. Pregnancy can cause low hemoglobin. Although this is fairly common during pregnancy, the result is significant. The client will likely be treated with an oral iron supplement.

    4.   A hemoglobin result of 10 gm/dl is below the normal hemoglobin, which is 12–16 gm/dl for females.

#43. 2.   **When the heart is not able to pump enough blood, there is a**   Dc   Ph/10   1
decreased blood flow resulting in a decrease in blood pressure.

    1.   Congestive heart failure is characterized by an inability of the heart to pump enough blood. Low cardiac output is indicated by a decrease in blood flow to the kidney, causing a decrease in urine output. If the client's condition were getting worse, the urine output would decrease.

    3.   When a client is in congestive heart failure the heart rate increases in an attempt to compensate for the low cardiac output. If the client's condition were getting worse the heart rate would increase.

    4.   When a person is in congestive heart failure the skin is usually cool and moist. If the client's condition were getting worse the skin would be cool and moist.

#44. 4.   **The nurse should start the supplemental oxygen. This action must**   Im   Ph/10   1
be followed by a repeat of the pulse oximetry to ensure this
measure is effective and determine if further action is needed.

    1.   The physician has already given an order addressing the action to take in this situation. If the supplemental oxygen does not raise the oxygen saturation to above 90% the physician should be contacted.

    2.   The LPN/LVN can carry out a physician's PRN order without first checking with the registered nurse when the parameters are clear; in this case oxygen for an oxygen saturation less than 90%.

    3.   Starting oxygen is appropriate, but the best action is to start oxygen and check the pulse oximetry to ensure the client is responding to the oxygen.

#45. **1.** **This comment suggests the child's mother believes there is a desired or a maximum number of times that the child should be suctioned. Although suction should be used only when necessary, a person should be suctioned when needed. This comment suggests further instruction is needed.**   Ev   Ph/10   1

2. The child should be suctioned when he cannot cough up sputum. This comment indicates a correct understanding of indications for suctioning.

3. Recognizing that the child will not need the same amount of suctioning each day indicates an understanding that suctioning should be done as needed, not on a set schedule.

4. Stating that she will suction the child only if necessary indicates an understanding that suctioning can be traumatic and should be done only if necessary.

#46. **1.** **Support from significant others is likely to be most helpful because the significant others will be with the client for the longest periods of time.**   Pl   Ps/6   2

2. Support from a counselor may be helpful, but time spent with the client is limited.

3. Support from friends may be helpful, but is probably not the most important.

4. Support from coworkers is helpful, but these people are there only for a limited time. This is not the most helpful.

#47. **4.** **If abuse has occurred, the abuser often will not leave the child in a situation where the child may talk to a health care worker and tell them what happened. A 10-year-old child will be able to cope with being left by parents, so continuous contact by the parents is not necessary.**   Dc   Ps/6   4

1. Having friends visit is typical for a 10-year-old. Peer acceptance is important at this age.

2. School is very important to the 10-year-old who is meeting the developmental stage of industry.

3. A parent leaving to be with the child's siblings is appropriate. A 10-year-old child can manage in the hospital without constant parental attention. He does not need to be the center of attention and learn how to manipulate the parents.

#48. 3. **The best place for the pillow is at the head of the bed. This prevents the client's head from striking the top of the bed.**   Im   Ph/7 1

   1. The best place for the pillow is at the head of the bed. This prevents the client's head from striking the top of the bed.

   2. The best place for the pillow is at the head of the bed. This prevents the client's head from striking the top of the bed.

   4. The best place for the pillow is at the head of the bed. This prevents the client's head from striking the top of the bed. Placing the pillow under the client's head increases friction and makes the move more difficult.

#49. 1. **An on-again, off-again pattern of snoring suggests periods of not breathing-a defining characteristic of sleep apnea.**   Dc   Ph/7 1

   2. Napping alone is not indicative of a serious sleep disorder. Afternoon naps may make it more difficult to fall asleep.

   3. Early rising may be normal or it may suggest depression. It is not a sign of a serious sleep disorder.

   4. Muscle jerking is common during NREM (non rapid eye movement) sleep.

#50. 2. **The most important action for the nurse to take is to immobilize the leg to prevent further injury. A painful extremity that is out of alignment may be broken.**   Im   Ph/10 1

   1. The nurse might give the client pain medication if ordered. However, the most important nursing action is to immobilize the leg. The findings suggest the leg is broken.

   3. The nurse or someone else should gather client records. However, the priority action is to immobilize the leg. The findings suggest the client may have a broken leg.

   4. At some point the nurse will complete an incident report. However, this is not the priority action. The findings suggest the client may have a fractured leg. Keeping the leg in alignment is top priority.

#51. 1. **Asking the client what he knows allows the nurse to assess the client's understanding of the procedure about to be done before giving the client pre-operative sedation. If the client does not understand the surgery that was on the consent form, then it is not truly informed consent, and the surgeon must be notified. The surgeon may need to discuss the planned operation further with the client to ensure that he understands what is to be done. This explanation is not the nurse's responsibility; it is the surgeon's.**   Im   Sa/1   1

2. Telling the client not to worry does not answer the client's question and is patronizing. The nurse needs to assess whether the client actually understands the surgery planned and if informed consent was obtained.

3. Telling the client he/she is nervous does not answer the client's question and is patronizing. The nurse needs to assess whether the client actually understands the surgery planned and if informed consent was obtained. Furthermore, if there is any question about proper consent, no medication should be given until the matter is clarified.

4. This answer is technically correct. However, the client's question indicates the client may not understand the surgery that consent was signed for. The nurse needs to assess whether the client actually understands the surgery planned and if informed consent was obtained.

#52. 3. **Ineffective therapeutic regimen management applies when a client has difficulty integrating the treatment plan into his or her activities of daily living. This is the problem the client describes.**   Dc   Ph/10   1

1. Impaired adjustment requires the client to verbalize that he doesn't accept his health problem. There is no evidence of that in this case. The client is having difficulty integrating the treatment plan into his ADLs: ineffective therapeutic regimen management.

2. Impaired home maintenance refers to the inability to keep the home clean and safe and the inability to pay for a place to live. There is no evidence of those problems in this case. The client is having difficulty integrating the treatment plan into his ADLs: ineffective therapeutic regimen management.

4. Noncompliance applies when a factor interferes with the client's ability to follow the treatment plan, such as not having transportation to the clinic for follow-up appointments, or not having money to purchase medications. That is not evident in this case. The client is having difficulty integrating the treatment plan into his ADLs: ineffective therapeutic regimen management.

#53. 3. Because the client is not on antibiotics, the physician must be notified immediately so the appropriate antibiotic can be ordered.   Im   Ph/9   1

  1. Documenting the results in the chart is not sufficient. Because the client is not on antibiotics, the nurse's first action should be to place a call to the physician and then document the lab results and the call to the physician.

  2. Discussing lab results with the client is not a priority. The nurse's first priority is to place a call to the physician and document the call and the lab results.

  4. The formal results from the laboratory should be recorded. Because the client is not on antibiotics, the nurse's first action should be to place a call to the physician and document the call and the lab results.

#54. 2. Charting a late entry helps to provide thorough and accurate documentation of the event concerning a client in the nurse's care. You should also sign the entry with your full name and credentials, or as directed by the facility policy.   Im   Sa/1   1

  1. Charting should not be delegated to another nurse. Date and time the entry for 3:15 P.M., then write "Late entry (date-10:30 A.M.) before making the addition. The nurse should also sign the entry with full name and credentials, or as directed by the facility's policy.

  3. The nurse should never omit information from a chart. This is not a situation requiring an incident report.

  4. The information should be recorded in the nursing record as well. Date and time the entry for 3:15 P.M., then write "Late entry (date-10:30 A.M.) before making the addition. The nurse should also sign the entry with full name and credentials or as directed by facility policy.

#55. 1. An incident report is required when a medication error occurs. In the nursing documentation, the nurse should record the error, the client's response, and any treatment the client receives as a result of the medication error. An incident report should never be mentioned in the client's record.   Im   Sa/1   1

  2. Although the nurse should complete an incident report, the nursing documentation should record the error, the client's response, and any treatment received as a result of the medication error. An incident report should never be mentioned in the client's record.

  3. An incident report is required when a medication error occurs. The nursing documentation should record the client's response, and the physician must be notified.

  4. Although the nursing supervisor and the physician should be notified, an incident report is required when a medication error occurs. The nurse should record the error, the client's response, and any treatment received as a result of the medication error in the nursing documentation.

#56. 3. **Adults who cannot read are often embarrassed about their illiteracy. They devise ways to cover up their disability. Typical explanations are not having glasses and stating that another person "takes care of those things." These statements by the client may mean he is unable to read. The client has worked in a job where he may be able to function without being able to read.**   Dc   Ph/9   2

  1. There is no evidence the client is in denial. Statements such as "I don't need to learn anything new" would suggest denial. The client is trying to facilitate education by referring the nurse to his wife. It is likely that he cannot read.

  2. There is no evidence that the client is not willing to take responsibility. He is trying to facilitate education by referring the nurse to his wife. It is likely that he cannot read.

  4. There is no evidence that the client is anxious. It is likely that he cannot read.

#57. 2. **Children of preschool age work out learning and anxiety through play.**   Pl   He/3   4

  1. This child is old enough to conceptualize ideas through play. While this approach might be appropriate for a younger child, this child can be prepared through the use of dolls and through play.

  3. This child is too young to understand a complex explanation, and this might be frightening for him. The best approach is to use play to explain things to the child.

  4. This approach would be more appropriate for a teenager whose physical appearance is very important to his or her self-concept. The best approach is to use play to explain things to this child.

#58. 1. **A mechanical soft or edentulous (without dentures) diet is appropriate for a client who has difficulty chewing. This is the first priority to address the client's immediate nutritional needs and combat his weight loss. Correcting the problem with the dentures can follow.**   Pl   Ph/7   1

  2. Although a dental consult is indicated to improve the fit of the dentures, the first priority is appropriate nutrition for the client, which can be immediately through a mechanical soft or edentulous diet.

  3. There is no indication that the client does not make educated food choices. He has clearly indicated that dentures and chewing are the main concern. A mechanical soft or edentulous diet is appropriate for a client who has difficulty chewing, to meet his immediate nutritional needs.

  4. Although client teaching about denture use may be indicated, the first priority is the client's nutritional status, which can be met through a mechanical soft or edentulous diet.

#59. 2. Fruits, especially oranges, bananas, and prunes, are high in potassium, which would help correct the potassium deficit of hypokalemia.   Im   Ph/7   6

1. Eggs and cheese are high in sulfur, which would not help correct the potassium deficit of hypokalemia. Fruits, especially oranges, bananas, and prunes, are the best choice.

3. Green leafy vegetables are high in magnesium, which would not help correct the potassium deficit of hypokalemia. Fruits, especially oranges, bananas, and prunes, are the best choice

4. Breads and cereals are not high in potassium. Bread and most cereals contain significant amounts of sodium, which would not help correct the potassium deficit of hypokalemia.

#60. 4. The nicotine in cigarettes is a stimulant and can interfere with sleep.   Dc   Ph/7   1

1. Eating a large meal before bedtime could interfere with sleep, but a light snack generally does not interfere with sleep. For this client the cause of insomnia is most likely the nicotine in cigarettes.

2. Some medications, such as those used to treat high blood pressure, asthma, or depression, can cause sleeping difficulties. Aspirin does not have this effect. For this client the cause of insomnia is most likely the nicotine in cigarettes.

3. A relaxing bedtime ritual, such as reading in bed before going to sleep, can enhance the ability to sleep. For this client the cause of insomnia is most likely the nicotine in cigarettes.

#61. 4. Self-care deficit is the most appropriate nursing diagnosis for this client because of his inability to perform one or more ADLs.   Dc   Ph/7   1

1. Although not bathing or getting the dressings on his hands wet could increase the risk for infection, self-care deficit is the most appropriate nursing diagnosis for this client because of his inability to perform one or more ADLs.

2. There is no evidence that the client has deficient knowledge. Self-care deficit is the most appropriate nursing diagnosis for this client because of his inability to perform one of more ADLs.

3. Although not being able to bathe could be related to pain or a disease process, there is no data to support this. Self-care deficit is the most appropriate nursing diagnosis for this client because of his inability to perform one of more ADLs.

#62. **3.** **Finishing a statement or thought for a client is rude and can block communication. This action would be least helpful in facilitating communication with the client.** Pl Sa/1 1

1. Background noises such as radios and television make it difficult for a client to hear information. Reducing background noise would be helpful in facilitating communication.

2. Adjusting a hearing aid can help a client hear better. This action would be helpful in facilitating communication.

4. Facing the client allows the client to read lips and makes words clearer. This action would be helpful in facilitating communication.

#63. **4.** **Child abuse is a learned behavior. If the mother was abused as a child, she will be more likely to abuse her own child.** Dc Ps/6 2

1. Age is not an indicator of potential for child abuse.

2. Although there is more responsibility and stress for the single mother, this is not the greatest indicator for potential child abuse.

3. There may be more economic stressors for a 16-year-old mother. However, this is not the greatest indicator for potential child abuse.

#64. **3.** **Checking gastric contents for residual is the most important information to include. Aspirating gastric contents does give an indication of tube placement. Measuring gastric contents tests for gastric emptying and should be done before giving a feeding.** Im Ph/7 1

1. Aspirating gastric contents tests whether there is any left in the stomach. If the nurse can aspirate contents, the tube is patent. However, this is not the most important information to include when responding.

2. Aspirating gastric contents does give an indication of the placement of the tube. Measuring gastric contents must be done before giving more feeding.

4. Aspirating gastric contents is not done to clear the line.

#65. **1.** **The normal serum potassium is 3.5–5 mEq/L. A finding of 3.2 mEq/L is of concern in a person who is taking a potassium depleting diuretic such as furosemide (Lasix).** Dc Ph/9 5

2. 3.7 mEq/l is within the normal range of 3.5–5 mEq/L.

3. 4.1 mEq/l is within the normal range of 3.5–5 mEq/L

4. 4.9 mEq/l is within the normal range of 3.5–5 mEq/L.

#66. 3. Outbreaks of head lice are common in schools and institutions and are not the result of a dirty house. Ev He/4 4

1. Washing bedclothes in hot water indicates understanding of how to prevent spreading of the lice or reinfestation of the child.

2. The school nurse should be notified of this very contagious condition so the other children can be assessed for head lice.

4. Head lice are often spread when children try on each other's hats or use each other's combs or brushes. This response indicates understanding of how the condition is spread.

#67. 1. Immobilization, advancing age, and hip fracture put this client at high risk for a pulmonary embolism. Tachypnea and chest pain with a sense of impending doom are signs she may be experiencing a severe blockage of the pulmonary artery. One of the immediate actions for this medical emergency is to start oxygen. Im Ph/10 1

2. Taking vital signs is not the best immediate action for the nurse. The nurse should start oxygen and notify the physician. Vital signs can be taken after starting oxygen.

3. Elevating the head of the bed will not assist in the management of a client who has a pulmonary embolism.

4. Although aspirin is both an anticoagulant and an analgesic, it is not the first action the nurse should take when a pulmonary embolism is suspected. The nurse should start oxygen and notify the physician. After establishing an IV line, the client will be treated with morphine to relieve pain and anxiety and IV heparin for anticoagulation. She might be given streptokinase, a thrombolytic agent.

#68. 2. Symptoms of anaphylactic shock must be recognized early and treatment initiated immediately. Death can occur within minutes if left untreated. Joan is already having dyspnea and must be treated immediately. The nurse should administer the epinephrine in the anaphylactic kit. Im Ph/10 1

1. Joan should be seen by a physician, but treatment should be initiated immediately. After receiving treatment she can be evaluated in the emergency room.

3. Calling for help may be appropriate but the nurse should immediately administer the medications. Calling the floor is a poor choice of help.

4. An anaphylactic reaction is a medical emergency. Joan must be treated, not monitored. Death can occur within minutes if not treated.

#69. 3. **Parenteral nutrition is the infusion of a solution directly into the vein to meet the client's daily nutritional requirements. The client's post-surgical status and the fact that he will remain NPO for only a few days make parenteral nutrition the best choice.**   Pl   Ph/7   6

   1. Diet therapy is the treatment of a disease or disorder with a special diet. Parenteral nutrition is the best choice to meet this client's post-surgical nutritional needs.

   2. Enteral feedings may be given to a client who cannot take food by mouth. However, this client needs parenteral nutrition to meet his post-surgical nutrition needs for a few days. Clients who have had bowel surgery must rest the bowel post-op, so enteral feedings would be contraindicated.

   4. Although enteral feedings via a nasogastric tube may be given to a client who cannot take food by mouth, this client needs parenteral nutrition to meet his post-surgical nutrition needs for a few days. The client may or may not have a nasogastric tube post-operatively, depending on the surgeon's preference, but it would not be used for feeding, as the bowel must be rested.

#70. 2. **This client requires droplet precautions to prevent spreading his disease to others and needs to wear a surgical mask during transport to the radiology department.**   Pl   Sa/2   1

   1. A face shield would protect the client from splashes or sprays of body fluid from other people. This client requires droplet precautions to prevent spreading his disease to others and needs to wear a surgical mask during transport to the radiology department.

   3. An N 95 respirator is used for airborne precautions and is worn by anyone entering the room of a person who has tuberculosis. This client requires droplet precautions to prevent spreading his disease to others and needs to wear a surgical mask during transport to the radiology department.

   4. Gloves and gown would not prevent droplet transmission. This client requires droplet precautions to prevent spreading his disease to others and needs to wear a surgical mask during transport to the radiology department.

#71. 3. **This client should be on contact precautions, which require the caregiver to wear a gown to protect from wound drainage and to wear gloves to prevent contact with materials such as dressings that may contain infective material. In addition, the nurse should wash hands with antimicrobial soap after glove removal before leaving the client's room.**   Pl   Sa/2   1

    1.   An N 95 respirator is worn to care for a client on airborne precautions. This client should be on contact precautions, which require the caregiver to wear a gown to protect from wound drainage and to wear gloves to prevent contact with materials such as dressings that may contain infective material. In addition, the nurse should wash hands with antimicrobial soap after glove removal before leaving the client's room.

    2.   Eye protection and a facemask would be worn to protect the caregiver from splashes or sprays of body fluid, which are not expected from this client. This client should be on contact precautions, which require the caregiver to wear a gown to protect from wound drainage and to wear gloves to prevent contact with materials such as dressings that may contain infective material. In addition, the nurse should wash hands with antimicrobial soap after glove removal before leaving the client's room.

    4.   A gown alone is not sufficient. This client should be on contact precautions, which require the caregiver to wear a gown to protect from wound drainage and to wear gloves to prevent contact with materials such as dressings that may contain infective material. In addition, the nurse should wash hands with antimicrobial soap after glove removal before leaving the client's room.

#72. 2. **Gown, gloves, mask, and goggles are all part of standard precautions when there is risk of splashing or spraying of body fluids.**   Im   Sa/2   1

    1.   Gloves alone are not sufficient. Gown, gloves, mask, and goggles are all part of standard precautions when there is risk of splashing or spraying of body fluids.

    3.   Mask and gown do not provide sufficient protection. Gown, gloves, mask, and goggles are all part of standard precautions when there is risk of splashing or spraying of body fluids.

    4.   Gown, gloves, mask, and goggles are all part of standard precautions when there is risk of splashing or spraying of body fluids. Even in emergency situations, proper precautions must be worn. It is essential for the nurse to know where protective equipment is located at all times.

#73. 2. Hypomagnesemia is characterized by low serum calcium and potassium levels. The nurse would suspect low serum potassium levels because the client is taking Lasix, a potassium-depleting diuretic. The nurse would suspect hypocalcemia because the client has hyperreflexia as evidenced by muscle cramps, facial tics, and positive Chvostek's and Trousseau's signs.

Dc   Ph/10   5

   1. Hypomagnesemia is characterized by low, not high, serum calcium and potassium levels.

   3. Altered acid-base balance does not usually occur with hypomagnesemia.

   4. ECG changes are not typically associated with hypomagnesemia.

#74. 3. The client has a low chloride level. Normal is 95 to 106 mEq/L. Anions (negative ions) such as chloride are excreted in combination with cations (positive ions) such as sodium during massive fluid losses from the GI tract. This helps maintain osmotic balance. The nurse should suspect a low serum sodium just on the basis of extensive vomiting.

Dc   Ph/10   1

   1. Chloride and sodium function in combination in this clinical situation to maintain osmotic balance. For example, when the chloride level is high (normal range is 95 to 106 mEq/L), the sodium level is also high. In this scenario, the chloride level is low. The nurse should suspect a low serum sodium just on the basis of extensive vomiting.

   2. Sodium level can usually be predicted from chloride level in this clinical setting. Sodium and chloride function in combination to maintain osmotic balance. The nurse should suspect a low serum sodium just on the basis of extensive vomiting.

   4. When chloride level is low (normal range is 95 to 106 mEq/L) sodium level is also low in this clinical setting. This is not a normal chloride level. The nurse should suspect a low serum sodium just on the basis of extensive vomiting.

#75. 4. **The order is incomplete. It does not contain a route of administration, the dosage units are not specified (milligrams), and the frequency of administration is not specified. The order must be clarified before medication can be administered.**   Im   Ph/8   5

1. The order is incomplete. It does not contain a route of administration, the dosage units are not specified (milligrams), and the frequency of administration is not specified. The order must be clarified before medication can be administered.

2. The order is incomplete. It does not contain a route of administration, the dosage units are not specified (milligrams), and the frequency of administration is not specified. The order must be clarified before medication can be administered.

3. The order is incomplete. It does not contain a route of administration, the dosage units are not specified (milligrams), and the frequency of administration is not specified. The order must be clarified before medication can be administered.

#76. 3. **The Sim's position, with the client lying on her side, relaxes rectal muscles and is the optimal position for examination and client comfort.**   Dc   He/4   1

1. The dorsal recumbent position is to examine the head, neck, anterior thorax, lungs, breast, axillae, and heart. The Sim's position, with the client lying on her side, relaxes rectal muscles and is the optimal position for examination and client comfort.

2. Although the knee-chest position can be used for rectal examination, it could be very uncomfortable for a client with severe inflammation. The Sim's position, with the client lying on her side, relaxes rectal muscles and is the optimal position for examination and client comfort.

4. The lithotomy position is used for examining the female genitalia, rectum, and genital tract and provides maximum exposure of the genital area. However, the Sim's position, with the client lying on her side, relaxes rectal muscles and is the optimal position for examination and client comfort.

#77. 3.   **A pulse deficit indicates blood flow too low to initiate a peripheral**   Dc   He/4   1
             pulse. This serious finding must be reported to the physician
             immediately.

   1.   This is not a normal finding. A pulse deficit indicates blood flow too
        low to initiate a peripheral pulse. This serious finding must be
        reported to the physician immediately.

   2.   A pulse deficit indicates blood flow too low to initiate a peripheral
        pulse. This serious finding must be reported to the physician
        immediately.

   4.   A pulse deficit indicates blood flow too low to initiate a peripheral
        pulse. This serious finding must be reported to the physician
        immediately.

#78. 2.   **Due to the unique nature of pain experience, the analgesic**   Im   Ph/8   3
             regimen needs to be titrated until the desired effect (pain
             reduction) is achieved. A client must always be reassessed after
             administering pain medication to see if he experiences relief of
             his discomfort.

   1.   Analgesics need to be titrated until the desired effect (pain reduction)
        is achieved. The most appropriate action would be to administer the
        minimum dose of medication, reassess his level of pain 30 minutes
        after administration, and reassess again at the minimal time interval
        for repeat dosing. A client must always be reassessed after
        administering pain medication to see if he experiences relief of his
        discomfort.

   3.   Although vital signs are normal, the client reports pain and is
        sweating, another physiologic indication of pain. The most
        appropriate action would be to administer the minimum dose of
        medication, reassess his level of pain 30 minutes after administration,
        and reassess again at the minimal time interval for repeat dosing. A
        client must always be reassessed after administering pain medication
        to see if he experiences relief of his discomfort.

   4.   The most appropriate action would be to administer the minimum
        dose of medication, reassess his level of pain 30 minutes after
        administration, and reassess again at the minimal time interval for
        repeat dosing. A client must always be reassessed after administering
        pain medication to see if he experiences relief of his discomfort. In the
        post-operative period, addiction should be of no concern.

#79. **1.** **Fear is a feeling of emotional distress related to a specific source that can be identified. This client can clearly express that her distress is related to watching her mother die of ovarian cancer. Therefore, fear is the appropriate diagnosis.**   Dc   Ps/5   2

   2. Anxiety is a sense of uneasiness to a vague, nonspecific threat. This client can clearly express that her distress is related to watching her mother die of ovarian cancer. Therefore, fear is the appropriate diagnosis.

   3. There is no evidence of lack of support from family members. This client can clearly express that her distress is related to watching her mother die of ovarian cancer. Therefore, fear is the appropriate diagnosis.

   4. In spiritual distress, the client expresses a disturbance in his or her belief system. There is no evidence of that in this scenario. This client can clearly express that her distress is related to watching her mother die of ovarian cancer. Therefore, fear is the appropriate diagnosis.

#80. **4.** **Public health is at risk when infected clients enter the community without proper treatment. Therefore, ineffective therapeutic regimen management, which means the client is not following the treatment plan, presents the greatest risk to public health.**   Dc   He/4   1

   1. Public health is at risk when infected clients enter the community without proper treatment. Therefore, ineffective therapeutic regimen management, which means the client is not following the treatment plan, presents the greatest risk to public health.

   2. Public health is at risk when infected clients enter the community without proper treatment. Therefore, ineffective therapeutic regimen management, which means the client is not following the treatment plan, presents the greatest risk to public health.

   3. Public health is at risk when infected clients enter the community without proper treatment. Therefore, ineffective therapeutic regimen managementn, which means the client is not following the treatment plan, presents the greatest risk to public health.

#81. 4. **Palpating and recording pulses is a key component of assessing a client with numbness and coldness of an extremity. These symptoms suggest poor circulation. Because these symptoms may indicate an emergency situation, this assessment should be done before a comprehensive history is taken. If pulses are absent, the physician should be called immediately.**

Dc Ph/10 1

1. Because these symptoms may indicate an emergency situation, a prompt, quick, focused priority assessment of palpating and recording of the femoral, popliteal, posterior tibial, and dorsalis pedis pulses should be done first before a comprehensive history is taken.

2. Because these symptoms may indicate an emergency situation, a prompt, quick, focused priority assessment of palpating and recording of the femoral, popliteal, posterior tibial, and dorsalis pedis pulses should be done. The assessment findings will indicate if a physician is needed immediately. If pulses are absent, the physician should be called immediately.

3. Because these symptoms may indicate an emergency situation, a prompt, quick, focused priority assessment of palpating and recording of the femoral, popliteal, posterior tibial, and dorsalis pedis pulses should be done first before a full history is taken.

#82. 1. **If the pulse rhythm is irregular, assessment must occur for 60 seconds rather than 30. An apical pulse provides more information than a radial pulse.**

Dc He/4 1

2. Carotid pulse generally assesses cranial circulation. There is no indication from the client's vital signs that cranial circulation is impaired. Temperature is normal. Assessment of the apical pulse takes priority and occurs for 60 seconds because the pulse rhythm is irregular.

3. There is no indication in the client's vital signs of respiratory distress. Assessment of the apical pulse takes priority and occurs for 60 seconds because the pulse rhythm is irregular.

4. The client's blood pressure is within an acceptable range. Assessment of the apical pulse takes priority and occurs for 60 seconds because the pulse rhythm is irregular.

#83. 3.   **Because the nurse has autonomy in deciding which medication**   Dc   Ph/8   5
and route have the most efficacy, it is essential for the nurse to
gather enough data to make the best decision. In this case,
determining the location and degree of pain is essential for
choosing the most effective pain medication. Different clients have
different levels of pain post-operatively.

   1.   Because the nurse has autonomy in deciding which medication and
        route have the most efficacy, it is essential for the nurse to gather
        enough data to make the best decision. In this case, determining the
        location and degree of pain is essential for choosing the most
        effective pain medication. Different clients have different levels of
        pain post-operatively.

   2.   Because the nurse has autonomy in deciding which medication and
        route have the most efficacy, it is essential for the nurse to gather
        enough data to make the best decision. In this case, determining the
        location and degree of pain is essential for choosing the most
        effective pain medication. Different clients have different levels of
        pain post-operatively.

   4.   Because the nurse has autonomy in deciding which medication and
        route have the most efficacy, it is essential for the nurse to gather
        enough data to make the best decision. In this case, determining the
        location and degree of pain is essential for choosing the most
        effective pain medication. Repositioning and relaxation methods may
        be part of an overall pain control program, but they do not substitute
        for the administration of pain medications, particularly on the day of
        surgery.

#84. 2.   **The client is exhibiting signs of anxiety. Allowing her to talk about**   Im   Ps/5   2
her feelings will provide the nurse with additional assessment
data about her emotional status. Then the nurse can make the
decision about whether the surgeon needs to be notified, or if the
client will calm down with nursing interventions.

   1.   The assessment findings are outside the normal limits. Additional
        assessment is needed before proceeding with care.

   3.   The client is anxious and will not be able to process any pre-operative
        teaching at this time. Additional assessment is needed before
        proceeding with care or teaching.

   4.   A more extensive nursing assessment needs to be done to determine
        the cause of the client's anxiety before the surgeon is called.

#85. 4. **The response indicates the client lacks self-efficacy, the belief that he or she will succeed.**   Dc   Ps/5   2

1. Maturation means the client is developmentally able to learn. There is no indication from the client's response that he lacks sufficient maturation to learn. This response indicates that the client lacks self-efficacy, the belief that he or she will succeed.

2. Organization depends on the nurse who is providing the teaching. He or she should incorporate previously learned information and provide a sequence from simple to complex or familiar to unfamiliar. This response indicates that the client lacks self-efficacy, the belief that he or she will succeed. There is nothing in the question that indicates the client cannot organize his own care at home.

3. Readiness to learn means that the client is able and willing to learn. Some indications of lack of client readiness are anxiety, avoidance, denial, or lack of participation. This client's response does not indicate lack of readiness to learn but a lack of the belief that he will succeed.

#86. 1. **This answer is culturally sensitive and allows the client to discuss her tradition.**   Im   Ps/5   1

2. Telling the client that no one her age should be drinking at bedtime could be interpreted as a judgmental, ageist response.

3. Dismissing the client's traditions as an old wive's tale is not appropriate.

4. Simply telling the client that alcohol is not permitted in the hospital could be interpreted as culturally insensitive and also would not encourage further communication with the client.

#87. 3. **Keeping the bed in low position and the call bell within reach are primary interventions for any client to protect them from the risk of falling. There is no evidence that this client needs any additional interventions at this time. She has no cognitive defects and is receiving epidural analgesia, which means she is alert.**   Pl   Sa/2   1

1. Restraints should be used only as a last resort when other measures have failed to protect the client. This intervention is not the most appropriate for this client, who is alert. She needs to have the bed in low position and access to the call bell so she can call for help if she needs to get up.

2. While it would be nice for a client to always have someone present in the room for assistance, this is unrealistic and not necessary for this client. This client needs to have the bed in low position and access to the call bell so she can call for help if she needs to get up.

4. Rearranging room assignments is done for clients who have a particular risk of falling. This is not the most appropriate intervention for this client, because there is no evidence that this client has a high risk for falling. She needs to have the bed in low position and access to the call bell so she can call for help if she needs to get up.

#88. 3. **Guidelines for the safe administration of medications state that medications prepared by one nurse should be administered only by that nurse.**   Im   Ph/8   5

    1. Guidelines for the safe administration of medications state that medications prepared by one nurse should be administered only by that nurse.

    2. Guidelines for the safe administration of medications state that medications prepared by one nurse should be administered only by that nurse.

    4. Guidelines for the safe administration of medications state that medications prepared by one nurse should be administered only by that nurse.

#89. 3. **Substance abuse is characterized by recurrent ingestion of a substance in situations in which it is detrimental to the client's physical or mental health or the welfare of others. He has been arrested twice for driving while intoxicated.**   Dc   Ps/6   2

    1. Withdrawal symptoms begin to appear within 6–12 hours of the cessation of long-term drinking. This client has no physical symptoms. This behavior fits the criteria for substance abuse.

    2. Bad judgment syndrome is not a substance abuse or dependence category. This behavior fits the criteria for substance abuse.

    4. Substance dependence is characterized by increasing use of the substance and withdrawal symptoms if intake is reduced or stopped. Because the client restricts his drinking to weekends, he has not reached this level. He may progress to this level if he begins to drink greater amounts of alcohol more days of the week. His current behavior fits the criteria for substance abuse.

#90. 1. **Because the MRI exam uses a powerful magnet, clients with implanted metal devices should have other types of medical imaging exams.**   Dc   Ph/9   1

    2. Because the MRI exam uses a powerful magnet, clients with implanted metal devices should have other types of medical imaging exams. A ceramic hip would not affect the exam.

    3. A history of claustrophobia may make the MRI difficult for some people because the client is placed in a tube. Asthma is not related to complications with MRI. Clients with implanted metal devices should have other types of medical imaging exams.

    4. Not every MRI requires dye. Clients with implanted metal devices should have other types of medical imaging exams.

#91. 3. **The clients in all of the choices have some risk factors for osteoporosis. This client has the most risk factors (5): advanced age, lack of estrogen, reduced mobility, steroids, and excessive alcohol intake.**   Dc   Ph/9   1

   1. Men are at less risk than women are for osteoporosis. This man has three risk factors: decreased activity, low calcium intake, and steroids.

   2. This client has two risk factors for osteoporosis: the eating disorder and amenorrhea. Bone strength is at its highest in young adults.

   4. This client has two risk factors: advanced age and anticonvulsant therapy. In addition, her active youth helped build bone density.

#92. 1. **The client should be informed prior to the time for the medication that she will soon be medicated and will not be able to get out of bed after receiving the medication. This gives the client time to wash her hands. The hand washing ritual helps lessen her anxiety. She should be allowed to do this prior to surgery.**   Pl   Ps/6   2

   2. The nurse should inform the client in advance about the need to stay in bed after receiving the medication. This would allow the client time to perform her anxiety-reducing rituals. Informing when giving the medication does not give her time to perform her ritual and is likely to cause great anxiety.

   3. It would be better to give the client time to perform her washing ritual before medicating her than to try to accommodate the ritual at the bedside. After receiving pre-operative medication, the client should be encouraged to rest and may go to sleep.

   4. It would be better to give the client time to perform her washing ritual before medicating her than to try to accommodate the ritual at the bedside. After receiving pre-operative medication, the client should be encouraged to rest and may go to sleep.

#93. 1. **Encouraging the client to discuss the effects of lupus on her lifestyle helps uncover how the unpredictability of the illness and the changes in appearance are affecting the client. By understanding the underlying reasons for the frustration, the nurse can help the client develop adaptive strategies that may alleviate some of the frustration.**   Im   Ps/5   2

2. Explaining to the client that things could be worse is patronizing, blocks communication, and does not constructively assist the client in dealing with her frustration. A more appropriate intervention would be to help uncover how the unpredictability of the illness and the changes in appearance are affecting her day-to-day life so that she can develop adaptive strategies.

3. Frustration with her condition does not mean there are conflicts in her personal life. There are no data to support this intervention. A more appropriate intervention would be to help uncover how the unpredictability of the illness and the changes in appearance are affecting her day-to-day life so that she can develop adaptive strategies.

4. There is no evidence that the client has a lack of knowledge; her problem is frustration with the unpredictability of her disease and her change in appearance. A more appropriate intervention would be to help uncover how the unpredictability of the illness and the changes in appearance are affecting her day-to-day life so that she can develop adaptive strategies.

#94. 1. **This information is correct and complete and worded in a way that avoids medical jargon that may be confusing to the child's parents.**   Im   Ph/10   4

2. Debriding in a whirlpool bath is done to prevent infection and tissue sloughing and to keep tissue healthy for skin grafts-not to prevent contractures.

3. Hydrotherapy does not provide complete information about the reasons for debriding, which are to prevent infection and keep tissue healthy for skin grafts. In addition, the wound may or may not be dressed, depending on the individual client's treatment plan.

4. The debriding bath is not an antibiotic solution. Debriding in a whirlpool bath is done to prevent infection and tissue sloughing and to keep tissue healthy for skin grafts.

#95. 4. **The response is empathic and attempts to verify and reflect**   Im   Ps/6   2
what the client said. Such responses build trust and rapport between
the nurse and client. In addition, this response allows the nurse
to assess how much danger the client believes himself to be in and
what actions he might be considering to protect himself.

   1.   Confronting this client's belief system could cause him to become
         even more adamant about this belief. The best response would be
         empathic, verifying or reflecting what the client said, such as "You
         think someone is coming after you?"

   2.   Although the client's response should be documented, calling the
         physician is not appropriate because this remark is consistent with
         his admitting diagnosis. The best response would be empathic,
         verifying or reflecting what the client said, such as "You think
         someone is coming after you?"

   3.   Ignoring the comment or changing the subject could heighten his
         anxiety or make him even more adamant about this belief. The best
         response would be empathic, verifying or reflecting what the client
         said, such as "You think someone is coming after you?"

#96. 2. **The client is experiencing moderate anxiety, which is**   Dc   Ps/5   2
characterized by difficulty concentrating and learning new
material.

   1.   Clients experiencing mild anxiety are still able to concentrate and
         focus. This client is experiencing moderate anxiety, which is
         characterized by difficulty concentrating and learning new material.

   3.   While clients with severe anxiety are not able to concentrate, they are
         also are significantly impaired with pronounced physiological
         symptoms. This client is experiencing moderate anxiety, which is
         characterized by difficulty concentrating and learning new material.

   4.   Clients with panic anxiety experience psychosis, delusions, and
         hallucinations. There is no evidence of these symptoms in this client.
         This client is experiencing moderate anxiety, which is characterized
         by difficulty concentrating and learning new material.

#97. 3. **The nurse should assess the client's mental status. She was**   Im   Sa/2   1
admitted with dehydration, which can cause disorientation. The
family may be observing behaviors that make her a danger to
herself.

   1.   The nurse should assess the client's need for restraints before
         contacting the physician.

   2.   This is a true statement but does not address the concerns the family
         has. The nurse should assess the client's mental status and possible
         need for restraints.

   4.   This is not true. The nurse should not tell the client's family to restrain
         the client.

#98. 4. **Both the wife and pregnant daughter should be asked to leave the room to prevent exposing them to radiation.**   Im   Sa/2   2

1. The wife should not be asked to assist in holding the client. This unnecessarily exposes her to radiation. The pregnant daughter should be asked to leave the room.

2. The client should not be asked to wear a lead apron over his chest when a chest x-ray is done. That would make taking the chest x-ray impossible.

3. Closing the door to the room during the x-ray might be done for the client's privacy. Closing the door does not significantly reduce radiation exposure to others. This action is not the most important action for the nurse. The nurse should ask the wife and daughter to leave the room to prevent unnecessary exposure to radiation.

#99. 4. **There is not enough data to determine that the woman is being abused. The client's complaints should be taken seriously and should be investigated. Elderly persons bruise easily. One ecchymotic area does not confirm elder abuse. The best action for the nurse is to report the client's remarks and the nurse's findings to the nursing supervisor.**   Im   Ps/6   2

1. There is not enough data to warrant calling the police. A woman with senile dementia has made an accusation that is so far not supported by data.

2. Asking the daughter why she abuses her mother is making the assumption that the daughter does abuse her mother. This is not justified.

3. There is not enough data to justify asking the physician to order long bone x-rays.

#100. 4. **The best choice in this situation is to ask the adults beside the child's bed the name of the child.**   Im   Sa/2   4

1. A two-year-old child cannot be relied upon to give his name accurately.

2. Giving the medication to the child in the bed on the medication card without identifying the child is dangerous. Sometimes children get in the wrong bed.

3. The nurse should make every effort to identify the client before refusing to give medication.

Appendices

Symbols & Abbreviations

Symbol	Meaning
~	similar
≅	approximately
@	at
√	check
Δ	change
↑	increased
↓	decreased
=	equals
#	pounds
>	greater than
<	less than
%	percent
+	positive
−	negative
♀	female
♂	male
△1 △2 △3	trimester of pregnancy (one triangle for each trimester)

Abbreviation	Meaning
a.c.	before meals
ad lib	freely, as desired
b.i.d.	two times a day
$\bar{c}$	with
cap	capsule
DC	discontinue
elix	elixir
h	hour
hrly	hourly

Abbreviation	Meaning
h.s.	at bedtime
ID	intradermal
IM	intramuscular
IV	intravenous
IVPB	intravenous piggyback
OD	right eye
od	every day
OS	left eye
OU	each eye
p.c.	after meals
po	by mouth
per	by
PRN	as needed
q	every
qd	every day
q2h	every 2 hours
q.i.d.	four times a day
qod	every other day
qs	sufficient quantity
SC	subcutaneous
Stat	immediately
supp	suppository
susp	suspension
tab	tablet
t.i.d.	three times a day
Tr or tinct	tincture

Appendix B

Metric System Equivalents

Liquid Measure (Volume)

Metric		Apothecary		Household
5 ml	=	1 fluid dram	=	1 teaspoonful
10 ml	=	2 fluid drams	=	1 dessertspoonful
15 ml	=	4 fluid drams	=	1 tablespoonful
30 ml	=	1 fluid ounce	=	1 ounce
60 ml	=	2 fluid ounces	=	1 wineglassful
120 ml	=	4 fluid ounces	=	1 teacupful
240 ml	=	8 fluid ounces	=	1 tumblerful
500 ml	=	1 pint	=	1 pint
1000 ml	=	1 quart	=	1 quart
4000 ml	=	1 gallon	=	1 gallon

Weight

Metric		Apothecary
1 mg	=	$\frac{1}{60}$ grain
4 mg	=	$\frac{1}{15}$ grain
10 mg	=	$\frac{1}{6}$ grain
15 mg	=	$\frac{1}{4}$ grain
30 mg	=	$\frac{1}{2}$ grain
60 mg	=	1 grain
1 g	=	15 grains
4 g	=	1 dram
30 g	=	1 ounce
500 g	=	1.1 pound
1000 g (1 kg)	=	2.2 pounds

Temperature Conversions

Fahrenheit to Celsius
C = (F − 32) × 5/9

97	36.1
98	36.6
98.6	37.0
99	37.2
100	37.7
101	38.3
102	38.8
103	39.4
104	40.0
105	40.5
106	41.1

Medical Prefixes and Suffixes

a-, an-	negative, without	cav-	hollow
ab-	away from	cent-	hundred
acou-	hear	-centesis	puncture
ad-	to, toward	cephalo-	head
adeno-	gland	cerebro-	brain
alb-	white	cervico-	neck
-algia	pain	cheilo-	lips
alve-	channel, cavity	cholecyst-	gallbladder
ambi-	both	chondro-	cartilage
amphi-	both	chrom-	color
amyl-	starch	cili-	eyelid
andr-	man	circum-	around
angio-	vessel	-cis-	incision
ankyl-	crooked, growing together	-clasia	breaking
ante-, anti-	before	colo-	large intestine
antr-	chamber	colp-	hollow, vagina
apo-	detached	corpora-	body
arachn-	spider	cortico-	bark, rind (outside covering)
arthro-	joint	costo-	rib
articul-	joint	cranio-	skull
auri-	ear	cry-	cold
		crypt-	hide, conceal
bi-	two	cune-	wedge
blasto-	bud, embryonic form	cut-	skin
brachi-	arm	cyan-	blue
brachy-	short	cyc-	circle
brady-	slow	cysto-, vesico-	bladder
broncho-	windpipe	cyto-	cell
bucca-	cheek		
		dactyl-	finger, toe
capit-	head	de-	down from
carcin-	cancer	dec-	ten
cardi-, cordi-	heart	dent-	tooth
cata-	down, negative	derm-	skin
caud-	tail	dextr-	right-handed

di-	two	hom-	same
diplo-	double	hyper-	above, elevated
dis-	apart	hypo-	under, below
-docho-	common bile duct	hystero-	uterus
dors-	back		
-duct	lead, conduct	-iasis	condition
duodeno-	duodenum	itro-	physician
dys-	bad, painful	idio-	peculiar
		ileo-	ileum
e-	apart, away from	infra-	beneath
ect-	outside	inter-	between
-ectasis	dilation	intra-	inside
-ectomy	excision	is-	equal
ede-	swell	-itis	inflammation
-emia	blood		
endo-	inside	jejuno-	jejunum
entero-	small intestine		
epi-	upon, after	kerato-	horny
eso-	inside	kil-	one thousand
estho-	perceive, feel	kine-	move
en-	normal		
eu-	normal	labi-	lip
exo-	outside	lact-	milk
		lapar-	flank
fasci-	band	laryngo-	throat
fauci-	throat	later-	side
febr-	fever	-lep-	take, seize
ferr-	iron	leuko-	white
for-	door, opening	lipo-	fat
-form	shape	lithio-	stone or calculus
fract-	break	lumb-	loin
		lute-	yellow
galact-	milk	-lysis	break down
ganglio-	swelling, plexus		
gastro-	stomach	macro-	long, large
gingive-	gums	mal-	abnormal
gloss-	tongue	-malac-	soft
glott-	tongue, language	masto-	breast
glyc-	sweet	mammo-	breast
gno-	know, discern	medi-	middle
gyn-	woman	mega-	great, large
gyr-	ring, circle	melan-	black
		men-	month
hemi-	half	mening-	membrane
hemo-	blood	ment-	mind
hemato-	blood	meso-	middle
hepato-	liver	meta-	beyond, after
histo-	tissue	metro-	uterus

micro-	small	phob-	fear, dread
mill-	one thousand	phot-	light
morph-	shape, form	-plasty	shape, repair
muco-	mucus	pleuro-	membrane encasing lungs
-myces	fungus	pne-	breathing
myco-	fungal	pneumo-	lungs
myelo-	bone marrow	-pole-	made, produce
myo-	muscle	poly-	much, many
myx-	mucus	procto-	anus and rectum
naso-	nose	pseudo-	false
nephro-	kidney	psych-	mind
neuro-	nerve	pto-	fall
nod-	knot	-ptosis	prolapse
nos-	disease	pulmo-	lungs
		pyelo-	kidney, pelvis
ocul-	eye	pyo-	pus
-odynia	pain		
oligo-	few, little	quadr-	four
-ology	study of		
-oma	tumor, swelling	recto-	rectum
onphal-	navel	ren-	kidney
onych-	nail	retro-	backward
oophoro-	ovary	rhino-	nose
ovari-	ovary	-rrhagia	break, burst
optic, opth-	eye	-rrhaphy	suture, sew
orchi-	testicle	-rrhea	flowing
orth-	straight	-rrhexia	break, rupture
-osis	condition, state resulting		
oss-, ost-	bone	salpingo-	fallopian tube
osteo-	bone	sanguin-	blood
-ostomy	new, opening	schis-	split
-otomy	incision	sclero-	hardening
oto-	ear	scop-	look at, observe
ov-	egg	-sect	cut
pancreato-	pancreas	semi-	half
para-	beside	sens-	perceive, feel
-pathy	sickness, disease	sep-	decay
-pepsia	digestion	septo-	infection
ped-	child	sial-	saliva
pend-	hang down	somat-	body
pept-	digest	-some	body
peri-	around, surrounding	spher-	ball
pha-	say, speak	spirat-	breathe
phag-	eat, swallow	spondyl-	vertebra
pharyngo-	throat	stear-	fat
phil-	affinity for	sten-	narrow
phlebo-	vein	-sthen-	strength

stomato-	mouth	trop-	turn toward
splanchc-	entrails, viscera	-trophy	nurture, nutrition
sub-	under	typ-	type
super-, supra	above, extreme		
syn-	together	un-	one
		uria-	urine
tact-	touch	uro-	urine
tax-	arrange, order	utero-	uterus
tens-	stretch		
tetra-	four	vas-	vessel
thel-	nipple	vene-	vein
thermo-	heat	vesic-	bladder
thoraco-	chest	vit-	life
thromb-	clot, lump		
-toc-	childbirth	xanth-	yellow, blond
-tomy	cutting		
tors-	twist	zo-	life
tracheo-	windpipe	zyg-	yoke, union
tri-	three	zym-	ferment
tricho-	hair		

Appendix E

NANDA Nursing Diagnoses

Activity intolerance
Activity intolerance, Risk for
Adjustment, Impaired
Airway clearance, Ineffective
Allergy response, Risk for latex
Anxiety
Anxiety, Death
Aspiration, Risk for
Body image, Disturbed
Body temperature, Risk for imbalanced
Bowel incontinence
Breastfeeding, Effective
Breastfeeding, Interrupted
Breathing pattern, Ineffective
Cardiac output, Decreased
Caregiver role strain
Caregiver role strain, Risk for
Communication, Impaired verbal
Communication, Readiness for enhanced
Confusion, Acute
Confusion, Chronic
Constipation
Constipation, Perceived
Constipation, Risk for
Coping, Community, Ineffective
Coping, Community, Readiness for enhanced
Coping, Defensive
Coping, Family, Compromised
Coping, Family, Disabled
Coping, Family, Readiness for enhanced
Coping, Ineffective
Conflict, Decisional (specify)
Conflict, Parental role
Denial, Ineffective
Dentition, Impaired

Development, Risk for delayed
Diarrhea
Disuse syndrome, Risk for
Diversional activity, Deficient
Dysreflexia, Autonomic
Dysreflexia, Autonomic, Risk for
Energy field, Disturbed
Environmental interpretation syndrome, Impaired
Failure to thrive, Adult
Falls, Risk for
Family processes, Dysfunctional: Alcoholism
Family processes, Interrupted
Fatigue
Fear
Fluid volume, Deficient
Fluid volume, Excess
Fluid volume, Readiness for enhanced
Fluid volume, Risk for deficient
Fluid volume, Risk for imbalanced
Gas exchange, Impaired
Grieving, Anticipatory
Grieving, Dysfunctional
Growth and development, Delayed
Growth, Risk for disproportionate
Health Maintenance, Ineffective
Health-seeking behaviors (specify)
Home maintenance, Impaired
Hopelessness
Hyperthermia
Hypothermia
Identity, Disturbed personal
Incontinence, Functional urinary
Incontinence, Reflex urinary
Incontinence, Stress urinary
Incontinence, Total urinary

Incontinence, Urge urinary
Incontinence, Urge urinary, Risk for
Infant behavior, Disorganized
Infant behavior, Readiness for enhanced organized
Infant behavior, Risk for disorganized
Infant feeding pattern, Ineffective
Infection, Risk for
Injury, Perioperative positioning, Risk for
Injury, Risk for
Intracranial adaptive capacity, Decreased
Knowledge, Deficient
Knowledge, Readiness for enhanced
Loneliness, Risk for
Memory, Impaired
Mobility, Impaired bed
Mobility, Impaired physical
Mobility, Impaired wheelchair
Nausea
Noncompliance (specify)
Nutrition, Imbalanced: Less than body
   requirements
Nutrition, Imbalanced: More than body
   requirements
Nutrition, Imbalanced: More than body
   requirements, Risk for
Nutrition, Readiness for enhanced
Oral mucous membrane, Impaired
Pain, Acute
Pain, Chronic
Parenting, Impaired
Parenting, Impaired, Risk for
Parenting, Readiness for enhanced
Peripheral neurovascular dysfunction, Risk for
Poisoning, Risk for
Post-trauma Syndrome
Post-trauma Syndrome, Risk for
Powerlessness
Powerlessness, Risk for
Protection, Ineffective
Rape-trauma Syndrome
Rape-trauma Syndrome, Compound reaction
Rape-trauma Syndrome, Silent reaction
Relocation stress Syndrome
Relocation stress Syndrome, Risk for
Role performance, Ineffective
Self-care deficit, Bathing/hygiene
Self-care deficit, Dressing/grooming
Self-care deficit, Feeding

Self-care deficit, Toileting
Self concept, Readiness for enhanced
Self-esteem, Low, Chronic
Self-esteem, Low, Situational
Self-esteem, Low, Situational, Risk for
Self-mutilation
Self-mutilation, Risk for
Sensory perception, Disturbed (specify)
   (Visual, auditory, kinesthetic, gustatory, tactile,
   olfactory)
Sexual dysfunction
Sexuality patterns, Ineffective
Skin integrity, Impaired
Skin integrity, Impaired, Risk for
Sleep deprivation
Sleep pattern, Disturbed
Sleep, Readiness for enhanced
Social interaction, Impaired
Social isolation
Sorrow, Chronic
Spiritual distress
Spiritual distress, Risk for
Spiritual well-being, Readiness for enhanced
Sudden Infant Death Syndrome, Risk for
Suffocation, Risk for
Suicide, Risk for
Surgical recovery, Delayed
Swallowing, Impaired
Therapeutic regimen management, Effective
Therapeutic regimen management, Ineffective
Therapeutic regimen management, Ineffective
   community
Therapeutic regimen management, Ineffective
   family
Therapeutic regimen management, Readiness for
   enhanced
Thermoregulation, Ineffective
Thought process, Disturbed
Tissue integrity, Impaired
Tissue perfusion, Ineffective (specify type)
   (Renal, cerebral, cardiopulmonary,
   gastrointestinal, peripheral)
Transfer ability, Impaired
Trauma, Risk for
Neglect, unilateral
Urinary elimination, Impaired
Urinary elimination, Readiness for enhanced
Urinary retention

Ventilation, Impaired spontaneous
Ventilatory weaning response, Dysfunctional
Violence, Risk for other-directed

Violence, Risk for self-directed
Walking, Impaired
Wandering

Source: North American Nursing Diagnosis Association. (2003). *Nursing Diagnoses: Definitions and Classifications, 2003–2004.* Philadelphia, PA: Author.

License Agreement for Delmar Learning, a division of Thomson Learning, Inc.

Educational Software/Data

You the customer, and Delmar Learning, a division of Thomson Learning, Inc. incur certain benefits, rights, and obligations to each other when you open this package and use the software/data it contains. BE SURE YOU READ THE LICENSE AGREEMENT CAREFULLY, SINCE BY USING THE SOFTWARE/DATA YOU INDICATE YOU HAVE READ, UNDERSTOOD, AND ACCEPTED THE TERMS OF THIS AGREEMENT.

Your rights:

1. You enjoy a non-exclusive license to use the software/data on a single microcomputer in consideration for payment of the required license fee, (which may be included in the purchase price of an accompanying print component), or receipt of this software/data, and your acceptance of the terms and conditions of this agreement.
2. You acknowledge that you do not own the aforesaid software/data. You also acknowledge that the software/data is furnished "as is," and contains copyrighted and/or proprietary and confidential information of Delmar Learning, a division of Thomson Learning, Inc. or its licensors.

There are limitations on your rights:

1. You may not copy or print the software/data for any reason whatsoever, except to install it on a hard drive on a single microcomputer and to make one archival copy, unless copying or printing is expressly permitted in writing or statements recorded on the diskette(s).
2. You may not revise, translate, convert, disassemble or otherwise reverse engineer the software/ data except that you may add to or rearrange any data recorded on the media as part of the normal use of the software/data.
3. You may not sell, license, lease, rent, loan or otherwise distribute or network the software/data except that you may give the software/data to a student or and instructor for use at school or, temporarily at home.

Should you fail to abide by the Copyright Law of the United States as it applies to this software/data your license to use it will become invalid. You agree to erase or otherwise destroy the software/data immediately after receiving note of termination of this agreement for violation of its provisions from Delmar Learning.

Delmar Learning, a division of Thomson Learning, Inc gives you a LIMITED WARRANTY covering the enclosed software/data. The LIMITED WARRANTY follows this License.

This license is the entire agreement between you and Delmar Learning, a division of Thomson Learning, Inc. interpreted and enforced under New York law.

LIMITED WARRANTY

Delmar Learning, a division of Thomson Learning, Inc. warrants to the original licensee/purchaser of this copy of microcomputer software/data and the media on which it is recorded that the media will be free from defects in material and workmanship for ninety (90) days from the date of original purchase. All implied warranties are limited in duration to this ninety (90) day period. THEREAFTER, ANY IMPLIED WARRANTIES, INCLUDING IMPLIED WARRANTIES OF MERCHANTABILITY AND FITNESS FOR A PARTICULAR PURPOSE, ARE EXCLUDED. THIS WARRANTY IS IN LIEU OF ALL OTHER WARRANTIES, WHETHER ORAL OR WRITTEN, EXPRESS OR IMPLIED.

If you believe the media is defective please return it during the ninety day period to the address shown below. Defective media will be replaced without charge provided that it has not been subjected to misuse or damage.

This warranty does not extend to the software or information recorded on the media. The software and information are provided "AS IS." Any statements made about the utility of the software or information are not to be considered as express or implied warranties.

Limitation of liability: Our liability to you for any losses shall be limited to direct damages, and shall not exceed the amount you paid for the software. In no event will we be liable to you for any indirect, special, incidental, or consequential damages (including loss of profits) even if we have been advised of the possibility of such damages.

Some states do not allow the exclusion or limitation of incidental or consequential damages, or limitations on the duration of implied warranties, so the above limitation or exclusion may not apply to you. This warranty gives you specific legal rights, and you may also have other rights which vary from state to state. Address all correspondence to: Delmar Learning, a division of Thomson Learning, Inc., 5 Maxwell Drive, P.O. Box 8007, Clifton Park, NY 12065-8007. Attention: Technology Department

Set-Up Instructions

1. Insert the *Delmar's Practice Questions for NCLEX-PN* CD-ROM.
2. Double-click on your My Computer icon on the desktop, then double-click on the CD-ROM drive icon.
3. Double-click on the *setup.exe* file to start the installation.
4. Follow the on-screen prompts from there.

System Requirements

Operating System: Microsoft® Windows® 98 or later.
Processor: Pentium or faster
Memory: 32 MB of RAM or more
Hard disk: 50 MB free space
CD-ROM drive: 4x or faster
Graphics: minimum 800×600 resolution w/256 color capabilities